Contents

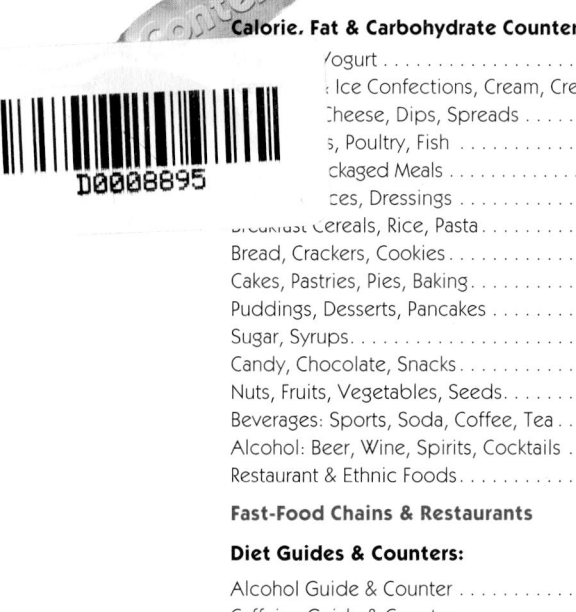

Weight Control Tips

Eat Sensibly

- Avoid fad diets. Eat 3 sensible meals daily.
- Limit fats and fatty foods, sugar, soda and alcohol.

(Sample Diet Plan, Page 11)

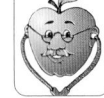

Exercise Daily

- Get active and exercise every day!
- Include muscle-strengthening exercises. You'll lose more fat and keep it off. You'll also feel and look better, and you can eat a little more food. *(Exercise Guide, Page 12)*

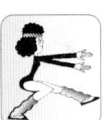

Reshape Eating Behaviors

- Be aware of eating and shopping behaviors that lead to overeating.
- Also focus on social and emotional situations that make you snack compulsively.

(Extra notes - Page 14)

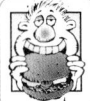

Keep a Food & Exercise Diary

- A diary helps you see exactly what you eat and drink, and how much you really exercise.
- An excellent motivator.
- Keeps you honest! *(Page 15)*

Arrange Moral Support

Gain the support of family and friends. Get extra professional help if required, from your doctor, dietitian, psychologist, exercise trainer, or slimming group. Beware of family saboteurs who discourage you from adopting a healthier lifestyle!

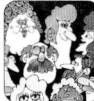

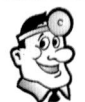

DOCTOR CHECK-UP
Ask your doctor to check you for high blood pressure, diabetes, and high blood cholesterol.

HEALTHY WEIGHTS
for Men & Women
(Over 18 years)

Based on weights with least risk of disease or death from heart disease, diabetes, stroke and cancer.

Based on Body Mass Index - range 20-25.

BMI calculated as: $\dfrac{\text{Weight (kg)}}{\text{Height (m)}^2}$

Height (No Shoes)	Healthy Weight Range
Ft Ins	Pounds
4'7"	86-108
4'8"	88-110
4'9"	92-114
4'10"	97-121
4'11"	99-123
5'0"	101-127
5'1"	105-132
5'2"	110-136
5'3"	112-140
5'4"	114-145
5'5"	119-149
5'6"	123-156
5'7"	127-158
5'8"	129-162
5'9"	134-167
5'10"	138-173
5'11"	143-178
6'0"	145-182
6'1"	149-187
6"2"	156-193
6'3"	158-198
6'4"	162-202
6'5"	170-211
6'6"	172-215
6'7"	175-220

Body Fat Distribution & Health

Fat above the hips carries a far greater health risk than fat on or below the hips - better to be a **'pear-shape'** than an **'apple-shape'**.

Abdominal obesity greatly increases the risk of developing diabetes, heart disease, high blood fats, hypertension, stroke and some cancers. So-called **'cellulite'** carries no extra health risk.

Waist Measurement (High Health Risk)

Men: Over 39 inches **Women:** Over 34 inches

Women who become obsessed with dieting away their thighs and buttocks on an otherwise lean body, are fighting mother nature and may well be inviting health problems.

If you are within a healthy weight range, it is better to exercise regularly to maintain body shape, rather than to be constantly dieting and lacking in energy. Accept your body shape and focus on other pursuits and enjoying life!

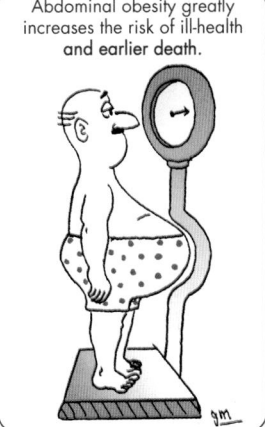

Abdominal obesity greatly increases the risk of ill-health and earlier death.

Estimating Body Fat Percentage

Body fat percentage is a better indicator of health than total weight.

Bioelectric impedance analysis (BIA) is gaining support as a practical and economical method for estimating body fat in both clinical and home settings.

BIA measures the resistance of a weak electrical current that is passed through the body. A computer within the body fat analyzer calculates the amount of body water, fat and muscle.

More Information: www.calorieking.com

BODY FAT & OBESITY

Men:	Above 25% body fat
Women:	Above 32% body fat

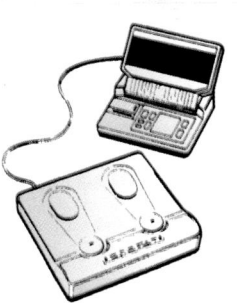

Tanita Body Fat Analyzer
With Built-In Scale

HEALTHY BODY FAT RANGES

Men:	Under 30 years	~	14 - 20%
	Over 30 years	~	17 - 23%
Women:	Under 30 years	~	17 - 24%
	Over 30 years	~	20 - 27%

Note: Less than 13% body fat in women can be unhealthy.

Unexplained Weight Gains

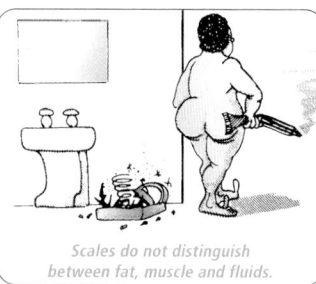

Scales do not distinguish between fat, muscle and fluids.

Body Fluid Changes

Body weight fluctuates from day to day. This is mainly due to changes in body fluids which make up around 70% of total body weight. It can be affected by changes in hormone levels, dietary factors such as salt and carbohydrate, and even exercise.

Weight change over several weeks is more likely to reflect changes in levels of fat and muscle rather than fluid. Unfortunately, the scales do not distinguish between weight changes due to water, fat or muscle. This is why **we shouldn't allow every fluctuation in weight to rule our lives.**

To limit fluid retention, avoid salty foods and go easy on the salt shaker. Eating sufficient fruit and vegetables supplies extra potassium which counteracts sodium and encourages fluid loss. However, **do not limit water intake.** Be sure to drink at least 6-8 glasses of water and other fluids per day.

When dining out, be aware that the extra pound or two that might show on the scales the next morning is not the result of a small dietary indiscretion. It is more likely due to fluid retention resulting from more highly seasoned and salty food.

Monthly hormonal changes in women can also account for a build-up of fluids of several pounds prior to menstruation.

Menopausal Weight Gains

Most women gain an average of 4-5 pounds in the years leading up to the menopause - usually in their middle to late 40's. This can occur even when exercise and eating habits have not changed significantly.

With hormonal changes occurring at that time, body fat also tends to be redistributed from thighs, buttocks and hips to the breast and stomach areas (a greater health risk).

Be sure to eat wisely and continue daily physical activity including strength-training to maintain or build muscles - and to boost metabolism and self-esteem.

Underactive Thyroid

Thyroid hormone is secreted into the bloodstream by the thyroid gland in the neck. When insufficient thyroid hormone is made, metabolism and body processes slow down and weight gain can occur.

Symptoms of hypothyroidism can be subtle and easily overlooked as signs of normal aging. **Early symptoms** may include fatigue, muscle weakness, sluggishness, a swollen tongue that you keep biting, and a puffy face. As metabolism continues to slow, **further signs can include** chronically cold hands and feet, slow reflexes, constipation, dry skin and coarse hair, brittle nails, heavy menstrual periods, slower pulse, and a husky voice.

Depression-like symptoms may also develop such as forgetfulness, loss of interest, mood swings and irritability.

Weight gains of as much as 10-20 pounds (mainly fluid) can occur, as well as a **raised blood cholesterol level.**

The condition is more common in women, especially following pregnancy, around menopause, or after age 60.

A simple blood test through your doctor can detect hypothyroidism. It is easily treated in most cases with thyroid hormone pills.

Adults 35 and older should have a TSH (thyroid stimulating hormone) test every 5 years. Testing when pregnant is also wise.

Calories in Food

Calories in food are derived from protein, fat and carbohydrate. Alcohol also provides calories. Vitamins, minerals and water provide no calories.

Calorie Values Per Gram

Fat/Oil	~	9 Calories
Carbohydrate	~	4 Calories
Protein	~	4 Calories
Alcohol	~	7 Calories

Note that fats have over double the calories of protein and carbohydrate. The higher the fat content of food, the higher the calories.

Sample Calculation

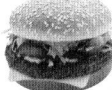

QUARTER POUNDER® WITH CHEESE has 534 calories derived from:

30g Fat (x 9 cals/gram)	=	270
38g Carbohyd.(x 4 cals/gram)	=	152
28g Protein (x 4 cals/gram)	=	112
Total Calories	=	**534**

Calorie Levels for Weight Loss

Commence with a calorie-controlled diet that allows a moderate weight loss of $^1/2$ - 1 pound per week. Weight loss is usually much larger in the first few weeks due to extra fluid losses.

Note: It is better to increase exercise rather than lessen food calories too drastically.

Suggested Calories for Weight Loss

Women:	Non-active	1000 - 1200
	Active	1200 - 1500
Men:	Non-active	1200 - 1500
	Active	1500 - 1800
Teenagers:		1200 - 1800

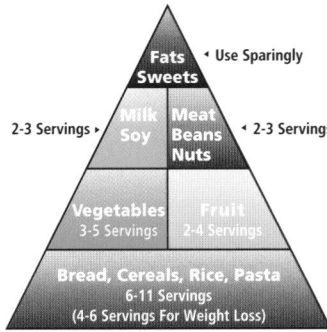

Fats Sweets — ◄ Use Sparingly

Milk Soy — 2-3 Servings ►

Meat Beans Nuts — ◄ 2-3 Servings

Vegetables 3-5 Servings

Fruit 2-4 Servings

Bread, Cereals, Rice, Pasta 6-11 Servings (4-6 Servings For Weight Loss)

The Food Guide Pyramid emphasizes eating a wide variety of foods from the 5 major food groups. For weight loss, make lowfat choices and eat the lower number of servings.

Examples of Serving Size

Bread & Cereal Group:
- 1 slice bread
- $^1/2$ bun, bagel or English muffin
- 4 small crackers or 1 tortilla
- 1 oz ready-to-eat cereal
- $^1/2$ cup cooked cereal, rice, pasta

Fruit Group:
- 1 medium apple, orange, banana
- $^1/2$ cup canned fruit
- $^1/4$ cup dried fruit
- $^3/4$ cup fruit juice
- $^1/4$ medium avocado

Vegetable Group:
- 1 cup raw leafy vegetables
- $1^1/2$ oz raw chopped vegetables
- $^1/2$ cup cooked vegetables
- $^1/2$ - $^3/4$ cup vegetable juice

Meat & Alternatives Group:
- 2-3oz (cooked) lean meat/poultry/fish
- 2 eggs **or** 7oz tofu **or** $^1/2$ cup nuts
- 1 cup (cooked) dried beans or chickpeas
- 4 Tbsp peanut butter

Milk & Alternatives Group:
- 1 cup (8 fl.oz) milk, soy drink, yogurt
- $1^1/2$ oz cheese or $^1/2$ cup cottage cheese

Recommended Fat Intake

Recommended Fat Intake

Americans consume too much fat with many having over 40% of total calories from fat - either as fat or oil, or as fat in foods and drinks. A range of 20-30% is healthier.

Fat Intake - Healthy Ranges

Children	30-60g
Teenagers (Active)	40-80g
Women	30-60g
Men: Active	40-80g
Heavy Activity/Athlete	80-120g

The chart below recommends maximum fat intake for different calorie levels.

MAXIMUM DESIRABLE FAT INTAKE (Daily)

Calories	Fat	% Fat Cals
1200 cals	30g fat	23%
1500 cals	40g fat	24%
1800 cals	50g fat	25%
2000 cals	60g fat	27%
2200 cals	70g fat	28%
2500 cals	80g fat	29%
2800 cals	90g fat	29%
3000 cals	100g fat	30%
3500 cals	117g fat	30%
4000 cals	135g fat	30%

Infants Fat Intake

Infants and toddlers under 3 years should not be restricted in their fat intake because much larger volumes of food would be required to guarantee adequate calorie intake and growth. Whole milk should be used rather than light milk(1%) or nonfat milk.

Similarly, a high fiber diet is also not suitable for infants.

Calories Versus Fats

For successful weight control it is important to be aware of both fats and calories in foods. It widens your choices at the supermarket and when eating out.

While choosing more lowfat foods is wise, it does not guarantee that total calories will be reduced, particularly if portion size is not limited.

It is a mistake to think that eating lowfat or fat-free foods allows you to eat double the quantity.

Be aware that lowfat and fat-free cakes, cookies and ice cream are **not calorie-free.** Nor are soda drinks, fruit juices, beer, alcoholic spirits, sugar and sugar candy which are also fat-free. Bread, rice and pasta also have negligble fat.

Carbohydrate Calories Count

It is also a fallacy that carbohydrate calories don't count. Carbohydrates in excess of body needs can still be converted to and stored as body fat - particularly in women in their child-bearing years.

Total Calories Count!

Ultimately, **it is food portion size and total calories that count** whether from fat, carbohydrate or protein. Remember, cows get fat on grass!

FOOD LABEL MEANINGS
FDA Nutrition Claim Definitions
(All are on a Per Serving Basis.)

Low Calorie: 40 calories or less
Light or Lite: One third fewer calories or, 50% or less fat than regular product
Fat-Free: Less than half a gram of fat
Low-Fat: 3 grams or less of fat
Reduced-Fat: 25% less fat than regular product
Fewer or Less Calories: At least 25% fewer calories than regular product

Percent Fat Calories
(Percentage of Calories from Fat)

While health authorities recommend that not more than 30% of our total food calories should come from fat, it is not implied nor even recommended that you eat only those foods with less than 30% calories from fat.

Our normal diet is made up of foods that are either well above or below 30%. Only on average should the total diet be less than 30% calories from fat.

Some higher fat foods such as avocados, nuts and seeds, are highly nutritious and favor lower blood cholesterol levels. **Moderation is the aim . . . not elimination.**

Nevertheless, knowing the percentage of calories from fat can be useful in spotting high-fat foods and drinks.

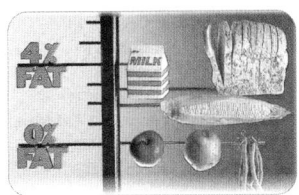

Fat Percentage Content
(Percentage of Fat in Food)

Don't be fooled by promotion of foods claiming to have a low percentage of fat. It's **serving size and total grams of fat that count.**

For example, whole milk with 3.5% fat sounds low (3.5g fat/100ml) but an 8fl.oz cup contains 8g fat (and 2 cups contain 16g fat).

Icecream with 10% fat seems high, yet a large scoop (3fl.oz) has only 5g fat. (Low-fat icecream has less than 2g fat/serve.)

❖　❖　❖

Also note that the percentage of fat in a food is not the same as the percentage of calories derived from fat.

Foods with a low percentage of fat can still have a high percentage of calories derived from fat - as shown below.

For example, around 50% of total calories in whole milk comes from fat - yet whole milk has less than 4% fat. Low fat/light milk with less than 1% fat has only 18% of total calories from fat - a much better choice.

FORMULA FOR CALCULATING PERCENTAGE CALORIES FROM FAT

$$\frac{\text{Grams of Fat/Serve} \times 9}{\text{Total Calories/Serve}} \times \frac{100}{1}$$

EXAMPLE:

Mars Bar (11g fat, 240 cals)

Percentage Calories from Fat
$$= \frac{11 \times 9}{265} \times \frac{100}{1} = 37\%$$

FAT CONTENT & PERCENTAGES OF MILK

	Whole Milk	Reduced Fat	Low-Fat (light)	Non-Fat Skim
Percentage Fat ▶	3.5%	2%	1%	0%
Fat (Grams) in 8 fl.oz Cup ▶	8g	5g	2g	0g
Calories ▶	150	120	100	95
Percent Calories From Fat ▶	48%	38%	18%	0%

Hints to Reduce Fat

Meats & Poultry

- **Choose lean cuts** of meat with little marbling. Choose the white meat of chicken and turkey, and extra lean ground beef.
- **Trim all visible fat** from meat and remove the skin from poultry. Removal of fat after cooking is okay (to prevent dryness).
- **Eat modest portions** (3-4 oz cooked weight) of meat, poultry or fish. **Add extra** beans, lentils, tofu, tempeh, vegetables, potatoes, rice, pasta, bread, or tortillas.
- **Avoid high-fat meat products** such as salami, bacon, sausage and franks. Choose lowfat and fat-free brands. Choose lean luncheon meats (90% or more fat-free).
- **Broil or bake. Avoid frying.** Allow casseroles to cool and skim off surface fat.

Fish & Seafood

- **Choose fresh or frozen fillets**, and canned fish (in water pack).
- **Avoid fried fish**, frozen fish in batter, canned fish in oil.

Fats & Oils

- **Use minimal amounts** of all types of fat and oil. All are high in calories.
- **Choose** 'light' and 'reduced fat' spreads but still use sparingly. Check the Fats and Spreads section of this book for lower fat brands.
- Use minimal amounts of oil when stir-frying. Use no-stick sprays like *Pam*.

Salad Dressings & Sauces

- **Avoid regular mayonnaise and oil dressings.** Choose 'light', 'reduced fat' or 'fat-free' brands (Check salad dressings section of this book).
- **Choose** lowfat or fat-free sauces. Most tomato-based pasta sauces are low fat but avoid 'pesto', 'alfredo', cheese and 'creamy' sauces.

Milk, Dairy, Soy Drinks

- **Choose** lowfat or skim milks and yogurts. **Avoid** full-cream milk, cream, *Half & Half* coffee creamers.
- **Soy Drinks:** Choose lowfat brands.
- **Cheese:** Choose fat-free, lowfat and fat-reduced (e.g. cottage, part-skim ricotta). Cheese substitutes can still be high in fat.
- **Icecream:** Choose lowfat and fat-free brands, frozen yogurt, sorbet, sherbet and ices. Limit regular icecream to a small serving. Avoid rich high-fat icecreams.

Frozen Meals & Entrees

- **Choose low fat varieties** such as *Lean Cuisine, Healthy Choice* and *Weight Watchers*. Add extra vegetables.

Soups

- **Choose low fat brands.** Avoid high-fat ramen noodle blocks/soup.

FRYING ADDS FAT

The greater the surface area of potato exposed to fat or oil, the higher the fat content.

Whole Potato (3 oz)
Nil Fat, 65 Cals
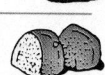

Roast Potato (3 oz)
5g Fat, 155 Cals
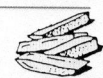

Fries (Large, 3 oz)
12g Fat, 220 Cals

Fries (Small, 3 oz)
15g Fat, 265 Cals

Potato Chips (3 oz)
30g Fat, 450 Cals

Bread, Bagels, Crackers

- **All breads are suitable** as well as pita, bagels, English muffins and rice cakes. Avoid croissants, sweet rolls, danish pastry and doughnuts. **Avoid** fat-soaked toast and garlic bread.
- **Choose lowfat crackers** such as graham, saltines, matzo, bread sticks, crispbreads. **Avoid** regular cheese or butter crackers.

Cereals, Pasta, Noodles, Rice

- **Most cold and hot cereals** are low in fat and nil in cholesterol. Avoid granola made with hydrogenated oils.
- **Choose** plain pasta or rice. Avoid dishes made with cream, butter or cheese sauces. **Avoid** high-fat ramen noodle blocks/soups.

Fruits & Vegetables

- **Choose all types.** (Note: Avocados contain no cholesterol. Their fat and fiber can help lower blood cholesterol.) Use mashed avocado on bread in place of fat.
- **Choose** dried beans, lentils, chick peas, baked beans.
- **Avoid** french-fried potatoes and regular potato salad. Avoid vegetables made in butter, cream or sauce.
- **Avoid** deli-style salads made with high fat dressings. Choose low-fat brands. Use low fat and fat-free salad dressings.

Snacks, Cookies, Candy

- **Avoid** high-fat snacks such as potato chips, corn/tortilla chips, cheesy balls, buttered popcorn, chocolate and carob bars.
- **Choose** fat-free potato chips and tortilla chips made with *olestra* (such as *Wow!* brand) but still limit quantity.
- **Choose** plain popcorn, lowfat cookies and muffins, hard candy, jelly beans, fruit rolls and frozen fruit bars and popsicles.
- **Choose** fresh and dried fruits, vegetables. Limit nuts and seeds if overweight.

Desserts/Sweets

- **Avoid high-fat desserts,** such as fruit pies, pastries, cheesecake, cheese board.
- **Choose** fresh fruits, fresh fruit salad, low fat custard and low fat yogurt. Use yogurt in place of cream or ice cream.
- **Avoid** regular icecream. *Choose* low fat brands but still limit quantity.
- **Choose** sugar-free gelatin desserts such as *Jell-O* (sugar-free package).

Fast-Foods & Take-Out

(Check the Fast-Foods Section of this book for actual fat counts and wise selections.)

- **Delis:** Choose sandwiches/bread rolls, pitas with lowfat fillings and plain salad. Limit meat/cheese to small portions. Request half quantities.
- **Avoid high-fat deli salads.** Choose plain salads and add your own lowfat dressing. Eat more fruit.
- **Chicken & Fish:** Avoid deep-fried chicken or fish, BBQ chicken with fat or skin, chicken nuggets. Choose broiled or baked chicken breast without fat or skin.
- **Hamburgers:** Choose medium size, lower fat burgers. Avoid bacon. Have a side salad (without dressing).
- **Pizzas:** Avoid sausage/pepperoni. Choose vegetarian topping and modest quantity of cheese. Eat a moderate serving. Eat extra salad and fruit.
- **Desserts:** Avoid apple pie, danish, choc chip cookies. Choose low fat muffins (e.g. *McDonald's*), fresh fruit or fruit salad.
- **Avoid regular shakes and sundaes.** Choose lowfat milk, lower fat shakes (such as *McDonald's*), and orange juice, but choose smaller sizes.

Hints to Reduce Sugar

• While reducing the amount of fat is an important dietary focus for weight control, sugar intake also needs to be watched.

• Many overweight, inactive persons consume over 500 calories of refined sugars per day (equivalent to over 30 level teaspoons) - a significant amount in weight control terms. Halving this amount would be reasonable and worthwhile.

Note: Naturally occurring sugars in fruits, vegetables and milk are fine when consumed in normal recommended amounts.

• Most sugar in our diet is 'hidden' in processed foods such as soft drinks, fruit drinks, candy, cookies, cake, jam, sauces, icecream, desserts, canned foods, and breakfast cereals.

Certainly enjoy moderate quantities of these foods, but for serious weight control, look for 'low calorie', 'diet' or sugar-free alternatives. Be careful not to substitute sugar-rich foods with high-fat foods which might boost calories even more!

• Sweeteners such as *Equal, NutraSweet, Sweet'n Low* and *Stevia* make it easy to cut back or eliminate sugar in drinks and recipes. (Most recipes can be adapted to contain less sugar with little effect on taste or quality.)

• The body can obtain sufficient sugar for its needs from carbohydrate-rich foods such as bread, rice, spaghetti and other pasta, potatoes, corn, fruit, vegetables, beans, nuts, seeds and lactose in milk.

These foods are also rich in other nutrients. Refined sugar is referred to as 'empty calorie' because it supplies calories but negligible nutrients and no fiber.

DIFFERENT FORMS OF SUGAR

Be aware that sugar comes in different forms. Check the label.

· Sugar	· Sucrose
· Brown Sugar	· Confectioners' Sugar
· Dextrose	· Glucose
· Fructose	· Malt, Maltose
· Corn Syrup	· High-Fructose Corn Syrup
· Honey	· Molasses
· Maple Syrup	· Turbinado Sugar

SUGAR CONTENT OF SOME COMMON FOODS

Teaspoons of Sugar

Coca Cola or *Pepsi*, 12 oz	10
20 oz size	17
Iced tea, sweetened, 12 oz	8
Choc malted Milk, 12 oz	4.5
Honey Smacks Cereal, 1 oz	4
Popcorn, caramel, 1 cup	3.5
Chocolate Bar, 1.5 oz	6
M&M's, 1.7 oz pkg	7
Cake, sponge, jam-filled	8
Choc Chip Cookie, 1 oz	2
Donut, iced	6
Apple Pie, 1 piece	7
Jell-O, 1/2 cup	4.5
Jam, 1 Tbsp, 20g	2.5
Syrup, maple, 1 Tbsp	3

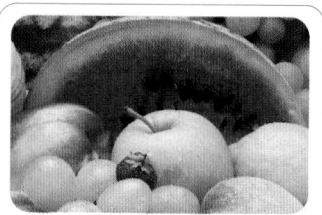

Reach for fresh fruit when you want to snack instead of candy or snack products rich in sugar and fat.

Sample Diet Plan - 1200 Calories

For Overweight Persons. Please Check With Your Doctor.
(Menu contains approximately 30-35 Grams Fat)

 ### Breakfast (approx. 250 cal)
1 Small Fruit or ½ oz Dried Fruit

Plus Cereal: 1½ oz Dry (high fiber)
or 1 cup cooked Oatmeal

Plus Milk (from daily allowance)

 ### Breakfast ~ Choice 2
1 Small Fruit

Plus 1 Toast (no added fat)
or ¾ oz Cheese
or 2 oz Cottage Cheese
or ¼ cup Baked Beans

Plus 1 Toast or ½ Muffin (English)

Milk Allowance (160 calories)
2 cups Skim Milk or 1½ cups Low Fat Milk
or equivalent Soy Drink, Yoghurt, Cheese, Tofu

Fat Allowance (140 calories; 15g Fat)
4 tsp Fat or 6-8 tsp Diet Margarine or 3 tsp Oil
or 1½ Tbsp Mayonnaise or ½ medium Avocado
or 1½ Tbsp Peanut Butter or 30g Nuts/Seeds

 ### Lunch (approx. 440 calories)
2 slices Bread (2 oz) or 1 medium Roll or Bagel
or 4 Crispbreads/Crackers or 6" Pita

Plus 2 oz lean Meat, Chicken or Turkey
or 3½ oz Tuna (in water) or 2½ oz Salmon
or 1 oz Cheese or 3 oz Cottage Cheese
or 2½ oz Ricotta Cheese
or ½ cup, 4 oz Fruit Yoghurt (lowfat)
or ½ cup (4 oz) Baked Beans or Bean Salad

Plus Large Salad (Oil-free dressing)
Plus 1 small Fruit or ½ oz Dried Fruit

 ### Dinner (approx. 360 Calories)
Soup (fat-free)

Plus 3 oz lean Meat (cooked weight)
or 4 oz Chicken Breast (no skin)
or 3 oz Chicken Thigh/Leg (no skin)
or 5 oz Fish (grilled, no fat)
or ¾ cup (6 oz) Beans (Soy, Baked, Haricot etc)/Lentils
or Low Fat Recipe Dish (e.g. Lean Cuisine)

Plus 1 small Potato or ½ cup Rice/Pasta or 1 slice Bread
Plus 2-3 servings Vegetables/Salad
Plus 1 small Fruit + Diet Gelatin Dessert

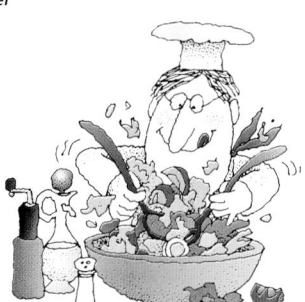

 ### Between Meals: Water, Coffee, Tea, Diet drinks,
Fruit from main meals; Raw vegetable pieces, Milk from Allowance

Note: Take a multivitamin/mineral supplement daily while dieting.

Exercise & Weight Control

- Persons who exercise regularly **lose more weight** and keep it off longer than non-exercisers.

- Exercise also improves general health and well-being. **Mood, confidence and self-esteem** are enhanced by a sense of control and accomplishment.

- **Exercise increases the metabolic rate** of the body even for hours after exercise - a good way to 'wake up' a sluggish metabolism and burn extra fat.

  Exercise compensates for any decrease in metabolic rate with increasing age and also in some heavy smokers who stop smoking.

- **Strength training** further builds muscle and aids body reshaping. You can also eat more food!

Note: It is muscle which burns fat. Each extra pound of muscle burns an extra 100 calories daily ~ even while you sleep! Weight from exercised muscles is okay. It is surplus fat that is potentially harmful.

- **Avoid injury** by beginning with walking, low impact aerobics, or weight-supported exercise (e.g. swimming, cycling). Avoid competitive sports.

- **How Much?** Start with 10 - 20 minutes/day and progress to 30-45minutes/day - even if broken into 5-10 minute lots. It all adds up! **Aim to achieve 250-500 calories of exercise daily.**

  Also walk up stairs instead of using lifts. Take a brisk walk at lunch. Use an exercise bike, treadmill or stair machine while watching TV.

- **How Often?** While aerobic fitness requires only 3 - 4 sessions weekly, **weight control is a daily event which requires daily exercise.**

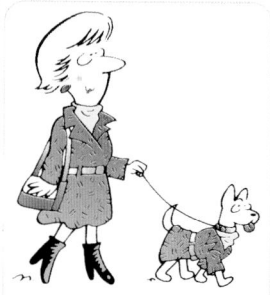

Brisk walking each day is a safe and effective way to keep trim and fit. Try it - you'll like it!"

Strength-training with light weights helps to retain or rebuild muscle tissue and enhances weight control.

TV CAN BE FATTENING!

Many adults and children watch over 20 hours of television per week and indulge in high-fat snacks at the same time - potent contributors to obesity.

Are you a TV couch potato? Limit your TV hours and plan healthy physical activities. At least use an exercise bike or treadmill while watching TV!

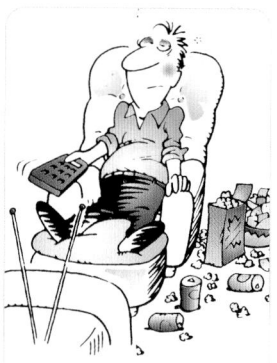

Middle-age spread has little to do with getting older. Too little exercise is the main culprit.

Daily exercise and sensible eating can minimize middle-age spread.

Calories Used in Exercise

LIGHT
4 Calories/Minute

Walking, slow
Cycling, light
Gardening light
Golf, social
Tennis, doubles
Housework, cleaning
Callisthenics, Yoga
Ten Pin Bowls
Ping-pong, social
Ice Skating
Aquarobics
Skate Boarding
Line/Square Dancing

MODERATE
7 Calories/Minute

Walking, brisk
Cycling, moderate
Swimming, crawl
Weight-training, light
Tennis, singles
Racquetball, beginners
Aerobics, light
Football, Grid Iron
Basketball, Baseball
Walking Downstairs
Snow Skiing (downhill)
Shoveling snow
Dancing (vigorous)

HEAVY
10 Calories/Minute

Walking (power), Jogging
Cycling (vigorous), Spinning
Swimming, strenuous
Weight-training, heavy
Wrestling/Judo, advanced
Racquetball, advanced
Tae Bo, Kick Boxing
Football, training
Basketball (Pro)
Climbing Stairs, Skipping
Skiing (cross country)
Aquarobics, advanced
Dancing (strenuous)

Note: Only those sports or activities that are sustained over a period of time (e.g running) qualify for heavy exercise. Stop-start sports such as tennis are considered 'moderate'.

BE A GROOVY GRANNY!

You are never too old to start a fitness and strength-training program. See your local fitness center or personal trainer.

June McClean (85 y.o) is America's fittest granny - also known as the 'Groovy Granny'.

Check out her video: 'Low Impact Aerobics For Seniors'.

(Order Details ~ Page 287)

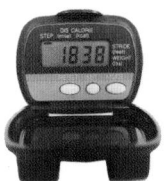

10,000 STEPS PER DAY

A pedometer can motivate you to be more active everyday. It counts steps, miles and even calories used (some models). It clips to your belt or waist band.

Aim for 10,000 steps per day, instead of an average 3,000-4,000 steps.

(Order Details ~ Page 287)

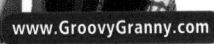
www.GroovyGranny.com

Reshape Eating Behaviors

- Eating is a behavior that is largely controlled by people with whom we live or socialize, places in which we carry out our lives, and our emotions. Become aware of those situations that commonly lead to extra food being eaten.

- We may also be unaware of 'bad' eating habits that can lead to excess calorie intake; e.g. eating quickly, large mouthsful, eating when tense or bored, finishing a large serving of food when not hungry.

Hints to help uncover and correct those 'bad' eating habits include:

- **Don't eat while engaged in other activities;** e.g. watching TV, reading. Eat only at the table, not at the fridge or while standing.

- **Don't eat quickly.** Chewing slowly allows time to register a feeling of fullness. Don't use fingers, only utensils. Cut food into smaller pieces. Don't load your fork until the previous mouthful is finished.

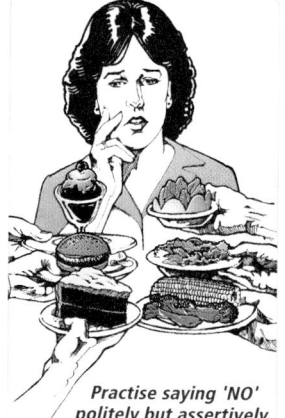

Practise saying 'NO' politely but assertively.

- **Don't purchase problem high calorie foods.** Shop from a set list to prevent impulse buying. Avoid shopping with children.

- **Buy snack foods** in the smallest package. The larger the serving size or package, the more you are likely to eat or drink.

- **Plan meals in advance. Stick to a set menu.**

- **Plan a strategy to avoid uncontrolled eating** and drinking at social events, or when your emotions urge you to binge.

  Rehearse repeatedly in your mind exactly what you will do in such situations. Remind yourself several times each day that you are in charge of your actions and that you can be strong-willed. Seek counseling or coaching on various strategies.

- **Promise yourself** that when you feel the urge to snack, you will engage in some activity that will distract you away from food (e.g. go for a walk, brush your teeth, phone a friend.)

  If you eat out of boredom, find some new hobby or interest that gets you out of the house. Even enrol in an adult education class.

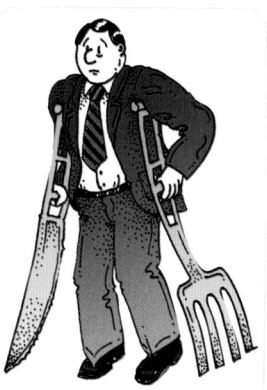

Do you use food as an emotional crutch? If so, professional counseling may be helpful.

The food diary is the most powerful proven aid for dieters. Persons who keep a food and exercise diary not only lose more weight they also keep it off. Here are some of the reasons:

- Recording your eating and exercise habits jolts you into realizing just what you do eat and drink each day; and also whether you exercise sufficiently.

- **Helps you identify problem foods** and drinks with excessive calories and fat.

- **Helps identify moods**, situations and events that lead to excessive eating of unwanted calories. You can then plan to overcome or avoid them.

- **Prevents 'calorie amnesia'**, the forgetfulness that leads to rebound weight gain after successful weight loss. Recording puts you back on the right track.

- **Helps you develop greater self- discipline.** You will think twice about over indulging if you have to record it - especially if someone checks your diary regularly. It certainly keeps you honest!

- **Motivates you** to carefully plan your meals and to exercise each day.

- **Serves as a check system** for your doctor, dietitian or counselor to assess your progress and make recommendations.

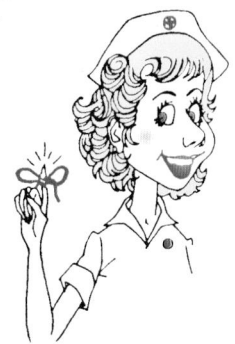

"Keeping a diary gives me feedback on exactly what I eat each day.
It helps prevent 'calorie amnesia' and reminds me to exercise each day.
It's a must for successful weight control!"

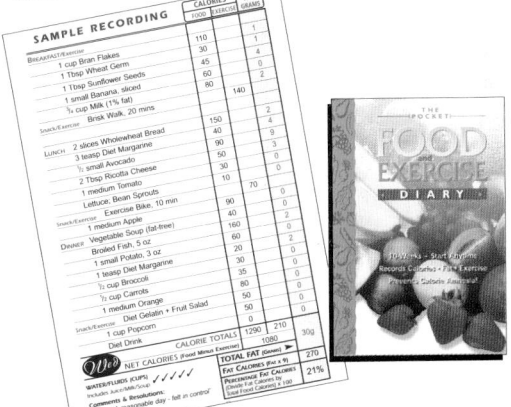

SAMPLE RECORDING

	CALORIES FOOD	CALORIES EXERCISE	FAT GRAMS
BREAKFAST/Exercise			
1 cup Bran Flakes	110		1
1 Tbsp Wheat Germ	30		1
1 Tbsp Sunflower Seeds	45		4
1 small Banana, sliced	60		0
½ cup Milk (1% fat)	80	140	1
Brisk Walk, 20 mins			
Snack/Exercise			
LUNCH 2 slices Wholewheat Bread	150		2
3 teasp Diet Margarine	40		4
½ small Avocado	90		9
2 Tbsp Ricotta Cheese	50		3
1 medium Tomato	30		0
Lettuce, Bean Sprouts	10	70	0
Exercise Bike, 10 min			
Snack/Exercise 1 medium Apple	90		0
DINNER Vegetable Soup (fat-free)	40		0
Broiled Fish, 5 oz	160		2
1 small Potato, 3 oz	60		0
1 teasp Diet Margarine	20		0
½ cup Broccoli	30		0
½ cup Carrots	35		0
1 medium Orange	80		0
Snack/Exercise Diet Gelatin + Fruit Salad	50		0
1 cup Popcorn	50		0
Diet Drink	0		0
CALORIE TOTALS (Food Minus Exercise)	1290	210	30g

Water/Fluids (Cups) ✓✓✓✓

Includes Juice/Milk/Soup

NET CALORIES (Food Minus Exercise) ▶ 1080

TOTAL FAT ▶ 30g

TOTAL CALORIES (Fat x 9) 270

PERCENTAGE FAT CALORIES (Divide Fat Calories By total Food Calories) x 100 = **21%**

Comments & Resolutions: A reasonable day - felt in control

PAGE #

Sample page from The Pocket Food & Exercise Diary, a 10-week diary to record food and exercise.

At day's end, exercise calories are deducted from food calories.

Includes Weekly Summary Page & Progress Checklist.

EXTRA DETAILS ~ SEE PAGE 288

What is Diabetes?

Diabetes is a disorder in which the body cannot make proper use of carbohydrates (sugar and starches).

- After digestion, sugar and starches are changed into **glucose** - the simplest form of sugar that is vital to body cells for energy and growth.

- **Insulin** is the hormone which acts like a key that opens the door to body cells and allows glucose to enter.

- **Without sufficient insulin**, unused glucose builds up in the blood and passes into the urine. This produces symptoms of frequent urination, continual thirst and tiredness.

- **Untreated diabetes** increases the risk of damage to nerves and blood vessels. This, in turn, increases the risk of heart disease, stroke, blindness, kidney damage, foot ulcers and gangrene, impotence and other complications.

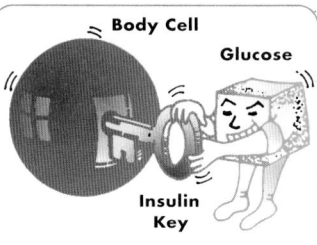

Insulin acts like a key. It opens the door to body cells and allows glucose to enter.

Some persons with diabetes (Type 1) have too few or no keys and require insulin injections.

Others (Type 2) have ample keys but 'mis-shapen' key holes (insulin resistant) - particularly if obese and inactive.

TYPE-1 DIABETES

Insulin-Dependent Diabetes

- Occurs in 10% of diabetes cases.

- Usually children and young adults.

- Pancreas gland produces little or no insulin. Daily insulin injections are necessary, plus:

- Regular meals with even carbohydrate distribution to match insulin dosage. Regular exercise and weight control are also important.

WARNING SIGNALS

- Frequent urination
- Continual thirst
- Rapid weight loss
- Unusual hunger
- Extreme weakness/fatigue
- Nausea, vomiting, irritability

TYPE-2 DIABETES

Non-Insulin Dependent

- Occurs in 90% of diabetes cases.

- Occurs mainly in adults - particularly in overweight and inactive persons.

- Insulin is produced but body cells resist its action and glucose cannot enter cells.

- Usually treated with diet and exercise. Sometimes requires medication (pills or insulin injections).

WARNING SIGNALS

- Any Type-1 symptom
- Blurred vision
- Excessive itching
- Skin infections with slow healing
- Tingling/numbness in feet

Importance of Weight Control

- **Type-2 diabetes** occurs 2-3 times more often in overweight persons - particularly if inactive.

- Such persons do not usually lack insulin. Rather, their insulin is less effective. As obesity develops, muscle and other body cells may resist insulin in varying degrees. The resultant build-up of blood glucose may lead to diabetic symptoms.

- **Weight loss alone** often corrects this condition in Type-2 diabetes. If overweight, try a moderate diet of 1200-1500 calories **plus daily exercise**.

  Within several weeks, body cells can lose their resistance and become sensitive once again to the effects of insulin. Insulin and blood glucose levels may normalise, and symptoms may disappear.

  Further, the need for oral antidiabetic drugs might be prevented or much lessened in dosage. **So, give diet and exercise a fair go** - and maintain them to keep symptoms under control.

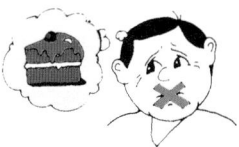

Modest weight loss and daily exercise can greatly improve control of Type-2 diabetes.

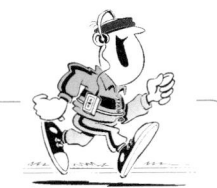

Get Moving! Everyday, do at least 30 minutes of moderate intensity exercise. It's the key to improving insulin sensitivity.

Add strength-training 3-4 times a week to double the benefits.

Managing Diabetes

Don't battle diabetes alone. Establish a partnership with your doctor, dietitian, nurse educator and pharmacist. For extra support, contact the *American Diabetes Association* 1-800-342-2383.

Hints to keep blood glucose within safe limits:

- **Control your diet.** Know what and when you will eat. Seek referral to a dietitian for expert advice.

- **Exercise regularly.** It assists weight control and can improve sensitivity of body cells to insulin. Plan exercise into your daily routine.

- **Monitor your blood glucose** at home and work - ideally with a portable blood glucose meter. It will help you become familiar with your blood glucose patterns, and the effects of diet, exercise and medication. **Insulin pumps** can also help control blood glucose levels around the clock.

- **Don't skip prescribed insulin or oral medication.** If on insulin, know what action to take if hypoglycaemia (low blood glucose) occurs. Also educate family and friends.

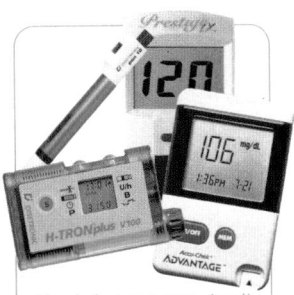

Blood glucose meters, insulin pumps and pens can greatly improve control of diabetes and lifestyle choices.

Guidelines for choosing a healthy diet apply equally to persons with or without diabetes. Eating a wide variety of foods with the emphasis on low-fat, high fiber and low in refined sugars, is recommended.

However, actual food quantities, as well as when you eat, will also influence control of blood glucose. Your dietitian will individualize a diet plan to suit your food preferences, lifestyle and medical status. Here are a few hints:

- **Maintain a healthy weight.** If overweight, even a modest weight loss plus daily exercise can help to normalise blood glucose in Type-2 diabetes.

- **Don't skip meals.** If you take insulin or an oral hypoglycemic agent, regular meals are important.

- **If on insulin**, eat meals at the same time each day. Eat a similar amount of food at each meal. An even distribution of carbohydrate over the day will make best use of the available insulin and prevent wide fluctuations in blood glucose levels. Leave an interval of about 30 minutes between insulin injection and breakfast.

- **Avoid sugars and foods high in added sugar** particularly if overweight. Small amounts of sugar as part of a meal may occasionally be okay. Check with your dietitian. Use *Equal*, *Splenda* and *NutraSweet*-sweetened foods and drinks.

- **Choose wholegrain breads, cereals and pasta.** Eat fresh fruits, vegetables and legumes. These foods contain more fiber and slow the release of glucose into your blood after a meal.

- **Limit foods high in saturated fat and cholesterol.** Enjoy fish, soy foods, and other foods rich in omega-3 fats. *(See Fats & Cholesterol Guide, Pages 246-252)*

- **Foods (and supplements) rich in antioxidant vitamins C, E and beta-carotene**, as well as omega-3 fats, magnesium, zinc and chromium may help prevent long-term complications of diabetes (such as damage to small blood vessels and nerves). Be sure to check with your doctor.

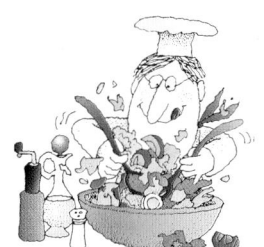

Eat a well-balanced diet, high in fiber-containing foods and low in fat.

NEW BLOOD SUGAR LEVEL FOR DIAGNOSING DIABETES
(Adopted by American Diabetes Assoc.)

Blood Sugar Levels
Previously: 140 mg/dL
New: 126 mg/dL

Everyone 45 and older should have a blood test every 3 years.

Excess Alcohol contributes to obesity, diabetes, and high blood pressure.

The risk of hypoglycemia (low blood sugar) and drug interactions with alcohol is also increased.

Carbohydrates & Diabetes

- Carbohydrate foods in their more natural forms are an important part of a healthy diet. They provide energy, fiber, vitamins, minerals, protein and water. Carbohydrates are found mainly in cereal grains, fruit, vegetables and milk. Animal flesh foods contain negligible amounts.

  A healthy diet of at least 2000 calories is based around carbohydrate foods and should provide over 50% of total calories - whether or not we have diabetes. Lower calorie diets for weight control will have as little as 40% carbohydrate calories.

- Carbohydrates include sugars, starches and fibers. Sugars and starch provide energy to body cells. Even though fiber is not digested, it benefits the body - more so in diabetes. *(See Fiber Guide ~ Page 262)*

  The various forms of carbohydrate affect blood glucose levels in different ways; and it is difficult to predict the effect of particular foods, sugars or meals, simply by their actual carbohydrate content.

  Thus, the same amount of carbohydrate from different foods may affect blood sugar differently. It depends on many factors.

  For example, fiber can slow digestion and absorption of sugars by acting as a physical barrier or by forming a gel. Both fiber and fat also slow the emptying rate of the stomach into the intestines where further digestion and absorption takes place. The physical form of food (solid, puree, liquid) also matters - the more natural the better.

  Generally, raw foods rather than cooked foods, and whole-foods rather than ground-up foods, are more slowly absorbed.

- Sugar: Small amounts eaten as part of a meal, may not adversely affect blood glucose in persons with good blood glucose control. Nevertheless, minimal amounts of sugar are encouraged for nutritional and weight control reasons.

Glycemic Index

- Glycemic index (GI) indicates how fast a carbohydrate containing food is digested and how much it causes blood glucose to rise (glycemic response).

LOWER GLYCEMIC FOODS

Slower Acting Carbohydrates

These foods are more slowly digested and absorbed. They help maintain more even blood glucose levels. Use these foods regularly. Examples:

- Dried beans, peas, lentils
- Nuts and seeds
- Wholegrain breads, pita
- Bran cereals, oats
- Barley, buckwheat, bulgur
- Spaghetti, pasta, Basmati Rice
- Fresh fruit: apples, avocados, bananas (firm), cherries, grapefruit, grapes, olives, oranges, peaches, pears, plums
- Vegetables: sweet corn, yam
- Milk, yogurt, soy drinks

HIGHER GLYCEMIC FOODS

Quicker Acting Carbohydrates

These foods more rapidly raise blood glucose levels. Eat in moderation.

- White/wholegrain bread, rice cakes, bagels, croissants, doughnuts
- Low fiber cereals: Cornflakes, *Rice Krispies, Froot Loops*
- White potato, white rice
- Watermelon, ripe bananas, cantaloupe, pineapple
- Glucose drinks and candy

(See Carbohydrate Distribution next page)

Diabetes & Carbohydrate Distribution

- For people with diabetes, regular meals with even distribution of carbohydrate over the day are important for good control of blood sugar levels.

- Smaller amounts of food eaten more frequently result in steadier, more even blood glucose levels. (Be sure to control your weight.)

  Recommended daily eating patterns for good blood glucose control:

  1. **Three Meals & Three Snacks ~**
     Best for persons on insulin (Type-1 diabetes) with normal blood glucose variations.

  2. **Three Meals ~**
     Best for Type-2 diabetes (especially if overweight).

  Note: If blood sugar levels show excessive variations see doctor and dietitian.

- Your doctor or dietitian will select the level of calories and carbohydrate most appropriate to your weight, medication and activity. (Regular blood glucose checks will provide feedback on the level of control.)

- **Amounts of carbohydrate** in the guide below provide an average of 50% of total calories. **A rough rule of thumb is:** 13 grams of carbohydrate per 100 calories. **At calorie levels above 2000,** carbohydrates approach 50-60% of total calories.

  At lower calorie levels used for weight loss (1200-1500 calories), carbohydrates account for as little as 40% of total calories. This is because protein has nutritional priority.

  These carbohydrate quantities (and percentages) apply equally to persons with or without diabetes.

IDEAL CARBOHYDRATE DISTRIBUTION
For Type-1 Diabetes (Insulin Dependent)
3 MEALS & 3 SNACKS
Balanced Blood Sugar Levels

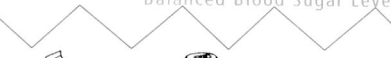
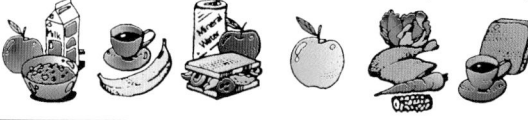

GUIDE TO CARBOHYDRATE DISTRIBUTION

Daily Total Calories		Daily Total Carbohyd.	Percent Carbohyd. Cals	Each Main Meal (3)	Between Meals (3)
1200 Cals	~	120g	40%	30g	10g
1500 Cals	~	170g	45%	40g	15g
2000 Cals	~	250g	50%	60g	25g
2500 Cals	~	345g	55%	70g	45g
3000 Cals	~	450g	60%	90g	60g

Notes, Abbreviations, Measures

- Calorie and fat values have been rounded off.
  Calories - to the nearest 5 or 10 calories.
  Fat - to the nearest half gram.
  Note: Trace amounts of fat (less than 0.3 grams per serving) have been treated as zero.

- Because manufacturer's figures on labels are rounded off, figures in this book may differ slightly from the label. Serving sizes may also vary.

- Food product formulations change from time to time, and hence the need to regularly update this type of publication. Many products also come and go. Check the food label for any changes.

- **Seek Professional Advice:** This book is intended for educational purposes only. It is not a substitute for professional advice.

- **Feedback Welcome:** Please contact the author directly with your queries, and suggestions for foods to be included in future editions. (Ideally, enclose the label with the manufacturer's details.)
  Write to: Allan Borushek,
  PO Box 1616, Costa Mesa CA 92628

- **Free Information Service:** Check the author's website for new food product updates.

  www.calorieking.com

C ~ **Calories**
F ~ **Fat (grams)**
Cb ~ **Carbohydrate (grams)**

Abbreviations

tsp	=	teaspoon
Tbsp	=	Tablespoon
oz	=	ounce(s)
c	=	cup
fl.oz	=	fluid ounce(s)
g	=	gram(s)
<1	=	less than 1

Volume Measures

3 tsp	=	1 Tbsp
2 Tbsp	=	1 fl.oz
1/2 cup	=	4 fl.oz
1 cup	=	8 fl.oz
		or 16 Tbsp
2 cups	=	1 Pint
2 Pints	=	1 Quart

(All measures are level)

Note: 8 oz weight is not the same as 8 fl.oz volume (space occupied). Dense foods weigh more per set volume. Examples:

  1 cup popcorn weighs 1/2 oz
  1 cup milk weighs 8 1/2 oz
  1 cup pudding weighs 10 oz

Metric Conversion

1/2 oz	=	14 grams
1 oz	=	28.4 grams
2 oz	=	57 grams
3 1/2 oz	=	100 grams
1 fl.oz	=	30 mls
1 cup (8 fl.oz)	=	240 mls
33 fl.oz	=	1 liter (volume)

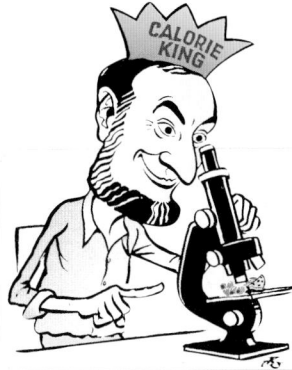

SOURCES OF INFORMATION

- U.S. Dept. of Agriculture
- Food Manufacturers
- Food Industry Boards & Councils
- Independent laboratory analysis
- Scientific publications
- Overseas food composition tables
- Author extrapolations

Milk

Quick Guide

C F Cb

Cow's Milk
Average All Brands

Whole (3.5% fat):

	C	F	Cb
2 Tbsp, 1 fl.oz	20	1	1.5
1 Glass, 6 fl.oz	110	6	8.5
1 Cup, 8 fl.oz	150	8	12
1 Pint, 16 fl.oz	300	16	23
1 Quart, 946 ml	600	32	46

Reduced-fat (2% fat):

2 Tbsp, 1 fl.oz	15	0.5	1.5
1 Glass, 6 fl.oz	90	4	8.5
1 Cup, 8 fl.oz	120	5	12
1 Pint, 16 fl.oz	240	10	23
1 Quart, 946 ml	480	20	46

Light/Lowfat (1% fat):

2 Tbsp, 1 fl.oz	12	0.3	1.5
1 Glass, 6 fl.oz	75	2	8.5
1 Cup, 8 fl.oz	100	2.5	12
1 Pint, 16 fl.oz	200	5	23
1 Quart, 946 ml	400	10	46

Fat Free/Skim:

2 Tbsp, 1 fl.oz	10	0	1.5
1 Cup, 8 fl.oz	90	0.5	12
1 Pint, 16 fl.oz	180	1	24
w. Replace (Oatrim Fiber): 1 cup	85	0	12

Protein-Fortified:

2% fat, 1 cup	140	5	14
1% fat, 1 cup	120	3	14
Skim, 1 cup	100	0.5	14

Acidophilus: *Average All Brands*

Reduced Fat (2%), 1 cup	130	5	13
Lowfat (1%), 1 cup	100	2	13

Buttermilk: *Average All Brands*

Reduced Fat (2%), 1 cup	120	5	10
Low Fat (1%), 1 cup	100	2.5	12
Oak Farms (1%), 1 cup	100	2.5	12

Lactose-Reduced:

Reduced Fat: *Lactaid*, 1 cup	130	5	12
Dairy Ease 100, 1 cup	130	5	12
Lowfat fat, *Lactaid*, 1 cup	110	2.5	12
Fat Free *Lactaid/Lucerne*, 1 cup	80	0	13

Soy & Non-Dairy Drinks
~ See Page 24 ~

Goat & Sheep Milk

Goat's Milk *(Meyenberg):*	C	F	Cb
Whole, 1 cup, 8 fl.oz	140	7	11
Light/Lowfat (1%), 8 fl.oz	90	2.5	9
Evaporated, reconst., 8 fl.oz	145	8	11
Kefir: *Alta Dena*, 1 cup	240	4.5	41
Steve's Kefir Peach, 1 cup	220	9	25
Sheep's Milk: Whole, 1 cup	265	17	13

Canned & Dried Milk

Average All Brands

Condensed: Reg. 2 Tbsp, 1 fl.oz	130	3	22
Lowfat (*Eagle*), 2 Tbsp	120	1.5	23
Fat Free (*Eagle*), 2 Tbsp	110	0	24
Evaporated: Whole, 2 Tbsp	40	3	3
Whole, 1/2 cup	170	10	13
Lowfat (*Carnation*), 2 Tbsp	25	1	3
1/2 cup	110	3	12
Light/Skim, 1/2 cup	100	0.5	14
Dried: Whole, 1/4 cup, 1 oz	150	8	11
Skim/Nonfat, 1/3 cup	80	0	12
Made-up, 1 cup, 8 fl.oz	80	0	12
Buttermilk, sweetcream, 1 oz	110	2	3
Nonfat, 1 Tbsp	25	0	3

Whey Drink

Acid: Dry, 1 Tbsp, 3g	10	0	2
Fluid, 1 cup, 8 fl.oz	60	0	13
Sweet: Dry, 1 Tbsp, 8g	25	0	6
Fluid, 1 cup, 8 fl.oz	65	1	13
Nutri Mil: Original, 8 fl.oz	80	3	11
Fat Free (Calcium Enriched)	60	0	11

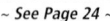

Quick Guide
Chocolate Milk

	C	F	Cb

Average All Brands: Per Cup, 8 fl.oz

	C	F	Cb
Whole Milk (3.3%): 1 cup	225	9	26
1 Pint	450	18	52
Reduced Fat (2%), 1 cup	190	5	26
Lowfat (1%), 1 cup	160	3	26

Brands ~ Chocolate Milk

Ready-To-Drink: Per 8 fl.oz Cup

Albertson's, lowfat	170	2.5	30
Bodywise, nonfat	180	0	35
Borden: Dutch Choc., 1 cup	220	8	28
Bosco	230	8	33
Brown Cow Farm, 1 cup	250	8	39
Deans'Chug': Regular	220	9	26
Lowfat, 1 cup	160	2.5	27
Dominick's Lowfat, 1 cup	170	2.5	28
Golden Guernsey, 1 cup	130	2.5	15
Grocers Pride Choc D'Lite, 1 cup	120	3	22
Hershey's: Lowfat (2%) Choc Milk	190	5	25
Whole Choc., 1 cup, 240ml	230	9	28
Hood, Lowfat (1%)	150	2	27
Horizon Organic	160	2.5	27
Knudsen	200	3	32
Kroger (3.25% milk)	220	9	28
Lactaid (1%)	160	3	26
Land O'Lakes, lowfat (0.5%)	150	1.5	35
Meadow Gold (3.5%)	210	8	25
Oak Farms , 1 cup	210	8	26
Parmalat (2%)	180	5	28
Quik: (*Nestle*) Chocolate Milk	230	8	30
Strawberry Milk	220	9	31
Ralph's	240	3	34
Yoo Hoo Choc Drink, 9 fl.oz	150	1	33

Bottled Coffee (Chilled)

Ready-To-Drink: Per bottle

Blue Luna: Per 12^{1}/$_{2}$ fl.oz			
Cafe Latte	195	3	36
Lite Cafe Mocha	114	3	15
Main St Cafe:			
French Van. Ice Latte, 12 fl.oz	190	33	31
Nescafe: Caffe Latte	140	3.5	23
Mocha	140	3	26
Starbucks: Coffee; Mocha	190	3	40

Shakes & Smoothies

Smoothies

	C	F	Cb

Made Up Ready-To-Drink
(8 fl. oz Milk/Soy + Fruit): Per 12 fl.oz

Average all types

with Whole Milk	300	8	50
+ Icecream, 1 scoop	400	13	62
with Nonfat Milk	240	0	50
Langers: 8 fl.oz, all flavors	135	0	34

Shakes

Regular: Chocolate, 10 fl.oz	360	11	58
Vanilla/Strawberrry, 10 fl.oz	320	9	53
McDonald's Reduced Fat,			
Small (14 fl.oz), all flavors	340	5	60
Burger King: Vanilla, medium	430	9	73
Chocolate w. Syrup, medium	560	10	105
Killer Shake (14oz): Choc./Van., 1 c	210	5	36

Cocoa-Chocolate Mixes

Add extra cals/fat/carbohydrate for milk

Alba '66 Milk Choc, 1 pkt	60	0	14
Carnation Cocoa Mixes:			
Chocolate Rich, 3 Tbsp/1 pkt	110	1	24
Milk Chocolate, 3 Tbsp	110	1	24
w.mini Marshmallows, 1 oz pkt	110	1	24
Malted Milk Original, 3 Tbsp	90	2	15
70 Calorie Cocoa Mix, 3 tsp	70	0.5	15
Fat-Free, 2 Tbsp/1 pkt	25	0	4
No Sugar, 1 pkt	50	0.5	8
Land O' Lakes: Per 1^{1}/$_{4}$ oz pkt			
Choc.Mint/Raspb./Supreme	160	5	25
Nestle Hot Cocoa Mix, 1 oz	110	1	23
w. Marshmallows, 1 oz	120	1	23
Ghirardelli: Per 2 heaping tsp			
Choc. Mocha/Hazelnut/Dble Choc	80	1.5	21
Pralines & Creme, 2 Tbsp	90	0	23
Ovaltine Cocoa Mixes, 4 tsp	80	0	20
Swiss Miss Cocoa Mixes:			
Milk Chocolate, 1 oz pkt	110	1.5	22
w. Marshmallows, 1.2 oz pkt	140	3	22
Choc. Sensation, 1.25 oz pkt	150	4	27
Lite, 1 pkt	70	0	18
Diet Cocoa Mix, 1 pkt	20	0	4
Sugar Free	60	0	10
Fat Free, 0.53 oz	50	0	9
Vending Machine, 1.34 oz pkt	145	2	24
Weight Watchers: Hot Cocoa Mix	70	0	10

Soy & Non-Dairy Drinks

Soy Non-Dairy Drinks

(Lactose & Cholesterol Free)

Per 1 Cup Serving (8 fl.oz)

	C	F	Cb
Cereal Match: Lowfat, 1 cup	100	3	17
Eden Blend: 1 cup	120	3	18
Edensoy (Organic): Carob	150	4	23
Extra Original	130	4	13
Vanilla; Extra Vanilla	150	3	23
Hain Soy Supreme: Original	80	3	9
Vanilla, 1 cup	100	3	12
Harmony Farms: Regular, 1 cup	80	3	10
Enriched; Vanilla, 1 cup	100	3	14
Health Source: All flavors	150	1.5	23
Health Source Plus	160	1	17
Health Valley: Soy Moo	110	0	21
Pacific: Original unsweetened	100	5	13
Enriched (Soy Isoflavin): Plain	90	2.5	14
Vanilla	110	2.5	16
Fat Free: Plain	70	0	14
Vanilla	90	0	14
Select (Soy Isoflavin), Plain	100	2.5	13
Silk (White Wave): Plain	80	2.5	9
Chocolate	108	2.5	14
SoyDream: Original, 8 fl.oz	140	5	14
Carob/Chocolate Enriched	210	4	37
Vanilla	160	5	21
Soy-Um (Trader Joe's): Original	100	3	13
Chocolate	160	3	27
Vanilla	110	3	15
Val/Shake: Regular	380	12	56
Vitamite: 1 cup	110	5	14
Vitasoy: Creamy, 1 cup	130	5	12
Carob	210	6	32
Light Original	90	2	15
Light Cocoa/Vanilla	110	2	20
Rich Cocoa: 8 fl.oz box	190	6	25
32 fl.oz size, 1 cup	210	6	32
Vanilla Delite	190	6	27
WestSoy: Plus, Plain	130	4	18
100% Organic: Original (2% fat)	140	5	18
Unsweetened	90	4.5	5
Nonfat: Plain	80	0	15
Vanilla	90	0	17
Lite: Plain	100	2	15
Cocoa	120	1.5	23
Vanilla	120	2.5	21
Lowfat: Plain	90	1.5	14
Vanilla	110	1.5	20

WestSoy (Cont):	C	F	Cb
Vigor Aid: Chocolate Mocha	240	6	38
French Vanilla	260	6	44

Soy Powder Mix

(1 oz mix makes 1 cup, 8 fl.oz)

	C	F	Cb
Better Than Milk: Original	100	2.5	16
Light	80	0.5	13
Soyagen, 1 oz	130	7	12
Soy Protein Isolate, 1 oz	95	1	0
Soy Quik (Ener-g), 1 oz	100	4.5	8

Rice & Cereal Drinks

	C	F	Cb
Almond Breeze: Original, 8 fl.oz	60	3	8
Vanilla, 8 fl.oz	90	3	16
Amazake: Almond Light, 8 fl.oz	110	2	20
Eden Blend: Rice & Soy, 1 cup	120	3	18
Eden Rice: 1 cup, 8 fl.oz	110	3	23
Hain Rice Supreme: Lowfat Orig.	100	3	16
Lowfat Cinnamon	130	3	22
Pacific Foods:			
Multigrain, 1 cup, 8 fl.oz	140	2	25
Naturally Oat: Original, 1 cup	110	1.5	21
Vanilla, 1 cup	130	1.5	24
Naturally Almond: 1 cup	70	2.5	10
Vanilla, 1 cup	90	2.5	15
Pacific Rice: Lowfat, Plain, 1 cup	90	2	17
Fat Free: Plain	70	0	17
Cocoa	90	0	20
Vanilla	110	0	24
Rice Dream: Carob, 1 cup	150	2.5	32
Chocolate; Choc. Enriched, 1 c.	170	3	36
Vanilla; Vanilla Enriched, 1 cup	130	2	28
Organic; Organic Enriched, 1 c.	120	2	25
Rice-Um (Trader Joe's): 8 fl.oz	120	2	26
Westbrae: Oat Plus, 1 cup	150	3	26
Original Vanilla, 1 cup	150	3	20

Rice/Nut Drink Mixes

Better Than Milk: Per 2 Tbsp Powder	C	F	Cb
Original, 23g	100	2.5	16
Light, 19g	70	0.5	14
Vanilla, 19g	90	5	10
Nut Quik, 2 Tbsp powder, 18g	110	9	3
Solait, 3 Tbsp powder, 22g	80	1.5	13
Sun's Up, 2 scoops, 40g powder	160	2	36
Rice Moo, 2 Tbsp powder, 19g	72	0	17

Quick Guide

Yogurt

Average All Brands: Per 8 oz

	C	F	Cb
Plain Yogurt: Whole, 8 oz	180	7	11
Lowfat	140	4	16
Nonfat	110	0	18
Fruit Flavored: Whole, 8 oz	250	6	38
Lowfat	230	3	32
Nonfat, regular	150	0	32
Nonfat, no sugar added	120	0	32
Goat's Milk Yogurt-Same as Regular			

Yogurt ~ Brands

	C	F	Cb
Alex Rod: Fat Free, all flav., 8 oz	70	0	12
Albertson's: Plain, lowfat, 8 oz	140	2.5	17
Fruit on the Bottom (lowfat):			
Average all flavors, 8 oz	220	2	42
Swiss (Nonfat), average, 6 oz	90	0	14
Indulgents (Lowfat), 6 oz	180	2	35
Alta Dena: Lowfat: Plain, 8 oz	170	4.5	13
Vanilla, 8 oz	260	3.5	44
Nonfat: Plain, 8 oz	110	0	17
Flavors, average	190	0	39
America's Choice: Swiss Style	210	2.5	41
Fruit on the Bottom: Cherry Van.	270	2.5	55
Other flavors, average	220	2.5	40
Nonfat, all flavors, 8 oz	100	0	15
Berkeley Farms (8 oz Cup)			
Lowfat: Boysenberry/Cherry	230	2.5	46
Raspberry	220	2.5	43
Strawberry, Lemon, Vanilla	270	2.5	52
Nonfat: Average all flavors	100	0	16
Breyers: Light n' Lively: 125g	130	1	25
Lowfat: 1% fat, all flavors, 8 oz	250	2.5	48
1.5% fat, plain	130	3	15
Flavors, average	220	3	38
Smooth & Creamy: 125g	130	1	25
Brown Cow Farm (Fat Free): Plain	120	0	18
Cappuccino/Maple Alm./Vanilla	170	0	33
Cherry Vanilla/Strawberry, 8 oz	190	0	39
Chocolate, 8 oz	220	0	45
Cabot: Plain, 8 oz	140	4	16
Flavors, 8 oz	220	3	42
Cascade Fresh: Lowfat, 6 oz	140	2	23
Fat Free, all flavors, 6 oz	110	0	20

	C	F	Cb
Colombo			
Light, all flavors, 8 oz	100	0	17
Classic (Fruit on the Bottom), 8 oz	200	4	43
Non Fat: Plain, 8 oz	110	0	17
Continental: Nonfat, 8 oz	190	0	36
Dannon			
Light: All flavors, 8 oz	100	0	16
Multipack, 4.4 oz	50	0	10
w. Crunchy Toppings, aver. 8 oz	140	0	25
Fruit on the Bottom (99% FF):8oz	240	3	42
Minipack, 4.4 oz	130	1.5	25
Fat Free: Plain, 8 oz	140	0	25
Blended, 125g	110	0	23
Chunky Fruit (Fat Free), aver., 6 oz	160	0	32
Low Fat: Vanilla, 8 oz	210	3	36
Double Delights Lowfat:			
w. Fruit Topping, aver., 6 oz	170	1	34
w. Choc./Caramel Topping, 6 oz	220	1	47
Light Duets:			
w. fruit topping, 6 oz	90	0	34
Danimals (lowfat), 4.4 oz	120	1	18
Sprinkl'ins: Rainbow Cryst., 4.1oz	130	1.5	24
Magic Crystals, 4.1 oz	110	1	21
Blended (multipack), 4.1 oz	110	0	23
Dominick's: Lowfat, 8 oz	230	2	40
Fruit on the Bottom, aver., 8 oz	230	2	40
Fat Free 80 Calories, 8 oz	80	0	13
Plain: Lowfat, 8 oz	130	2.5	15
Nonfat, 8 oz	120	0	17
Friendship: Fruit Flavors, 6 oz	190	5	31
Grocer's Pride: Lowfat, 4.4 oz	140	1.5	28
Hood: Fat Free, Plain, 8 oz	130	0	18
Average all flavors, 8 oz	190	0	40
Horizon Organic			
Nonfat: Cherry, 6 oz	140	0	28
Other fruit flavors, aver., 6 oz	120	0	22
Plain, 1 cup, 8 oz	170	0	32
Vanilla, 1 cup, 8 oz	110	0	15
Imperial Supreme: Lowfat, 6 oz	140	1.5	26
Jerseymaid (Vons)			
Fruit on the Bottom (lowfat), 8 oz			
Cherry	250	4	43
Other flavors, average	230	4	40
Prestirred (lowfat), average	240	4	40
Plain, lowfat, 8 oz	150	5	15

Jell-O	**C**	**F**	**Cb**
Kid Pack, all flav., 125g	130	1	25
Jewel: Lowfat, average, 8 oz	250	2.5	48
Knudsen: 70 Calories, 6 oz	70	0	11
Free, average, 6 oz	170	0	33
Cottage Doubles, 5.5 oz	140	2.5	18
Kroger		
Lowfat, average all flavors, 8 oz	210	1.5	40
Lite, average all flavors, 8 oz	100	0	14
Health Indulgence (Nonfat):		
Fruit on the Bottom, aver.	170	0	35
Fat Free: Plain, 8 oz	120	0	18
Vanilla, 8 oz	190	0	36
98% Fat Free: Plain, 8 oz	140	4	16
Vanilla, 8 oz	240	4	42
Lactaid: Lowfat Vanilla, 8 oz	240	2.5	45
La Yogurt		
Fruit Flavors, average, 6 oz	170	2	32
Light, average all flavors, 6 oz	70	0	12
Fruit La More, average, 6 oz	160	0	32
Light n' Lively		
Free 50 Calories, 4 oz	50	0	8
Free 70 Calories, 6 oz	70	0	11
Free (Regular) 6 oz: Vanilla	160	0	32
Strawb. Fruit/Peach/Lem./Berry	170	0	34
Strawberry/Raspberry	180	0	36
Kidpack/Multipack, aver. 4.4 oz	140	1	28
Meadow Gold: Plain, 8 oz	160	5	16
Flavors, average, 8 oz	250	4	42
Mountain High		
Original: Plain, 8 oz	190	8	18
Fat Free Plain, 8 oz	120	0	20
Fat Free: all flavors, 8 oz	170	0	33
Mystic Lake Dairy (Goat Milk Yogurt)		
Plain, 1 cup, 8 oz	120	6	9
Pavel's: Orig. Russian, 8 oz	140	8	10
Lowfat Vanilla, 8 oz	120	4	12
Nonfat Russian, 8 oz	110	0	15
Private Selection (Ralph's)		
Lowfat, average all flavors, 8 oz	220	2	43
Fat Free: Coconut Cream Pie, 6 oz	130	0	23
Other flavors, average, 6 oz	150	0	31

Publix	**C**	**F**	**Cb**
Light, average, 8 oz	130	0	21
Fruit on the Bottom, aver., 8 oz	250	2.5	43
Fat Free: Plain, 8 oz	140	0	23
Swiss Style (lowfat), 8 oz	240	2.5	41
Redwood Hill Farm (Goat Milk Yogurt)		
Fruit flavors, average, 8 oz	180	5	28
Vanilla, 8 oz	190	6	28
Plain, 8 oz	130	6	10
Select (Safeway): Fat Free, 8 oz	250	0	52
Snackwell's: Nonfat, 6 oz	160	0	36
Stonyfield Farm: Lowfat, 8 oz	120	1.5	20
Nonfat, aver. all flavors, 8 oz	160	0	31
"TCBY" Fat Free (Fantasies):		
Banana Creme Pie, 6 oz	110	0	18
White Chocolate, 6 oz	90	0	12
Trader Joe's: Nonfat, 8 oz	190	0	40
Lowfat, average, 8 oz	230	2.5	44
Yofarm: All flavors, aver., 8 oz	220	6	37
Yo Crunch, 6.5 oz (185g)	210	2	41
Yoplait: Light: All flavors 6 oz	90	0	16
Original Lowfat: C'nut Creme, 6oz	200	3	35
99% Fat Free, all flavors, 6 oz	180	1.5	34
Multipack, 4 oz	120	1	22
Go-Gurt: 64g tube	80	2	12
Custard Style: All flavors, 6 oz	190	3.5	32
Trix: Multipack, 4 oz	130	1.5	24

Soy/Non-Dairy Yogurt

	C	**F**	**Cb**
Health Source: Soy Nonfat, 6 oz	150	0	32
Nancy's Soy: Aver. all flav., 8 oz	210	4	37
Soy Nonfat, 8 oz	150	0	32
White Wave: *Per 6 oz*		
Silk Dairyless: Plain; Vanilla	105	2	16
Keylime; Lemon/Kiwi	160	2	17
Average other flavors	140	2	24

Yogurt Drinks

	C	**F**	**Cb**
Alta Dena: Yogurt Drinkables		
Average all flavors, 1 cup	220	0	46
Glen Oaks: All flav., aver., 1 cup	250	4	46
Yonique, 6 fl.oz: Pina Colada	190	4	30
Peach; Banana; Guava	170	2	30
Yo Soy, 8 fl.oz	80	4	4

Icecream & Frozen Yogurt

Quick Guide　C　F　Cb

Icecream

Vanilla: *Average All Brands*

Other flavors ~ See Brand Listings.

Regular Icecream (10% fat):
(Examples: *Borden/Breyers/Hood*)

	C	F	Cb
3 fl.oz scoop	100	5	12
1/2 cup, 4 fl.oz	130	7	16
1 Pint, 16 fl.oz	520	28	62
1/2 Gallon (4 Pints)	2100	112	248

Rich (16% fat): (*Baskin-Robbins*)

3 fl.oz scoop	130	8	12
1/2 cup, 4 fl.oz	170	10	17
1 Pint	690	40	68

Super-Rich (20% fat): (*Haagen-Dazs/Ben & Jerry's*)

3 fl.oz scoop	200	14	16
1/2 cup, 4 fl.oz	270	18	21
1 Pint	1100	72	84

Reduced Fat/Light (6% fat):
(*Breyer's Light/Hood Light*)

3 fl.oz scoop	100	3	14
1/2 cup, 4 fl.oz	140	4	18
1 Pint	560	16	72

Low Fat (less than 4% fat):
(*Healthy Choice/Weight Watchers/Snackwell's*)

3 fl.oz scoop	90	2	17
1/2 cup, 4 fl.oz	120	2.5	22
1 Pint	480	10	88

Fat Free: (*Baskin-Robbins FF/Borden FF/ Breyers FF/Dreyers FF/Hood FF)*)

3 fl.oz scoop	75	0	17
1/2 cup, 4 fl.oz	100	0	22
1 Pint	400	0	88

Soft Serve: Regular, 1/2 cup

Regular, 1/2 cup	140	5	20
1 cup	280	10	40
Nonfat, 1/2 cup	90	0	23
1 cup	180	0	46

Quick Guide　C　F　Cb

Frozen Yogurt

Average All Brands

Hard: Lowfat, 1/2 cup	140	3	26
Nonfat, 1/2 cup	110	0	29
Soft: Lowfat, 1/2 cup	120	2.5	28
Nonfat, 1/2 cup	100	0	30

Brands ~ See Icecream & Ices Section

Quick Guide　C　F　Cb

Gelato/Ices

Gelato: *Per 1/2 Cup*

	C	F	Cb
Milk base: Vanilla	200	15	18
Choc. Hazelnut	370	29	26
Water base: 1/2 cup	100	0	25

Ice (Milk base): *Average all flavors*

Hard (4% fat), 1/2 cup	100	3	15
Soft Serve (3% fat), 1/2 cup	110	2	19
Shaved Ice: Average, 12 fl. oz	160	0	40
Sherbet: Average, 1/2 cup	120	2	28
Sorbet: Fruit (no fat), 1/2 cup	120	0	30
Fruit Ice Pops	80	0	20

Tofu Frozen Desserts ~ Page 30

Sundaes

Denny's Sundaes:

Single Scoop, no topping	190	14	14
Double Scoop, no topping	375	27	29
Banana Split	895	43	121
Hot Fudge Cake	690	38	83

Toppings:

Blueberry, 2 oz	70	0	17
Chocolate, 2 oz	320	25	27
Fudge, 2 oz	200	10	20
Strawberry, 2 oz	80	1	17

McDonald's Sundaes:

Hot Fudge Sundae. 6.3 oz	340	12	52
Toppings: Nut/Sundae, 1/4 oz	40	3.5	2

~ Full Analysis: See Fast-Foods Section ~

Icecream Bars & Pops

See Pages 31 & 32

Icecream Cones & Cups

	C	F	Cb
Wafer Cone/Cup, average	20	0	4
Sugar Cone, average	40	0	9
Waffle Cone:			
Small	60	0	11
Large	100	1	22
Brands:			
Oreo Chocolate Cone	50	1	10
Comet Sugar Cone	50	0	11
Keebler Sugar Cone	45	0	11

Icecream & Ices

Brands | C | F | Cb

Alta Dena: Per 1/2 Cup
	C	F	Cb
Honey Chocolate	160	9	19
Golden Honey Vanilla	160	10	17

Baskin-Robbins
See Fast-Foods Section ~ Page 167

Ben & Jerry's: Per 1/2 Cup
	C	F	Cb
Butter Pecan	330	25	22
Cherry Garcia; Vanilla	260	16	23
Choc. Chip; Peanut Butter & Jelly	300	17	33
Choc. Fudge Brownie	250	15	32
Chubby Hubby	350	21	32
Chunky Monkey; Coffee Heath	310	19	32
Coffee Almond Fudge Chip	310	22	24
Coffee Coffey; Mint Choc. Cookie	285	18	27
Cool Britannia	270	16	29
New York Super Fudge Chunk	320	21	26
Peanut Butter Cup	380	25	32
Phish Food	300	14	41
Dilbert's World Totally Nuts	310	21	27
Vanilla Heath Bar Crunch	310	19	30
Vanilla Caramel Fudge	300	17	33
Wavy Gravy	340	20	33
Lowfat: Coconut Cream Pie	150	2.5	29
Average other flavors	190	3	35
Frozen Yogurt: Vanilla Heath	210	6	34
Choc. Cherry/Chip; Coffee	190	4	35
Choc. Fudge Brownie	190	2.5	36
Cherry Garcia; Peach Raspberry	175	3	32
Sorbet: Devil's Food Chocolate	170	2.5	36
Average other flavors	130	0	30
Pops: See Page 31			

Bon Bon's
	C	F	Cb
Vanilla w. choc. coating, 5 pieces	200	14	17
8 pieces	330	23	27

Bresler's: Per 1/2 Cup
	C	F	Cb
All Flavors Icecream: average	230	12	23
Royal Cremes, average	260	16	24
Royal Lites, average	220	0	49

Breyer's: Per 1/2 Cup
	C	F	Cb
All Natural: Butter Pecan	180	12	15
Cherry Vanilla; Coffee	150	7	17
Chocolate; French Vanilla	160	10	15
Choc. Chip; Mint Choc. Chip	170	10	18
Cookies 'n Cream	170	9	19
Peach; Strawberry	130	6	18
Vanilla; Van./Choc./Strawberry	150	8	16
Van. & Choc.; Van. Fudge Twirl	160	8	18
Homemade: Dble Choc Fudge	180	9	23
Butter Pecan; Van.; Neopolitan	150	8	16
Breyers Light: Average, 1/2 c.	140	4	19
Fat Free: Average	110	0	21
Reduced Fat: Average	160	6	19
Vienetta: All flavors, 1 slice	190	11	17
No Sugar Added: Vanilla	80	4	11
Vanilla Fudge Twirl	90	3.5	14
Vanilla Chocolate Strawberry	90	4	11
Mint Chocolate Chip	100	5	21
Sorbet: Average, 1/2 cup	160	7	26
Frozen Yogurt: Average, 1/2 cup	150	4	25

Colombo: Per 1/2 Cup
	C	F	Cb
Frozen, Soft Serve: Nonfat var.	100	0	22
Slender Sensations varieties	65	0	11
Lowfat: Old Worlde; P'nut Butter	120	2.5	20
Vanilla varieties	110	1.5	21

Dairy Queen/Brazier
See Fast-Foods Section ~ Page 179-180

Dannon Frozen Yogurt: Per 1/2 cup (4 fl.oz)
	C	F	Cb
Light Soft, all flavors, average	90	1	21
Light 'N Crunchy, all flavors, aver.	110	1	23
Pure Indulgence, all flavors, aver.	150	3	25

Dolewhip (Soft Serve): Per 4 fl.oz, 1/2 Cup
	C	F	Cb
Chocolate; Vanilla	100	3	18
Fruit flavors, average	80	0.5	16

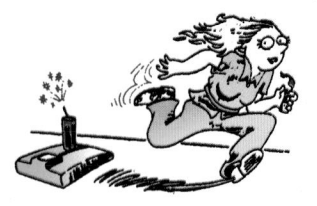

Being cheerful keeps you healthy. It is a slow death to be gloomy all the time.

Proverbs 17:22

Brands (cont)

	C	F	Cb
Dreyers: *Per 1/2 Cup*			
Grand Light: Vanilla	100	3	15
Cookie Dough; P'nut Butter Cups	130	5	17
Other varieties, average	120	4	18
Homemade: Butter Pecan, 71g	160	9	16
Banana Crunch, 1/2 cup, 71g	130	6	17
Chocolate Peanut Butter, 71g	200	12	18
Peaches & Cream, 65g	120	5	16
Strawberries & Cream, 71g	130	6	17
Vanilla, 1/2 cup, 71g	140	7	16
No Sugar Added: Aver. all flavors	90	3	12
Fat Free: Average all flavors	110	0	25
Fat Free - No Sugar Added	95	0	20
Edys: *Per 1/2 Cup*			
Banana Split; Choc. Fudge Mousse	160	8	19
Cherry Choc; Van./Choc.; Espresso	150	8	17
Choc. Fudge Sundae; Dble Fudge	170	9	19
Ice Cream Sandwich	140	8	14
Grand Light:			
Butter Pecan; Choc. Almond	120	5	16
Chiquita 'N Chocolate	110	5	13
Choc. Fudge Mousse	110	3	17
Cookie Dough; P'nut Butter Cups	130	5	18
Cookies 'n Cream; Rocky Road	110	4	16
French Silk	120	4	18
Vanilla	100	3	15
Fat Free: Average all flavors	115	0	25
Eskimo Pie: *Per 1/2 Cup*			
Butter Pecan	140	7	16
Praline/Choc. Marshmallow	130	4	23
Reduced Fat: Neopolitan; Fudge	110	4	18
Bars ~ See Page 31			
Friendly's: *Per 1/2 Cup*			
Icecream: Chocolate Almond Chip	170	10	18
Forbidden Chocolate	150	9	14
Fudge Nut Brownie	200	11	23
Vanilla	150	8	16
Vanilla Choc. Strawberry	150	8	16
Vienna Mocha Chunk	180	11	19
Frozen Yogurt: *Per 1/2 Cup (2.6oz)*			
Lowfat flavors, average	120	3	20
Regular flavors, average	150	4	24
Frostline (Soft Serve)			
Chocolate, 1/2 Cup	90	2	20
Vanilla, 1/2 Cup	90	3	18

	C	F	Cb
Frusen Gladje: *Per 1/2 Cup*			
Butter Pecan	280	21	16
Chocolate	240	17	17
Chocolate Choc. Chip	270	18	21
Mocha Chip; Praline & Cream	280	18	22
Strawberry	230	15	20
Swiss Choc. Candy Almond	270	19	18
Vanilla	230	17	16
Vanilla Swiss Almond	270	19	18
Good Humor			
Light: *Per 1/2 Cup*			
Choc. Chip, Toffee Bar Crunch	130	4	20
Coffee	110	3	18
Cookies n' Crm; Praline Alm. Crnch	130	3	21
Vanilla, Vanilla Choc. Strawb.	110	3	19
Bars/Ices/Sandwiches ~ Page 31 & 32			
Haagen-Dazs			
Per 1/2 Cup			
Brownies a la Mode	280	18	25
Butter Pecan	320	24	20
Cappuccino; Caramel Cone	310	21	27
Chocolate; Coffee	270	18	22
Choc. Choc. Chip; Cookie Dough	300	20	26
Cookies & Cream; Rum Raisin	270	17	23
Deep Choc Peanut Butter	370	25	27
Macadamia Nut	320	24	20
Strawberry	250	16	23
Strawb. Cheesecake; Vanilla Fudge	290	18	28
Triple Brownie Overload	300	20	26
Vanilla	270	18	21
Vanilla Chocolate Chip	290	20	24
Vanilla Swiss Almond	310	21	23
Icecream Bars ~ See Page 31 & 32			
Soft Serve: Nonfat Coffee	140	4	20
Chocolate Mousse	80	0	24
Full Listings ~ See Fast Foods Section			
Sorbets ~ See Fast Foods Section			
Frozen Yogurt: Vanilla Fudge	160	0	34
Vanilla Raspberry Swirl	130	0	28
Other flavors	140	0	30

See Full Listings - Fast-Foods Section
Continued Next Page

> '*Success is 1% Inspiration and 99% Perspiration.*'

Brands (Cont)

Healthy Choice: Per 1/2 Cup	C	F	Cb
Vanilla	100	2	18
Rocky Road	140	2	28
Other flavors, average	120	2	22
Lowfat: All varieties, average	110	1.5	21

Hood: Per 1/2 Cup			
Chocolate	140	7	17
Chocolate Chip; Maple Walnut	160	9	18
Cookie Dough; Cookies 'n Cream	160	8	21
Grasshopper Pie	160	7	22
Heavenly Hash; Vanilla Fudge	140	6	21
Strawberry	130	7	16
Vanilla; Van. Choc. Strawberry	140	7	16
Light: Almond Praline	110	5	23
Carrib. Coffee	110	5	18
Vanilla; Van.Choc.Strawberry	110	4	18
Other Flavors, average	140	5	22
Lowfat: (No Added Sugar)			
Average all flavors, 1/2 cup	115	3	18
Fat Free: Average all flavors	120	0	27
Icecream Bars ~ See Page 32			

I Can't Believe It's Yogurt
See Fast-Foods Section

It's Soy Delicious			
Chocolate	130	4	23
Vanilla	130	4	23

Jerseymaids (Vons): Per 1/2 Cup			
After Dinner Mint; Cookies & Crm	170	9	19
Choc Chip; Mint Choc Chip	160	9	17
Heavenly Hash; Nut Chunky Choc.	170	8	22
Mocha Almd Fudge; Rocky Road	160	7	20
Neopolitan; Vanilla	140	7	16
Strawberry	140	6	18

Luigi's Real Italian Ice			
Squeeze-Up Tube: 8 fl.oz each	150	0	37

Rice Cream (Non Dairy): Per 1/2 Cup			
Vanilla	150	6	23
Supreme: Average all flavors	150	6	23

Sealtest: Per 1/2 Cup			
Butter Pecan	160	9	16
Choc. Chip Cookie Dough	160	8	20
Fudge Royal; Heavenly Hash	150	7	20
Vanilla/Choc. Strawberry	140	7	16

Snackwell's: Per 1/2 Cup	C	F	Cb
Brownie; Rocky Road	130	2	26
Praline Caramel	140	2	28
Vanilla	100	2	18

Starbucks: Per 1/2 Cup			
Espresso Swirl	220	10	29
Biscotti Bliss	240	12	30
Cafe Almond Fudge	260	13	30
Chocolate Chocolate Fudge	290	17	28
Italian Roast	230	12	26
JavaChip	250	13	29
Vanilla MochaChip	270	14	31
Lowfat: Mocha Mambo; Latte	170	3	30
Bars ~ see Icecream Bars & Pops Section			

Stonyfield Farm

Chocolate; Raspberry; Vanilla	120	2	22

TCBY ~ See Fast-Foods Section

Tofutti Non-Dairy Dessert: Per 1/2 Cup			
Premium: Vanilla	190	11	20
Better Pecan; Alm. Bark	220	13	22
Choc. Cookie Crunch	210	11	26
Chocolate Supreme	180	11	18
Van. Fudge; Wildberry	190	9	24
Low Fat Supreme: Average	110	2	25
Cutie Pies: Average, 67g bar	250	19	18
Too Toos: Vanilla S'wich	215	10	28
Van. Choc. Swirl/Chip S'wich	230	11	30
Teddy Fudge: 52g bar	70	1	19

Turkey Hill: Per 1/2 Cup			
Black Cherry	140	7	18
Butter Pecan	170	11	16
Choco. Mint Chip, Cookies 'n Crm	160	10	17
Neapolitan, Vanilla & Choc.	150	8	18
Rocky Road	170	8	23
Vanilla, Vanilla Bean	140	8	16
Lite: Choco Mint Chip	140	5	19
Cookies 'n Cream	130	5	21
Vanilla & Choc., Van. Bean	110	3	18

Weight Watchers: Per 1/2 Cup			
Cookie Dough Craze	140	3.5	24
Oh! So Very Vanilla	120	2.5	18
Positively Praline Crunch	140	3	25
Reckless Rocky Road	140	3	23
Triple Chocolate Tornado	150	3.5	26
Bars ~ See Page 31-32			

Per Bar/Serving	C	F	Cb
Baby Ruth (*Nestle*)	180	12	15
Baskin Robbins: Tiny Toons	140	17	20
Cappuccino Blast, average	120	4	20
Sundae Bar: Pralines 'n Cream	280	17	28
Ben & Jerry's: Vanilla Pop	360	23	35
Choc Chip Cookie Dough Pop	450	28	48
English Toffee Crunch Pop	340	23	35
Big Bear: See Klondike	290	10	45
Big Ed's Super Saucer: 10 fl.oz	420	28	32
$^1/_2$ Sandwich, 5 fl.oz	210	14	16
Borden: Sundae Cone	210	10	27
Twin Pops	60	0	14
Bon Bons (*Nestle*): Milk Choc., (8)	330	23	27
Dark Chocolate, 8 pces	310	21	26
Bounty: all varieties	70	5	7
Butterfinger Icecream Bar, 2.5 oz	190	13	16
Breyers: Vanilla Bar	250	17	21
w. chocolate coating	230	15	20
Sandwich (Vanilla)	250	11	32
Carnation: Orange Sherbet, 3 oz	90	1	19
Icecream Cup: Choc., 3 fl.oz	140	8	16
Strawb., Vanilla, 3 fl.oz	100	6	12
Choc./Vanilla Malt, 12 oz	270	6	48
Sundae Cup, all types, 5 fl.oz	210	9	30
Chipwich Jr: Choc. Chip S'wich	240	10	35
Chiquita: Swirls, all flavors	80	3	12
Cool Creations: Mini Sandwich	110	5	16
Cookies & Cream Sandwich	240	11	34
Pops, all types, 2 oz	60	0	14
Mickey Mouse: 2.5 oz Bar	120	8	10
4 oz Bar	170	11	17
Creamsicle: Sugar-free pops	25	0	15
Orange, 2.8 fl.oz	110	3	20
Crunch (*Nestle*): King, 4 oz	270	19	21
Reduced Fat, 2.5 oz	130	7	14
Regular Icecream Bar, 3 oz	200	14	16
Crystal Light: Cool 'n Creamy	50	2	7
Dole Bars: Coconut, 4 oz	210	7	33
Fruit Juice, reg., 1.75 oz	45	0	11
No Added Sugar, 1.75 oz	25	0	6
Fruit 'n Juice: Small, 2.5 oz	70	0	16
Pine-Coconut, 4 oz	150	4	27
Other flavors, 4 oz	120	0	28
Dreyers: Icecream Bars, average	250	17	22
Fruit Bars, 3 fl.oz	90	9	23
Smoothie Bars: Average	95	0	21
Sundae Cone, 4 fl.oz	240	11	31

Per Bar/Serving	C	F	Cb
Dove Bar: Almond	340	22	30
Bite Size, 5 pces, average	350	22	36
Caramel Pecan	350	35	35
Mocha Cashew	260	17	25
Peppermint	390	17	31
Vanilla Dark Choc; Cookie	340	21	35
Single Vanilla Dark	200	12	24
Vanilla Milk Chocolate	350	24	29
Drumstick (*Nestle*): Chocolate	320	17	36
Choc. Dipped	320	16	40
Original Vanilla	340	19	35
Vanilla Caramel/Fudge	360	20	39
Eskimo Pie: Arctic Madness, 2.5 oz	230	15	23
Bars, 50g: Orig.; Van; Milk Choc	160	11	13
Butterscotch Crunch; Cherry	160	10	16
Big Bar, 99g	300	20	26
Icecream Sandwich, 66 g	160	4	28
Reduced Fat: Dark Choc., 49g	120	7	39
Crispy Bar, 47g	130	8	13
Pecan, 51g	190	15	12
Sundae Cones	240	15	24
No Sugar Added: Bar, 49g	120	8	13
Icecream Sandwich, 65g	160	4	27
Flintstones: Push Up Sherbet	100	2	20
Push Up Pebbles, 2.75 oz	120	6	15
Cool Cream, 2.75 oz	90	2	18
Froz-Fruit: Cherry	60	0	15
Strawberry	80	0	20
Frosty Dreams (*Nestle*)	100	2	19
Frosty Pops (*Nestle*)	40	0	11
Fruit A Freeze: Coconut	130	5	20
Lime	65	0	16
Banana; Strawberry	90	1.5	19
Dark Choc-Dipped Strawberry	90	3.5	14
Fudge Bar (*Nestle*)	110	1	23
Fudgesicle: Fudge Bar	90	1	17
Sugar-Free·	40	1	8
Fudgetastics: Sticks Sundae	220	15	17
Good Humor: Candy Crunch	280	21	21
Chocolate Eclair	170	9	21
Chocolate Taco	320	17	38
Classic Almond	210	12	21
Colonel Crunch	165	8	22
Dinosaur	110	2	25
Giant Sandwich, 5 fl.oz	240	10	38
Icecream Sandwich	190	8	28
King Cone	300	14	38

Per Bar/Serving	C	F	Cb
Good Humor (Cont):			
Strawberry Shortcake, 3.75 fl.oz	210	9	29
Cups: Sundae Twist	160	3	33
Combo (6 fl.oz)	200	10	25
Haagen-Daz Bars:			
Uncoated; Coffee; Vanilla	200	13	16
Vanilla & Dark Chocolate	400	27	33
Multipack, each	320	22	17
Sorbet Bars, average	90	0	22
Sorbet 'n Yogurt Bars, average	100	0	20
Also See Page 196			
Hood: Chocolate Eclair, 1 bar	150	10	14
Cooler Cup, 2.1 oz	80	1	18
Crispy Bar	180	13	15
Fabukous Fudgies, 1 bar	100	3	19
Fabulous Fudge P'nut Butter	110	4	17
Fudge Bar	100	1	21
Hendrie's Cherry Choc. Dips	120	9	11
Hoodsie Cup Van./Choc.	100	5	12
Orange Cream Bar	90	2	18
Rockets, each	120	5	18
Vanilla Bar	160	12	11
Icecream Sandwich *(Nestle)*	170	6	26
Jell-O: Pop Bars	31	0	7
Jigglers, all varieties, 6 oz	215	1.5	50
Pudding Bars	80	2	13
Klondike: Almond Bar	310	21	26
Big Bear Van. Icecream S'wich	290	10	46
Choc Chip Cookie Sandwich	520	21	77
Gold Bar	340	23	30
Krunch	200	13	17
Lite Bar	110	6	14
Original Vanilla; Chocolate	290	20	25
Sandwich: Chocolate	270	10	41
Lite	100	2	18
Vanilla	250	9	37
The One	290	20	25
Kool-Aid Pops	40	0	10
Krispy Frostick:	150	10	13
Juice Flavored Sticks	50	0	13
M&Ms: Cookie Icecream S'wich	240	12	32
Mars Almond Bar	210	14	20
Matterhorn: Cone, 10 fl.oz	510	38	19
Milky Way: Choc, Reduced Fat	140	7	19
Caramel Swirl, 1 bar	180	10	21
Snack Bar, Vanilla/Chocolate	70	4	9
Minute Maid: Fruit Juice Pops	60	0	15

Per Bar/Serving	C	F	Cb
Nestle Icescreamers: Push Up Pop	90	1.5	19
Shock Tarts, 1 pop	45	0	11
Tiger Tails, 1 pop	60	0	15
Oreo: Choc; Vanilla	160	9	19
Pathmark: Vanilla w. choc. coat.	150	10	14
Polar Bar: Vanilla w. choc. coat.	240	18	15
Choc. Chip Cookie Dough	450	28	48
Pops (water/juice), average	60	0	14
Popsicles: Fudgesicle Fudge Pop	90	1.5	16
Sugar-free Ice Pop	15	0	4
Reece's: Peanut Butter Icecream	160	11	22
Rice Dream: Cones, all types	270	14	37
Vanilla Bar, 1 bar	220	14	25
Vanilla Nutty Bar, 1 bar	260	18	23
Mocha/Vanilla Pie	290	15	37
Snackwell: Icecream Sandwich	100	1.5	20
Yogurt Bars, 1 bar, 80g	120	2	22
Snickers: Pralines n' Creme	220	13	22
Icecream Bar	180	11	18
Snack, 4 bars	390	25	38
Starbuck's:			
Coffee & Almond Bars, 81g	280	18	26
Coffee Frappuccino Bars	110	2	20
Java Ice Cream Bar	270	16	29
Mocha Frappuccino Bar	120	2	21
Starburst: Juice Bars	20	0	5
Super Sundae Bar, 86g	310	20	26
3 Musketeers, 2 fl.oz bars	170	10	21
Snack Bars, regular	60	4	16
Super Sundae Bar, 86g	310	20	26
Tandem *(Nestle)*: Sandwich	380	21	39
Twin Pop *(Nestle)*	60	0	14
Vitari, soft serve, 4 fl.oz, average	80	0	20
Welch's Fruit Juice Bars:			
All flavors,92g bar	45	0	11
54g bar	25	0	6
No Sugar Added, 1 bar	25	0	6
Fruit Smoothie, 1 ctn	240	0	59
Weight Watchers Bars:			
Chocolate Dip	100	6	11
Chocolate Mousse	40	1	9
Chocolate Treat	100	0.5	20
English Toffee Crunch	110	6	12
Orange Vanilla Treat	40	0.5	10
Vanilla Sandwich	150	3	28

Quick Guide   **C** **F** **Cb**

Cream

Average All Brands

	C	F	Cb
Half & Half Cream: 1 Tbsp	20	2	0.5
2 Tbsp, 1 oz	40	4	1
Light, coffee/table (20% fat): 1 T.	30	3	0.5
2 Tbsp, 1 oz	60	6	1
Medium (25% fat), 1 Tbsp	40	4	0.5
Sour Cream:			
Regular, 1 Tbsp	30	3	0.5
2 Tbsp, 1 oz	60	6	1
1 cup	490	48	8
Lowfat/Light, 1 Tbsp	20	2	1.5
2 Tbsp, 1 oz	40	2.5	2
Half & Half, 1 Tbsp	20	2	1
Fat Free: (*HeluvaGood*), 2 Tbsp	20	0	6
(*Kroger*), 2 Tbsp, 32g	25	0	5
(*Naturally Yours; Oak Farms*), 2 T.	20	0	3
(*Knudsen*), 2 Tbsp, 32g	35	0	6
Sour Cream Substitute:			
(*Albertson's/ IMO*), 2 T., 1 oz	50	5	2
(*Tofutti*) Sour Supreme, 1 oz	50	5	1

Whipping Cream:

	C	F	Cb
Heavy (37% fat):			
1 Tbsp fluid/2 T. whipped	50	5.5	1
1/4 cup whipped	100	11	2
1/2 cup fluid/1 c. whipped	400	44	8
Light (30% fat):			
1 Tbsp fluid/2 T. whipped	45	5	0.5
1/2 cup fluid/1 c. whipped	350	37	4

Whipped Toppings

	C	F	Cb
Cream (Pressurized): *Average All Brands*			
1 Tbsp	10	1	0.5
1/4 cup	40	4	2
Cream Toppings: *Jewel:* Lite, 2 T.	20	1	2
Cool Whip: Extra Creamy, 2 T.	25	1.5	2
Lite, 2 Tbsp, 9g	20	1	2
Free, 2 Tbsp, 9g	15	0	3
Non Dairy, 2 Tbsp	22	2	2
Kraft: Whipped, 2 Tbsp	20	2	1
Real Cream, 2 Tbsp	20	2	1
Reddi-Wip: Original Light, 2 T.	20	2	1
Deluxe, 2 Tbsp	30	3	0.5
1/4 cup/4 Tbsp	60	6	2
Fat Free, 2 Tbsp, 8g	10	0	2
Vetra: Light, sweetened, 2 T., 6g	15	1	1

Non-Dairy Coffee Creamers

Powder   **C** **F** **Cb**

	C	F	Cb
Coffee-Mate:			
Regular, 1 tsp	10	0.5	1
1 heaping tsp	15	1	2
Fat Free, 1 tsp	10	0	2
Lite, 1 tsp	10	0.5	2
Flavors: 1 1/3 Tbsp	60	3	9
Fat Free: Average, 1 1/3 Tbsp	50	0	11
Cremora: Same as *Coffee Mate*			
N-Rich: Same as *Coffee Mate*			

Liquid/Refrigerated: *Per Tbsp*

	C	F	Cb
Coffee-Mate Non-Dairy Creamer:			
Plain: Regular/Plain, 1 Tbsp	20	1	2
Fat Free, 1 Tbsp	10	0	2
Lite, 1 Tbsp	10	0.5	1
Flavors: All flavors, 1 Tbsp	40	2	5
Fat Free, all flavors, 1 Tbsp	25	0	5
Hood (Non Dairy), 1 Tbsp	25	0	5
International Delight:			
Regular/Flavors, 1 Tbsp	35	1.5	6
Fat Free flavors, 1 Tbsp	30	0	7
Mocha Mix: Original, 1 Tbsp	20	1.5	1
Fat Free, 1 Tbsp	10	0	1
Lite, 1 Tbsp	10	0.5	1
Morning Blend (Ralph's):			
Non-Dairy Creamer: Reg., 1 Tbsp	15	1.5	0
Fat Free, 1 Tbsp	5	0	2
Rich's Coffee Rich: Regular, 1 T.	25	1	2
Light	15	0.5	0.5
Rich's Farm Rich: Regular, 1 Tbsp	20	1	2
Light/Fat Free	10	0	0.5

Coconut Cream/Milk

	C	F	Cb
Coconut Cream (Canned),			
Plain/unsweetened, 2 Tbsp, 1 oz	70	6	4
1/2 cup	280	24	16
Sweetened: *Coco Lopez,* 1 oz	120	5	20
1/2 cup, 4 oz	480	20	80
Coconut Milk, can, 1/2 cup	225	24	3
Coconut Water (center), 1 cup	45	0.5	9

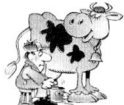

Fats, Spreads, Oils

Quick Guide C F Cb

Butter & Margarine
Butter, Margarine, Blends

Average All Brands

	C	F	Cb
Regular: 1 tsp (5g)	35	4	0
1 Pat (5g)	35	4	0
1 Tbsp, approx. 1/2 oz	100	11	0
2 Tbsp, 1 oz	205	23	0
1 Stick, 1/2 cup, 4 oz	810	92	0
1 Pound, 2 cups, 16 oz	3240	368	0
Light (Regular) 40% Fat:			
1 tsp, 5g	17	2	0
1 Tbsp, 1/2 oz	50	6	0
2 Tbsp, 1 oz	100	11	0
Whipped (Regular):			
1 tsp (4 g)	27	3	0
1 Tbsp (10g)	70	7.5	0
1 Stick, 1/2 cup, 2 2/3 oz	570	60	0
Light (Whipped) 40% Fat:			
1 tsp, 5g	10	1	0
1 Tbsp, 9g	35	3.5	0
2 Tbsp, 18g	70	7	0
Unsalted: Same as Salted			

Clarified Butter

	C	F	Cb
100% Fat: 1 Tbsp, 1/2 oz	130	15	0
2 Tbsp, 1 oz	260	30	0

Flavored Butter/Spread

Average All Brands

	C	F	Cb
Honey Butter (60% Fat):			
1 Tbsp, 1/2 oz	90	7	4
Downey's, 1 Tbsp, 1/2 oz	60	1	11
Garlic Butter (80% Fat):			
1 Tbsp, 1/2 oz	100	11	0
Sweet Cream Butter:			
Regular, 1 Tbsp	100	11	0
Stick (70% Fat), 1 Tbsp	90	10	0
Tub (60% Fat), 1 Tbsp	80	9	0

Other Spreads & Fats

	C	F	Cb
Copha, Dripping, Lard, Suet, Shortening:			
1 Tbsp, 1/2 oz	120	13	0
Chicken, Duck, Goose Fat:			
1 Tbsp, 1/2 oz	115	13	0

Light & Reduced Fat Spreads

Per 1 Tbsp (Unless Stated)

	C	F	Cb
Benecol: Regular, single serve, 8g	45	5	0
Light, single serve, 8g	30	3	0
Blue Bonnet: Lowfat Margarine	45	4.5	0
45% Veg. Oil Spread	70	7	0
Breakstone: Whipped Butter	60	7	0
Brummel & Brown: Spread	50	5	0
Chiffon: Whipped, 1 Tbsp	70	7	0
Country Crock: Regular	60	7	0
Light	50	5	0
Country's Delight (70% Veg.)	90	10	0
Country Morning: Light	50	6	0
Downey's Honey Butter	60	1	0
Dutch Farms: 52% Veg. Spread	70	7	0
Fleischmann's: Soft Spread	80	9	0
Original	90	10	0
Fat Free Spread	5	0	0
'I Can't Believe It's Not Butter': Reg.	90	10	0
Light	50	5	0
Imperial: Diet, 1 Tbsp	50	6	0
Jewel: Soft Spread	60	7	0
Unbelievably Butter	90	9	0
Kraft: 'Touch of Butter' (bowl)	50	6	0
Land O'Lakes: Tub	80	8	0
Honey Butter	90	7	4
Light Whipped Butter	35	3.5	0
Light Butter	50	6	0
Mazola: Diet	50	6	0
Mother's; Mrs Filbert's, 1 Tbsp	70	8	0
Miracle: Soft	60	7	0
Stick	70	7	0
Nucoa: HeartBeat Margarine	25	3	0
Olivio: Vegetable Spread	80	8	0
Parkay: Squeeze, 1 Tbsp	80	9	0
Stick, 1/3 Less Fat	70	7	0
Tub, 1 Tbsp	60	7	0
Tub, Light/Soft Diet	50	6	0
Whipped	70	7	0
Promise: Regular	90	10	0
Extra Light	50	6	0
Buttery Light	45	5	0
Ultra, w. canola oil	35	4	0
Smart Balance: Regular	80	9	0
Light, 1 Tbsp	45	5	0
Smart Beat: Fat Free	10	0	3
Take Control: Veg Oil Spread	50	6	0
Weight Watcher's: Light, all types	45	4	2

34

Butter Substitutes

	C	**F**	**Cb**
Bake It Perfect (Fat Free Spread), 1 T.	5	0	0
Best O'Butter, 1/2 tsp	4	0	0
Butter Buds: 1 serving, 1/2 tsp	4	0	0
Butterlike Saute Butter, 1 Tbsp	35	2	0
Butter Sprinkles (Watkins): 1 tsp	5	0	0
Molly McButter: 1/2 tsp	5	0	0
Mrs Bateman's Baking Buttter, 1 T.	35	1	0
(Direct 800 574 6822)			

Spreads Comparison

Mayonnaise: Regular, 1 Tbsp	100	11	0.5
Light, average, 1 Tbsp	50	5	1
Fat Free (e.g. *Wt. Watcher's*), 1 T.	12	0	3
Miracle Whip (Kraft):			
Regular, 1 Tbsp	70	7	2
Light, 1 Tbsp	40	3	3
Free, 1 Tbsp	15	0	3
SmartBeat Dressing: 1 Tbsp	12	0	2
Extra Listings for Mayonnaise & Dressings ~ See Page 82 ~			
Peanut Butter, 1 Tbsp	100	8	3.5
Avocado, mashed, 1 Tbsp	25	2.5	2
Birdseye:			
No Fat Veggie Dip, 2 T., 1.1 oz	25	0	5

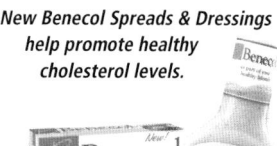

Animal Fats/Lards

Average All Types	**C**	**F**	**Cb**
Beef Tallow/Drippings, Lard (Pork), Chicken, Duck, Goose, Turkey.			
1 Tbsp (13g)	115	13	0
2 1/4 Tbsp, 1 oz	255	28	0
1 cup, 7 1/4 oz	1850	205	0
1/2 pound, 8 oz	2040	227	0
Ghee/Butter Oil: 1 Tbsp, 13g	110	13	0
2 1/4 Tbsp, 1 oz	250	28	0

Vegetable Shortening

Average All Types (example, *Crisco*)			
1 Tbsp	113	13	0
2 1/4 Tbsp, 1 oz	250	28	0
1 cup, 7 1/4 oz	1810	205	0

Vegetable Oils

Includes almond, avocado, canola, corn, coconut, flaxseed, grapeseed, linseed, mustard, olive, palm, peanut, rice-bran, safflower, sesame, sunflower, soybean, wheatgerm. Note: Oil is 100% fat.

1 tsp, 5g	45	5	0
1 Tbsp, 1/2 oz	120	14	0
2 Tbsp, 1 oz	250	28	0
1 cup, 7 3/4 oz	1930	205	0

Fish Oils

Average All Types (Includes cod liver, herring, salmon, sardine):			
1 Tbsp, 1/2 oz	125	14	0

Cooking Sprays

Cooking Sprays (*Pam, Mazola, Weight Watchers, Wesson*):			
Per serving	2	0	0
2-3 second spray	6	1	0
Parkay Buttery Spray	0	0	0

Olestra (Olean)

Olestra *(Olean)*	0	0	0

Olean is *Proctor & Gamble's* brand name for olestra - a no-calorie cooking oil that gives snacks (like potato chips, tortilla chips and crackers) taste and texture without adding fat or calories.

Cheese

C F Cb

Firm/Hard Cheeses
(American, Cheddar, Colby, Coon, Swiss)

Regular Cheese:

	C	F	Cb
1 oz slice/piece	110	9	0.5
8 oz package	880	72	4
16 oz (1lb) package	1760	144	8
Cubes: 1" cube, 3/4 oz	55	5	0.5
1 1/4" cube, 1 oz slice	110	9	0.5
Diced: 1 cup, 4 1/2 oz	500	40	2
Grated: 1 Tbsp, 1/4 oz	27	2	0
Shredded:			
1/4 cup, 1 oz	110	9	0.5
1 cup, 4 oz	440	36	4
Sliced: 1 thin (3 1/2" sq.), 3/4 oz	85	7	0.5
Rectangular (7"x 4"x 1/8"), 1 1/2 oz	165	14	1
Round (3 1/4" diam. x 1/8"), 3/4 oz	85	7	0.5
Semi-circular, 1 1/4 oz			
(5 1/2" long, 3 1/2" radius, 1/8"thick)	140	11	0.5
Light: Average All Brands, oz	70	4.5	1
Fat Free: Average All Brands, 1 oz	50	0	2
Lowfat: Average All Brands, 1 oz	50	1.5	1

Cheese

Per 1 oz Unless Indicated

	C	F	Cb
American:			
Regular, 1 slice, 1 oz	110	9	1
Kraft Deluxe, 0.7 oz slice	70	6	0.5
Grated, 1 Tbsp, 1/4 oz	23	2	0
Light (*Borden*), 1 oz	70	4	0.5
Land O'Lakes, 1 oz	70	5	0.5
Smart Beat, 0.6 oz slice	35	2	0
Fat Free: Single, 0.75 oz	30	0	3
Alpine Lace, 1 oz	45	0	2
HealthyChoice, Singles, 0.7 oz	25	0	2
Weight Watchers, all types, 3/4 oz	30	0	3
Babybel (Laughing Cow), 1 oz	90	7	0
Crumbled, 1/2 cup, 2 1/2 oz	250	20	1
Dorman's Castello, 1 oz	135	12	1
Bonbel (Laughing Cow), 1 oz	100	8	0
Mini, 3/4 oz	75	6	0
Brick, 1 oz	100	8	0
Brie, 1 oz	95	8	0
Camembert, 1 oz	90	7	0
Caraway, 1 oz	105	8	1

	C	F	Cb
Cheddar:			
Regular, 1 oz	110	9	0.5
(Also see 'Quick Guide')			
Reduced Fat/Light, 1 oz	80	5	0.5
Weight Watchers, 1 oz	80	5	1
Fat Free: *Alpine Lace,* 1 oz	45	0	2
Weight Watchers, 1 sl., 3/4 oz	30	0	3
Cheese Balls (Kaukauna), 1 oz	100	7	0.5
Cheese Nut, Average, 1 oz	100	7	2
Cheese Logs, Average, 1 oz	100	7	0.5
Cheshire, 1 oz	110	9	1.5
Colby, Regular, 1 oz	110	9	0.5
Reduced Fat (*Alpine Lace*), 1 oz	80	5	1
Colby-Jack, 1 oz	110	9	0.5
Cottage Cheese: *Average All Brands*			
Creamed: 2 Tbsp, 1 oz	30	1	1
1/2 cup, 4 oz	120	5	4
w. fruit, 1/2 cup, 4 oz	130	4	15
Reduced Fat (2%), 2 T., 1 oz	25	<1	1
1/2 cup, 4 oz	100	2	4
Low Fat (1%), 2 Tbsp, 1 oz	20	<1	1
1/2 cup, 4 oz	80	1	3
NonFat, 2 Tbsp, 1 oz	20	0	1
1/2 cup, 4 oz	80	0	3
Borden Dry Curd (0.5%), 1/2 c., 4 oz	80	0	0
Friendship: Low Fat P'apple, 4 oz	120	1	17
NonFat Plus Peach, 1/2 c., 4 oz	110	0	15
Pot Style, 1/2 cup, 4 oz	90	3	3
w. Pineapple, 4 oz	140	4	16
Knudsen: 1.5% Fruit, 4 oz	110	2	12
Free, 1/2 cup, 4.3 oz	80	0	4
Cottage Dbles, 1 ctn, 5.5 oz	140	2.5	18
On the Go!, 1 cup, 4 oz	110	1.5	13
Light N' Lively: Garden Salad, 4 oz	90	2	5
Peach and Pineapple,			
1/2 cup, 4.3 oz	120	1	14
Chevre: See Goat's Milk Cheese			
Cream Cheese: See Page 39			
Edam: Regular, 1 oz	100	8	0
Farmer (Friendship), 2 Tbsp, 1 oz	50	3	0
Feta: Regular, *Frigo,* 1 oz	100	8	1
Crumbled, 1/2 cup, 2 1/2 oz	190	15	2.5
Reduced Fat (*Alpine Lace*),	60	4	1
Fontina (Sargento/Classica), 1 oz	110	9	0.5
Gjetost (Goat's Milk, fresh), 1 oz	85	7	0.5
Sargento, 1 oz	130	8	12
Goat's Milk: Soft: *Chevre,* 1 oz	70	6	0.5
Chavril, 3 Tbsp, 1 oz	60	4.5	1

Goat's Milk Cheese (Cont)	C	F	Cb
Semi-Soft: 1 oz	100	8.5	1
Hard: Sargento, 1 oz	130	10	0.5
Gorgonzola: 1 oz	110	9	0.5
Galbani Dolcelatte: 1 oz	95	8	1
Gouda: 1 oz	100	8	0.5
Gruyere, 1 oz	115	9	0
Havarti, 1 oz	120	11	0
Italian (Classica Italiano), 1 oz	110	10	0
Jarlsberg, 1 oz	100	7	1
Jarlsberg Lite shredded, 1 oz	70	4	1
Kefir, 2 Tbsp, 1 oz	60	4	1
Limburger, 1 oz	90	8	0
Mascarpone, 1 oz	130	13	1
Mexican (Sargento Recipe Blend),			
Shredded, 1/4 cup, 1 oz	110	9	1
Monterey, 1 oz	105	8.5	0
Monterey Jack: regular, 1 oz	110	9	0
Light Naturals (Kraft), 1 oz	80	5	1
Alpine Lace , Monti-Jack Lo, 1 oz	80	5	1
Weight Watchers, 1 oz	90	6	1
Mozzarella:			
Regular, Kraft/Dorman's, 1 oz	90	7	0.5
Land O'Lakes/Polly-O, 1 oz	80	6	0.5
Shredded, 1/4 cup, 1 oz	80	6	0.5
Light: Polly-O Lite, 1 oz	60	2.5	0.5
Kraft Light Naturals, 1 oz	80	5	0.5
Sorrento Lite, 1 oz	60	3	0.5
Part Skim (Alpine Lace), 1 oz	70	5	0.5
Polly-O, 1 oz	90	6	0.5
Fat Free: Healthy Choice, 1/4 c.,1oz	45	0	1
Polly-O, 1 oz	35	0	1
Kraft, shredded, 1/4 cup, 1 oz	50	0	2
Muenster: regular, 1 oz	110	9	0
Reduced Fat: Dorman's, 1 oz	80	5	0
Neufchatel: Dominick's, 1 oz	70	6	2
Philadelphia, 1 oz	70	6	0.5
Flavored: Fruit/Herbs	80	7	1
Chocolate (Hickory Farms), 1 oz	110	8	1
Parmesan: Fresh/Block, 1 oz	110	7	0
Shredded/Grated, 1 Tbsp	22	1.5	0
Grated (Packaged): 1 Tbsp	26	2	0
1oz quantity	130	9	1
1/2 cup, 1 3/4 oz	230	16	2
w.Romano (Frigo), grated, 1 oz	130	9	1

Note: Packaged grated and shredded Parmesan have more calories (per unit weight) than block Parmesan due to a lower moisture content.

Pizza, shredded:	C	F	Cb
Frigo, 1/4 cup, 1 oz	90	7	1
1 cup, 4 oz	360	28	4
Lowfat (Frigo), 1 oz	65	3	1
Port Du Salut, 1 oz	100	8	0.5
Port Wine (Hickory Farms), 1 oz	100	7	2.5
Pot (Sargento), 1 oz	25	0	1
Provolone: Regular, 1 oz	100	8	1
Reduced Fat, Alpine Lace, 1 oz	70	5	1
Pub (Hickory Farms), 1 oz	95	7	1
Quark: 40% fat, 1 oz	47	3	1
20% fat, 1 oz	32	1.5	1
Skim, 1 oz	22	0	1.5
Queso: Anego/Asadero/Blanco	105	9	1
Queso Chichuahua/De Papa	110	9	2
Queso De Taco, 1 oz	105	9	1
Ricotta Cheese:			
Whole Milk, 2 Tbsp, 1 oz	50	3.5	1
1/2 cup, 4 1/2 oz	225	16	4.5
Part Skim, 2 Tbsp, 1 oz	40	2.5	1
1/2 cup, 4 1/2 oz	180	12	4.5
Light/Low Fat, 2 Tbsp. 1 oz	30	1.5	2
1/2 cup, 4 1/2 oz	140	6	9
Fat Free (Polly-O), 1/2 c., 4 1/2 oz	100	0	4
Baked Ricotta, 2 oz portion	130	9	3
Romano: Block/Loaf, 1 oz	110	8	1
Grated (Pkg), 1 oz	120	9	1
1 Tbsp	26	2	0.5
Roquefort, 1 oz	105	9	0.5
Slim Jack (Dorman's), 1 oz	90	7	1
Sheep's Milk (Hollow Rd Farm)	45	3	1
Smoked: Sargents Smokestick	100	7	1
Hickory Farm, Smoky Lyte, 1 oz	80	6	1
Stilton, 1 oz	118	9	1
String (Frigo/Kraft/Sargento), 1 oz	80	5	1
String Lite (Frigo), 1 oz	60	2	1
Mootown Light (Sargento), 1 stick	50	2.5	0.5
Swiss: Regular, 1 oz	110	9	1
Reduced Fat: Alpine Lace, 1 oz	90	6	1
Dorman's/Kraft Light Naturals, 1oz	90	5	1
Weight Watchers, 3/4 oz slice	30	0	2
Taco, shredded, 1/4 cup			
(Frigo/Kraft/Sargents)	110	9	1
Tilsit (Sargents), 1 oz	100	7	0.5
Tybo (Dorman's/Sargents), 1 oz	100	7	0.5
Vermont (Churny), 1 oz	100	9	1
Wensleydale, 1 oz	108	9	0
Whey Cheese, 1 oz	125	8	9

Cheese (Cont)

Cheese Products   **C** **F** **Cb**

Cheese Food:
	C	F	Cb
Average all flavors, 3/4 slice	70	5	1.5
1 oz slice	90	6	2
Alouette: Fr. Onion/Garl.,2 T., 0.8oz	70	7	1
Light Garlic, 2 Tbsp, 0.8 oz	50	4	1
Cracker Barrel, Cheddar, 1.1 oz	100	8	4
Delico: Alouette Cajun, 2 T, 0.8 oz	70	7	1
Garden Vegetable, 2 T, 0.8 oz	60	6	1
Handi-Snacks:			
Cheez 'n Breadsticks, 1 pkg	130	7	11
Cheez'n Pretzels, 1 oz pkg	110	6	11
Cheez'n Crackers, 1.1 oz pkg	130	8	10
Mozzarella Stringchse Stick, each	80	6	0.5
Healthy Choice: Amer. Singles, 1 sl.	30	0	2
Heluva Good Cheese: Amer., 1 sl.	45	5	2
Cheddar w. H/radish, 2 Tbsp, 1oz	90	7	3
Jalapeno: Aver., all brands, 1 oz	90	7	2
Kraft: American grated, 1T., 0.2 oz	25	2	1
Singles, 1 slice, 3/4 oz	70	6	1
Free Singles, 1 slice, 0.7 oz	30	3	3
Pimento Spread, 2 Tbsp, 1.1 oz	80	6	3
Velveeta (Process Cheese Spread)			
Regular, 3/8" slice, 1 oz	100	6	3
Light, 3/8" slice, 1 oz	60	3	3
Lifeway: Farmers Cheese, 2 oz	75	5	2.5
Roka Blue, 2 Tbsp, 1.1 oz	80	7	2
Rondele: Soft Spreadable, 2 T, 1 oz	100	9	1
Light, 2 Tbsp, 0.9 oz	60	4	1
SmartBeat: All flav., 1 sl., 0.6 oz	35	2	2
Spreadery: Vermont, 2 Tbsp, 1 oz	80	5	3
Neufchatel, all flavors, 2 T, 1 oz	80	7	1
Velveeta: Cheese, 1 slice, 1 oz	100	6	3
Light, 1 oz	60	3	3
Shredded, 1/4 cup, 1.3 oz	130	9	3
WisPride: Hickory Smoked Cup;			
Port Wine Ball/Cup, 2 T., 1.1 oz	100	7	4
Light, 2 T., 1.1 oz	80	3	5

Cheese Whiz (Sauce)

	C	F	Cb
Regular, 2 Tbsp, 33g	90	7	20
Light, 2 Tbsp, 33g	80	3	6
Squeezable, 2 Tbsp, 33g	100	8	4

Cheese Substitutes   **C** **F** **Cb**

Per 1 oz Unless Indicated
	C	F	Cb
Almond Rella (Nu Soya):			
Cheddar; Garlic & Herb, 1 oz	60	3	3
Borden: Taco-Mate, 1 oz	100	7	2
Delicia: American Colby	80	6	1
Dorman's Lo Chol: All types	100	7	1
Formagg:			
American Wh./Yellow, 1 sl. 0.7oz	60	4	0.5
Cheddar, 1 slice, 0.7 oz	60	4	0.5
Mozzarella (Old World), 1 oz	60	3	1
Parmesan Grated, 1 Tbsp, 1/4 oz	22	1.5	1.5
Provolone (Vintage), 1 oz	60	3	1
Swiss White, 1 slice, 0.7 oz	60	4	0.5
Frigo: Cheddar; Mozzarella, 1 oz	90	7	1
Georgia's: Imitation Cheddar;			
Mozzarella., shredded, 1/2 c., 1 oz	90	7	1
Golden Image:			
Amer.ican 1 slice, 0.7 oz	70	5	1
Mild Cheddar, 1 slice, 0.7 oz	70	5	1
Harvest Moon : Per 1/4 cup, 1.3 oz			
Shredded: American; Cheddar	120	9	3
Mozzarella	110	9	3
Nu Tofu: Mozzarella, 1 oz	70	4	2
Fat Free: Mozz./Ched./Jack, 1 oz	40	0	2
Sargento Classic Supreme:			
Cheddar, shredded, 1 oz	90	6	2
Mozzarella, shrd, 1/4 cup	80	6	0.5
Smart Beat, all variet. 0.6 oz sl.	35	2	2
Soya Kaas: Regular, 1 oz	70	5	1
Fat Free, all varieties, 1 oz	40	2	1
Soyco: Almond/Oat/Rice Slices			
1 slice, 0.7 oz	40	2	1
Veggy Singles, 1 slice, 0.7 oz	40	2	1
Grated Parmesan, 2 tsp, 5g	15	0.5	0
Tofu Rella : Per 1 oz			
Tofu Rella, average all varieties	180	2	39
Zero-Fat Rella, all varieties	45	0	3
Almond/Hemp/Rice Rella,			
average all varieties	70	3.5	3
Tofutti Better Than Cream Cheese	80	8	1
Weight Watchers: Fat Free Slices,			
All varieties, 3/4 oz slice	30	0	3
Grated Italian Topping, 1 Tbsp	20	0	2
White Wave, Soy A Melt:			
Cheddar/Mozz./Mont. Jack, 1 oz	80	5	1
Fat Free, 1 oz	40	0	3
Singles: Amer./Mozzrlla, 3/4 oz sl.	60	4	1

Snack & Cheese Dips, Spreads

Cream Cheese   Ⓒ Ⓕ Ⓒᵇ

	C	F	Cb
Regular/Soft:			
2 Tbsp, 1 oz	100	10	1
3 oz pkg	300	30	2
w. Chives/Herbs/Pimento, 1 oz	90	9	0.5
w. Fruit/Strawb./P'apple, 1 oz	90	8	5
Lox, 1 oz	90	9	0.5
Philadelphia Brand:			
Plain/Soft, 2 Tbsp, 1 oz	100	10	1
1/3 Less Fat, 1 oz	70	6	1
Light, 1 oz	70	5	2
Fat Free, 2 Tbsp, 1 oz	30	0	3
Flavor./Herbs/Fruit/Salmon, 1 oz	100	10	2
w. Smoked Salmon 1 oz	100	9	1
Light Blueberry, 2 Tbsp	70	4.5	5
Whipped, 3 Tbsp, 1 oz	110	11	1
Alpine Lace: Fat Free, 2 T., 1 oz	30	0	1
Dominick's: Fat Free, 2 Tbsp, 1 oz	35	0	4
Light, 2 Tbsp, 1 oz	60	5	3
Weight Watchers, 2 Tbsp, 1 oz	40	2.5	1

Dips/Spreads

Per 2 Tbsp (1 oz) Unless Indicated

	C	F	Cb
Avocado/Guacamole	50	4	4
Baba Ghannouj (Eggplant/Sesame)	70	6	2
Birdseye: No Fat Veggie Dip, 1.1 oz	25	0	5
Breakstone: Sour Cream, all flav.	50	4	2
Chalco: Quéso Quesadilla; Cotija	120	10	0
Fresco, 2 Tbsp, 1 oz	70	8	2
Chef's Kitchen (Jewel): Dilly Dip	150	16	1
French Onion/Quarter; Spinach	70	6	2
Chi-Chi's: Con Quéso, 2 Tbsp	90	7	4
Hot/Medium/Mild/Acante, 2 T.	10	0	2
Dominick's: Port Wine & Cheddar	100	8	4
Eagle: Bean	35	2	4
French Onion Dip, aver. all brands	60	6	3
Frito Lay: Chili Cheese	45	3	3
French Onion	60	5	3
Bean/Jalapeno Bean	40	1	6
Jalapeno & Cheddar	50	3	3
Guacamole, 2 Tbsp, 1 oz	50	4	4
Guiltless Gourmet: Nacho Dip	25	0	5
Other varieties	30	0	5
Heluva Good Cheese:			
Cheese 'N Salsa	80	3	3
Clam/French Onion	50	5	2
Bacon/Homestyle/Ranch	60	5	2
Light Fr. Onion/Jalapeno Cheddar	40	2	3

Dips/Spreads (Cont)   Ⓒ Ⓕ Ⓒᵇ

Per 2 Tbsp (1 oz)

	C	F	Cb
Hummus, 2 Tbsp, 1 oz	50	1	5
1/2 cup, 4.5 oz	220	4.5	23
Hy-Top: Pimiento, 1 oz	90	8	3
Kaukauna: Nacho Cheese	90	7	4
Knudsen: Nacho Cheese	60	4	3
Sour Cream Bacon & Onion	60	5	2
Sour Cream French Onion	50	4	2
Kroger: The Big Dipper; all flavors	60	5	2
Kraft: Average all flavors	60	5	4
Premium: Bac. & On./Nacho Ch.	60	5	2
Other flavors	50	4	2
Philly flavors: Pineapple	100	9	1
Chive & Onion; Salmon	110	10	2
Cheesecake; Strawberry	110	9	5
Fat Free: Strawberry	45	0	6
Garden Veges	30	0	3
Lay's: Lowfat Sr. Cream, Onion	40	1	0
Louise's: (Fat Free) Honey Mustard	40	0	0
Sour Cream & Onion/Wh.Cheese	25	0	0
Marzetti: Blue Cheese	200	21	1
Light Ranch Veggie	60	7	5
Other flavors, average	140	14	2
Nalley's: All flavors, average	120	12	3
Naturally Fresh: All flavors, 1 oz	80	0	19
Old Dutch: Cheddar, Nacho	35	3	3
Old El Paso:			
Black Bean	25	0	5
Cheese'n Salsa: Mild; Medium	40	3	3
Lowfat, medium	30	1.5	3
Chunky Salsa varieties	15	0	3
Jalapeno Dip	30	1	4
Olys Bagel Spread: Berry	100	8	5
Honey Cinnamon; Raisin	100	8	6
Garden Veg; Garlic & Herb	90	8	1
Prices: Orig. Pimiento Cheese Spr.	80	7	2
Ruffles: French Onion; Ranch	70	6	4
Sealtest: French Onion	50	4	2
Snyder's Mustard Pretzel	90	4	13
Supremo Chihuahua: Quéso Bianco	100	8	0
Quéso Fresco; Rancherito	80	6	0
Tostitos Dip: Con Quéso	40	2	5
Medium/Mild/Hot	15	0	3
Tzatziki (Cucumber/Yoghurt Dip)	40	3	1
Wise: Jalapeno Bean	25	0	5
Taco	12	0	3
Salsa: See Page 78			

39

Egg & Egg Dishes

Chicken Eggs C F Cb

Fresh Eggs
Raw (weight with shell):

	C	F	Cb
Small, 40g	65	4	0
Medium, 44g	70	4	0
Large, 50g	75	4.5	0
Extra Large, 56g	80	5	0
Jumbo, 63g	90	5.5	0
Egg Yolk, 1 extra large	63	5	0
Egg White, 1 extra large	16	0	0

Dried Egg Powder

	C	F	Cb
Whole Egg, 1/4 cup, 1 oz	170	12	0
1 Tbsp	30	2	0
Egg White, 1/4 cup, 1 oz	105	0	0
Egg Yolk, 1/4 cup, 1 oz	195	18	0
1 Tbsp	27	2.5	0

Egg Substitutes

1/4 Cup (Equivalent to 1 Egg) ~ Zero Cholesterol.

	C	F	Cb
Better 'n Eggs (Papetti), 1/4 cup, 2 oz	30	0	0
Egg Beaters (Fleischmann's):			
Regular, 1/4 cup	30	0	1
Cheese Omelete, 1/2 cup	110	5	2
Vegetable Omelete, 1/2 cup	50	0	5
Egg Watchers (Tofutti), 2 oz	30	0	1
Eggstra, 1/2 envelope	50	2	4
Healthy Choice, 1/4 cup, 2 oz	25	0	1
Egg Substitute (Jewel), 1/4 cup	30	0	1
Scramblers (Morn Star), 1/4 cup	35	0	4
Second Nature: Regular, 1/4 cup	60	2	3
Fat Free, 1/4 cup, 60ml	30	0	1
Simply Eggs, 1/4 cup	35	1	1

Other Eggs

	C	F	Cb
Duck, 1 large, 2 1/2 oz	130	9.5	0
Goose, 1 large, 5 oz	280	19	0
Quail, 3 eggs, 1 oz	42	3	0
Turkey, 1 large, 3 oz	135	9.5	0
Turtle, 1 egg, 1 3/4 oz	75	5	0

Omega-3 Fat Enriched

	C	F	Cb
Eggs Plus (Pilgrim's Pride): 1 large	70	4.5	0

Note: Cholesterol content same as regular eggs, but Omega-3 fats inhibit blood cholesterol increase.
(Also see Cholesterol ~ Page 249)

Cooked Eggs C F Cb

	C	F	Cb
Boiled Egg: Same as raw egg			
Fried Egg:			
With fat: 1 large egg	100	8	0.5
2 small eggs	175	13	1
No fat/nonstick pan, 1 large	80	5.5	0
Deviled Egg, 2 halves	145	13	0.5
Eggs Benedict (2) on toast			
or English muffin	860	56	25
Eggs Florentine (2) on toast			
or English muffin	890	59	25
Pickled Egg, 1 large	80	5.5	0
Poached Egg, 1 large	80	5.5	0
Scotch Egg, 1 egg	300	21	16
Scrambled Eggs: 1 large egg:			
w. 1 Tbsp milk + 1 tsp fat	120	9	1
w. 1 Tbsp skim milk/no fat	85	5.5	1
2 large eggs:			
w. 2 Tbsp milk + 2 tsp fat	260	20	2
w. 2 Tbsp skim milk/no fat	180	11	2

Omelets

	C	F	Cb
1 Egg: Plain (w. 1 tsp fat)	125	10	0.5
with 1/2 oz cheese	175	15	0.5
w. 1/2 oz cheese + 1/2 oz ham	200	16	0.5
2 Eggs: Plain (w. 2 tsp fat)	250	20	1
with 1 oz cheese	360	29	2
w. 1 oz cheese + 1 ham	410	32	2
3 Eggs: Plain (w. 1 Tbsp fat)	360	29	1.5
w. 2 oz cheese	580	47	2.5
w. 2 oz cheese + 2 oz ham	680	53	2.5
Extras: Tomato/Onion/Veges	20	0	4.5
Egg Substitute (Eggbeaters):			
2 eggs (1/2 cup) + 1 tsp fat	100	4	2
3 eggs (3/4 cup) + 2 tsp fat	160	8	3
Extras: 1 oz cheese	110	9	1
1 oz ham	50	3	1
Tom./Onion/Veges	20	0	4.5

Egg Nog

Per 1/2 Cup (4 fl.oz)

	C	F	Cb
Regular: *Borden*	160	9	16
Crowley	190	9	23
Hood (Goldeen)	180	8	22
Light: *Borden/Hood*	120	2	23
Fat Free: *Hood*	100	0	21

Breakfast Sides

	C	F	Cb
Toast: Plain, 1 thick slice	85	1	13
with 2 tsp butter/marg.	155	9	13
with 3 tsp/1Tbsp fat	190	13	13
English Muffin: Plain, 2 oz	130	1	26
with 3 tsp fat	230	12	26
Bacon, 2 strips	70	5	0
Ham: Lean, 2 oz	100	3	0
Hash Browns: 1/2 cup	125	6.5	14
1 cup serving	250	13	28
Sausages, 2 links (1 oz ea.)	180	16	1.5

Frozen Egg Dishes

	C	F	Cb
Downyflake: Scrambled Eggs			
w. Ham & Hash Browns, 1 pkg	360	26	17
w. Ham & Pecan Twirl	470	28	40
w. Hash Browns & Sausage	420	34	17
Pillsbury Toaster Scrambles, 1	170	11	14
Swanson Great Starts: Per Packet			
Scrambled Eggs: w. Burrito	200	8	25
w. Bacon & Home Fries	290	19	17
w. Home Fries	200	12	15
w. Sausage & Hash Browns	360	26	21
Low Fat	240	13	18
Low Fat/Chol Eggs: w. Pancakes	220	7	30
w. Canadian Bacon	240	6	33
Egg, Bacon, Cheese Muffin	290	15	25
Egg, Sausage & Cheese	460	28	37
French Toast Sticks w. Syrup	320	10	50
Pancakes w. Sausage	490	25	52
Sandwich Egg, Cheese	350	20	30
Sausage, Egg & Chse on Biscuit	460	28	37
Quaker Scrambled Eggs			
w. Cheese/Fried Potatoes	250	13	22
w. Sausage & Hash Browns	290	20	14
w. Sausage & Pancakes	270	14	21
Weight Watchers: Omelet	220	5	30

Frozen Egg Rolls

	C	F	Cb
Average All Brands (Chun King/La Choy)			
Chicken Egg Rolls: Mini, 5 rolls	165	6	24
Restaurant Style, 1 roll, 3 oz	170	5	25
Pork & Shrimp Egg Rolls:			
Mini, 5 rolls	175	5	23
Pork Restaurant Style, 1 roll	170	6	24
Shrimp Egg Rolls: Mini, 5 rolls	155	5	23
Restaurant Style, 1 roll	150	4	24

Fast Food/Restaurants

	C	F	Cb
Bojangles:			
Bacon/Egg/Chse S'wich	550	42	27
Burger King:			
Bisc. w. Bacon/Egg/Cheese	510	31	39
Croissan'wich Saus./Egg/Chse	550	42	22
Carl's Jr.: Scrambled Eggs	160	11	1
Denny's: Country Scramble	795	50	67
Eggs Benedict	860	56	55
Omelette: Ham 'n Cheddar	745	55	24
Veggie-Cheese	715	53	29
Farmer's	915	70	38
Steak & Eggs	885	66	21
Hardees: Bacon & Egg	570	33	45
Ham, Egg & Cheese	540	30	48
Ultimate Omelet	570	33	45
McDonald's: Egg McMuffin	290	12	27
Bacon, Egg & Cheese Bisc.	470	28	36
Scrambled Eggs (2)	160	11	1
Perkins: Country Club Omelet	930	79	6
Quincy's: Scrambled Eggs	95	7	1
Roy Rogers: Ham & Egg Bisc.	460	23	48

**New Diet Aid
– The Refrigerator Air-Bag!**

POOF!

Note: Cooking reduces weight of meat by 20-45% due to water and fat losses. Average weight loss is 30%. Actual loss depends on cooking method and cooking time. Examples:

4 oz raw wt. = approx. 3 oz cooked wt.
4 oz cooked wt. = approx. 5$^1/2$ oz raw wt.

What 3 oz Cooked Meat Looks Like

- Half the size of this book (4$^1/4$" x 3" x $^3/8$" thick)
- Rectangular piece (4" x 2$^1/2$" x $^1/2$" thick)
- Pack of cards (3$^1/2$" x 2$^1/2$" x $^5/8$" thick)

Quick Guide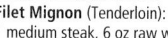

Steak

Sirloin (Choice Grade)
External fat trimmed to $^1/4$"
Broiled, Edible Portion (no bone)

Small Serving, 3 oz
(3 oz cooked, from 4-4$^1/2$ oz raw)

	C	F	Cb
Lean + fat ($^1/4$"), 3 oz	230	14	0
Lean + marbling, 3 oz	195	10	0
(External fat trimmed **before** cooking)			
Lean only, 3 oz	170	7	0
(No external fat or marbling)			

Medium/Regular Serving, 5 oz
(from approx. 7 oz raw)

Lean + fat ($^1/4$"), 5 oz	470	29	0
Lean + marbling, 5 oz	400	20	0
Lean only, 5 oz	350	14	0

Large Serving, 8 oz
(from 11-12 oz raw)

Lean + fat, 8 oz	610	38	0
Lean + marbling, 8 oz	520	26	0
Lean only, 8 oz	454	18	0

Extra Large Serving, 12 oz
(from approx. 16-17 oz raw)

Lean + fat ($^1/4$"), 12 oz	915	57	0
Lean + marbling, 12 oz	780	39	0
Lean only, 12 oz	680	27	0

Pan Fried
Sirloin (choice), medium serving:

Lean + fat ($^1/4$"), 5 oz	450	32	0
Lean only, 5 oz	330	15	0

Other Steaks C F Cb

Filet Mignon (Tenderloin)
1 medium steak, 6 oz raw wt.
Broiled, with $^1/4$" fat trim

	C	F	Cb
Lean + fat ($^1/4$"), 4 oz	340	24	0
Lean only, 3$^1/4$ oz	210	10	0
Broiled, ($^1/4$" fat removed before cooking)			
Lean + marbling, 3$^1/4$ oz	220	12	0
Lean only, 3 oz	180	8	0

New York/Club Steak:
Top Loin/Short Loin
1 steak, regular (9$^1/4$ oz raw, $^1/4$" fat)

Broiled: Lean + fat ($^1/4$"), 6$^1/4$ oz	510	35	0
Lean + marbling, 5$^1/2$ oz	330	16	0
Lean only, 5$^1/4$ oz	310	14	0

Porterhouse Steak:
1 medium, 6 oz raw wt. (no bone)
Broiled:

Lean + fat ($^1/4$"), 4$^1/4$ oz	370	27	0
Lean only, 3$^1/2$ oz	220	11	0

T-Bone Steak:
1 medium, 8 oz raw wt.

Broiled: Lean + fat	380	27	0
Lean only	220	10	0

Beef - Average All Cuts

Average All Retail Cuts C F Cb
Edible weight (no bone)

Raw
(1 lb raw yields approx. 11-12 oz cooked)

Lean + fat ($^1/4$" trim), 1 oz	70	5.5	0
$^1/2$ Pound, 8 oz	560	44	0
Lean only, 1 oz	40	2	0
$^1/2$ Pound, 8 oz	320	16	0
Fat only, 1 oz	190	20	0

Cooked (No Added Fat)

Lean + fat ($^1/4$"), 1 oz	86	6	0
Small serving, 3 oz	260	18	0
Lean + marbling, (no ext. fat), 1 oz	78	5	0
Small serving, 3 oz	235	15	0
Lean only, 1 oz	60	3	0
Small serving, 3 oz	180	9	0
Fat only, 1 oz	193	20	0

Beef - Individual Cuts

	C	F	Cb
Average All Grades			
Edible Weight (no bone)			
Brisket, whole, braised:			
Lean + fat (1/4"), 3 oz	330	27	0
Lean + marbling, 3 oz	250	17	0
Lean only, 3 oz	205	11	0
Chuck, blade, braised:			
Lean + fat (1/4"), 3 oz	290	22	0
Lean + marbling, 3 oz	285	20	0
Lean only, 3 oz	210	11	0
Flank: Raw, 4 oz	200	12	0
Braised, 3 oz	225	14	0
Broiled, 3 oz	190	11	0
Ribs, whole (ribs 6-12):			
Average all grades, roasted			
(1 lb raw yields 10 1/4 oz roasted)			
Lean + fat (1/4")			
(3.6 oz w. bone, 3 oz no bone)	300	25	0
Lean only, 3 oz (no bone)	200	11	0
Round, bottom, braised:			
Lean + fat (1/4"), 3 oz	235	14	0
Lean only, 3 oz	180	7	0
Round, eye/tip, roasted:			
Lean + fat (1/4"), 3 oz	200	11	0
Lean, 3 oz	150	5	0
Round, top: *Per 3 oz*			
Braised, Lean + fat	210	10	0
Lean only	175	5	0
Broiled, Lean + fat	185	8	0
Lean only	155	4	0
Pan-fried, Lean + fat	235	13	0
Lean only	190	7	0

Ground Beef

	C	F	Cb
Raw: Reg. (73% lean), 4 oz	350	30	0
Lean (80% lean), 4 oz	300	24	0
Extra lean (85% lean), 4 oz	250	17	0
Healthy Choice (97% lean), 4 oz	130	4	0
Baked/Broiled: Reg., 3 oz	250	18	0
Lean, 3 oz	230	16	0
Extra lean, 3 oz	200	12	0
Pan-fried: Regular, 3 oz	260	19	0
Lean, 3 oz	230	16	0
Extra lean, 3 oz	200	12	0
Ground Beef Patties: Average			
Frozen, raw, 4 oz	320	26	0
Broiled, 3 oz	240	17	0

Quick Guide
Roast Beef

	C	F	Cb
Round (Eye/Tip, average)			
Average All Cuts			
Small Serving, 3 oz			
(2 thin slices/1 thick slice)			
Lean + fat (1/4"), 3 oz	200	11	0
Lean only, 3 oz	150	5	0
Medium Serving, 5 oz, (3-4 thin slices)			
Lean + fat, 5 oz	330	18	0
Lean only, 5 oz	250	8	0
Large Serving, 8 oz, (3 thick slices)			
Lean + fat, 8 oz	530	29	0
Lean only, 8 oz	400	13	0

Roast Dinner Extras

	C	F	Cb
Gravy: Thin, 2 Tbsp	20	1	0.5
Thick, 2 Tbsp	50	2	0.5
1 Ladle/4 Tbsp	100	4	1
Veges: Beans, green, 1/2 cup	20	0	5
Cauliflower w. cheese sauce, 4 oz	135	9	15
Corn, kernels, 1/4 cup	35	0	9
Carrots, 1/4 cup	20	0	3
Peas, 1/4 cup	35	0	6
Pumpkin baked: w.fat, 4 oz	90	7	5
No added fat, 2 pces, 4 oz	25	0	5
Potato:			
Roasted w. fat, 1 small	155	8	30
Baked in Jacket, 1 large	220	0	50
with 1 Tbsp whipped butter	295	8	50
with Sour Cream, 2 Tbsp	270	6	51
Sweet Potato/Yam, 1 medium	80	0	20

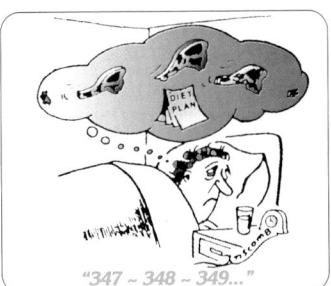

"347 ~ 348 ~ 349..."

Lamb

	C	F	Cb
Choice Grade			
Leg (Whole), roasted:			
Lean + fat, 3 oz	220	14	0
Lean only, 3 oz	160	7	0
Leg (Sirloin Half), roasted:			
Lean + fat, 3 oz	250	18	0
Lean only, 3 oz	175	8	0
Leg (Shank Half), roasted:			
Lean + fat, 3 oz	190	11	0
Lean only, 3 oz	155	6	0
Loin Chop, broiled:			
1 chop (raw wt., 4^1/4 oz):			
Lean + fat (2^1/4 oz edible)	200	15	0
Lean only (1.6 oz edible)	100	5	0
Rib Chop, broiled/roasted:			
1 chop (raw wt., 3^1/2 oz)			
Lean + fat (2^1/2 oz edible)	255	21	0
Lean only (1^3/4 oz edible)	120	7	0
Shoulder (Arm/Blade):			
Braised: Lean + fat, 3 oz	290	21	0
Lean only, 3 oz	240	14	0
Broiled: Lean + fat, 3 oz	240	16	0
Lean only, 3 oz	180	9	0
Roasted: Similar to Broiled			
Cubed Lamb (Leg/Shoulder):			
For stew or kabob			
Raw, lean only, 8 oz	310	12	0
Braised, lean only, 3 oz	190	8	0
Broiled, lean only, 3 oz	160	6	0
New Zealand Lamb (Imported):			
Similar calories and fat to domestic.			

Veal

	C	F	Cb
Edible Weights			
Leg (Top Round):			
Braised: Lean + fat, 3 oz	180	6	0
Lean only, 3 oz	170	5	0
Pan-fried, breaded:			
Lean + fat, 3 oz	195	8	9
Lean only, 3 oz	175	6	9
Pan-fried, not breaded:			
Lean + fat, 3 oz	180	7	0
Lean only, 3 oz	155	4	0
Roasted: Lean + fat, 3 oz	135	4	0
Lean only, 3 oz	130	3	0

Veal (Cont)

	C	F	Cb
Loin Chop: 1 chop, 7 oz raw wt.			
Braised: Lean + fat	230	14	0
Lean only	155	6	0
Roasted: Lean + fat	175	10	0
Lean only	125	5	0
Rib, roasted: Lean + fat, 3 oz	195	12	0
Lean only, 3 oz	150	7	0
Shoulder, Arm/Blade, roasted:			
Lean + fat, 3 oz	155	7	0
Lean only, 3 oz	145	6	0
Sirloin, roasted:			
Lean + fat, 3 oz	170	9	0
Lean only, 3 oz	145	6	0
Cubed for Stew, braised:			
Leg/Shoulder, lean only, 3 oz	160	4	0
(1 lb raw wt. yields approx. 9^1/4 oz cooked)			

Pork

	C	F	Cb
Figures based on NLMB data (1990)			
Fresh Pork (Cooked Wt., no bone)			
(4 oz raw wt. = approx. 3 oz cooked wt.)			
Blade Steak, broiled:			
Lean + fat, 3 oz	220	15	0
Lean only, 3 oz	190	11	0
Country Style Ribs, broiled:			
Lean + fat, 3 oz	270	22	0
Lean only, 3 oz	205	13	0
Leg (Ham), roasted:			
Lean + fat, 3 oz	250	18	0
Lean only, 3 oz	180	9	0
(Ham, cured ~ See Cold Meats)			
Loin Chops, broiled: Average			
(From 1 chop: 5 oz raw wt. w.bone			
or 4 oz raw wt., no bone)			
Lean + fat, 3 oz	200	11	0
Lean only, 3 oz	165	7	0
Rib Chops, broiled:			
Lean + fat, 3 oz	215	13	0
Lean only, 3 oz	180	7	0
Rib Roast, roasted:			
Lean + fat, 3 oz	210	13	0
Lean only, 3 oz	175	9	0
Loin Roast, roasted:			
Lean + fat, 3 oz	190	10	0
Lean only, 3 oz	160	7	0

Meat ✦ Bacon, Ham, Game

Pork (Cont) | C | F | Cb

	C	F	Cb
Sirloin Chop, broiled:			
Lean + fat, 3 oz	175	8	0
Lean only, 3 oz	155	6	0
Sirloin Roast, roasted:			
Lean + fat, 3 oz	215	14	0
Lean only, 3 oz	180	9	0
Tenderloin, roasted:			
Lean + fat, 3 oz	140	4	0
Lean only, 3 oz	135	4	0
Ground Pork			
Raw: Average, 1/4 lb, 4 oz	300	24	0
Broiled, 3 oz	245	18	0
Pan-fried, drained, 3 oz	250	19	0

Bacon

	C	F	Cb
Raw: 1 med. slice (20 lb), 3/4 oz	125	13	0
1 thick slice (12 lb), 1 1/3 oz	210	22	0
(1 lb raw yields approx. 5 oz cooked)			
Broiled/Pan-Fried: 1 med. sl., 6 g	36	3	0
3 medium slices, 18g	110	9	0
2 thin slices, 1/2 oz	80	7	0
1 thick slice, 12g	70	6	0
Canadian-style: Cooked, 1 slice	43	4	0
As purchased, 1 slice, 1 oz	45	4	1
Bacon Bits, 1 Tbsp, 1/4 oz	20	1	0
Breakfast Strips: Broil., 1 sl., 12 g	50	4	0

Ham

	C	F	Cb
Boneless Ham, cooked:			
Regular, (approx. 11% fat):			
Unheated (as purch.), 1 oz	52	3	0
Roasted, 3 oz	150	8	0
Extra Lean (5% fat):			
Unheated, 1 oz	37	2	0
Roasted, 3 oz	125	5	0
Whole Ham, cooked:			
Lean + fat (as purchased)			
Unheated, 1 oz	70	5	0
Roasted, 3 oz	345	26	0
Lean only, unheated, 1 oz	40	2	0
Roasted, 3 oz	135	5	0
Canned Ham: Similar to boneless ham			
Chopped, canned, 3 oz	260	21	0
Ham Patties, ckd, 1 pty, 2 1/4 oz	205	18	1
Ham Steak, extra lean, 2 oz	70	2	0
Luncheon Slices~ See Cold Meats: Page 48			

Game Meats | C | F | Cb

	C	F	Cb
Bison Steak, lean, 6 oz (raw)	160	6	0
Boar (wild), roasted, 3 oz	140	4	0
Caribou, roasted, 3 oz	140	4	0
Deer/Venison, roasted 3 oz	135	3	0
Rabbit: Roasted, 3 oz	130	6	0
Stewed, 1 cup, diced, 5 oz	300	14	0

Variety & Organ Meats

	C	F	Cb
Brains: Braised, 3 oz	130	9	0
Pan-fried, 3 oz	200	14	0
Chitterlings, pork, simmered, 3oz	260	25	0
Ears, pork, simmered, 1 ear	180	12	0
Feet, pork: Simmered, 3 oz	165	11	0
Cured, pickled, 3 oz	170	14	0
Hormel, 2 oz	80	6	0
Head Cheese (Pork Snouts/Ears/Vinegar/Spices):			
1 oz slice	50	4	0
Heart: Average, braised, 3 oz	140	5	0
Jowl, pork, raw, 4 oz	750	80	0
Kidneys, simmered, 3 oz	130	4	0
Liver: Raw, 4 oz	160	5	3
Braised, 3 oz	140	4	3
Pan-fried, 3 oz	200	9	3
Pancreas, braised, 3 oz	200	13	0
Pork Cracklins, 0.5 oz	80	6	0
Pork Hocks, 1 piece, 6 oz	340	23	0
Scrapple, pork, 1 oz	60	4	4
Spleen, braised, 3 oz	130	4	0
Stomach, pork, raw, 4 oz	180	11	0
Sweetbreads: Beef, ckd, 3 oz	270	20	0
Lamb, cooked, 3 oz	150	5	0
Tail, pork, simmered, 3 oz	340	31	0
Tongue, braised, 3 oz: Veal	170	9	0
Beef/Lamb/Pork, average	240	17	0
Tripe, beef, raw, 4 oz	110	5	0
Lean + fat	310	25	0

In eating, one third of the stomach should be filled with food, one third with drink, and the rest left empty.

~ Gitten, the Talmud

Sausages, Franks

Fresh Sausages

	C	F	Cb
Pork/Beef: *Average All Types*			
Small: Raw, 4" link, 1 oz	120	12	1.5
Broiled/Pan-fried	50	4	1.5
Medium: Raw, 2 oz	235	23	2.5
Broiled/Pan-fried	100	8	2.5
Large: Raw, 3 oz	360	36	3.5
Broiled/Pan-fried	150	12	3.5
Italian: Raw, 3.2 oz	315	28	1.5
Cooked, 2.4 oz	215	17	1.5

Note: Fat is lost in broiling/pan frying.
(Cooked wt. = approx. 60-70% raw wt.)

Franks & Weiners

	C	F	Cb
Beef: *Average All Brands*			
Regular/Smoked: *Per Frank*			
4 oz link	280	22	5
2.6 oz link	240	19	2
2 oz link (8/16 oz pkg)	180	17	2
1.6 oz link (10/16 oz pkg)	140	13	1
1.5 oz link (8/12 oz pkg)	135	12	1
1.2 oz link (10/12 oz pkg)	110	10	1
1 oz link (16/16 oz pkg)	90	8	0.5
Small/Cocktail (50/lb), each	30	3	0.5
Light/Fat Reduced:			
Best's Kosher, (97% FF), 1.7 oz	50	1	5
Oscar Mayer, 2 oz link	110	8	1
Hebrew National (97% FF), each	45	1.5	2
Healthy Choice (Jumbo Frank)	70	1.5	0
Pork: *Country Style,* 2 oz panfried	240	22	1
Chorizo, 5 sausages, 2.5 oz	280	26	3
El Popular, 2 oz cooked	210	17	3
Jimmy Dean, cooked, 2 oz	240	21	0
Oscar Mayer (2), 1.7 oz, ckd	170	15	1
Light, 2 oz link	110	8	2
Turkey Franks: *Ball Park,* 1.75 oz	40	0	6
Empire Kosher, 2 oz	90	6	1
Foster Farms, 2 oz	130	11	0
Louis Rich: Reg. (10/16 oz), 2 oz	110	8	2
(8/12oz pkg), 1½ oz	80	6	2
Mr Turkey, smoked, 2 oz	90	5	3
Shelton's: 1 frank, 1.2 oz	80	6	1
Chicken Franks *(Shelton's),* 1.2 oz	95	8	1
Empire Kosher, 2 oz	100	7	1
Foster Farms, 2 oz	140	12	0
Scott Petersen, 1.2 oz	80	6	1
Zacky Farms, 2 oz	150	13	0

Smoked Sausages

	C	F	Cb
Butterball (w. Turkey), 2 oz	60	0	4
Eckrich, 2 oz	180	16	4
Healthy Choice, 2 oz	70	1.5	6
Lemington Foods: 2 oz link	180	15	3
Skinless, 3 oz link	250	21	5
Bacon & Cheddar, 3 oz pce	250	20	7
Scott Petersen: Skinless, 3 oz link	280	24	5

Vegetarian Sausages

	C	F	Cb
Lightlife: Bkfst Links, 1 link, 35g	70	3	4
Lean Italian Links, 1 link, 40g	80	3	5

Breakfast Sausages/Biscuits

	C	F	Cb
Healthy Choice			
Breakfast Sausage, 2 patties, 1.6 oz	50	1.5	3
Jimmy Dean			
Sausage Biscuit 2	390	25	29
Mini Burgers, 2	270	14	23
Saus. Egg & Cheese, Biscuit, 1	390	27	28
Minyard: Pork Sausage Biscuit, 1	200	12	16
Owens Border Breakfast			
2 Sausages, Egg, Cheese, Tacos	330	11	42
2 Hot Sausages, Biscuits	370	23	26
Knob Sausages, 2 oz, ckd	210	18	0
Swift Premium			
Morning Makers: *Per 3.5 oz*			
Egg & Cheese, 1 pce	240	8	30
Ham, Egg & Cheese	250	10	31
Sausage, Egg & Cheese	250	8	32

WILL-POWER TONIC
~ RECIPE ~

- 1 Cup of Desire
- 1 Quart of Determination
- 1 Tbsp of Common Sense
- 1 Tbsp of Stick-to-itiveness
- 1 Tbsp of Foresight
- 1 Cup of Energy

Bagel, Corn & Hot Dogs

Hot Dogs, Ready-To-Go | C | F | Cb
(Includes Ketchup/Relish; No Mayo)

	C	F	Cb
Small (1 oz frank/ 1 oz roll)	200	8	24
Regular (1 1/2 oz frank/ 2 oz roll)	310	13	39
Large (2 oz frank/ 2 oz roll)	360	18	40
Super/Giant (3oz frank/3oz roll)	540	26	59

Corn Dogs
Beef/Pork Frank: Average, 2.6 oz	250	17	21
Mini, each	65	4.5	5
Turkey: *Gobblers! (Shelton's)*	220	11	27

Bagel Dogs
Best's Kosher: 1 dog, 1 oz	320	11	43
Mini, 1 piece, 0.8 oz	60	2	8
Vienna Beef: 1 piece, 1 oz	85	3.5	7

Weinerschnitzel (Franchise Outlets)
Carbohydrate figures ~ author estimates only.

Chili Dog, 1 serve	295	16	38
w. Lowfat Frank	230	5	38
Chili Cheese Dog	350	21	40
w. Lowfat Frank	280	9	40
Corn Dog	290	23	25
Deluxe Dog	275	14	38
w. Lowfat Frank	220	3.5	38
Kraut Dog	265	14	37
Mustard Dog	260	14	37
Relish Dog	280	14	37
Western Dog	380	23	40

Also See Fast-Foods Section

Toppings/Extras
American Chse, 1 slice, 1 oz	110	9	1
Catsup, 1 Tbsp	16	0	4
Chili (w. Beans), 1/4 cup	70	3.5	9
Mustard, 1 Tbsp	20	0	1
Pickle Relish, 1 Tbsp	20	0	5
Sauerkraut, 1/2 cup	20	0	5

Deli & Luncheon Meats

Beef Jerky: | C | F | Cb
	C	F	Cb
Bridgeford Beef Jerky, 1 oz	50	1	3
Beef Stick (5.5 oz stick), 1 oz	140	12	0
Beef Steak, 1 oz	50	1	0
Beef & Cheese (Giant Size), 1/2 pkg, 1.5 oz	170	14	1
Pepperoni Sticks, 2, 1 oz	140	12	0
Pepperoni (1" diam.), 1 oz	130	12	0
Teriyaki, 1.25 oz pkg	80	1	8
Original; Hot 'n Spicy	70	1	5
Berliner (pork/beef), 1 oz	65	4	0.5

Beerwurst (Beef):
Small (2.75"diam), 1/16" slice	20	2	0
Large (4"diam), 1/8" slice	75	7	0.5

Beerwurst (Pork):
Small (2.75"diam), 1/16" slice	15	1	0
Large (4"diam), 1/8" slice	55	4	0.5

Bologna, Beef & Pork:
Regular: 1 thin slice, 1 oz	90	8	1
1 thick slice, 1.6 oz	145	13	1
Light *(Oscar Mayer)*, 1 sl., 1 oz	60	4	2
Red. Fat *(Hebrew Nat.)*,1 oz	65	6	0
Fat Free *(Osc. M.)*, 2 sl., 1.6 oz	40	0	1
Healthy Choice, 1 oz	35	1	3
Weight Watchers, 2 sl., 3/4 oz	35	2	0
Turkey, average, 1 oz	60	5	0.5
Chicken *(Tyson)*, 1 slice	45	4	0.5
Ring *(Boar's Head)*, 2 oz	160	13	0.5
Blood Sausage, 1 oz	100	9	0.5

Bratwurst:
Average, 1 oz	90	8	0.5
Boar's Head, cook., 1 wurst, 4 oz	300	25	0
Bob Evan's, Beer, 2.6 oz link	270	21	1
Braunschweiger (Pork/Liver/Sausage), *Oscar Mayer*, 1 oz slice	100	9	1
Chicken, *Average All Brands*			
1 thick or 2 thin slices, 1 oz	30	1	1
Chicken Roll, 1 slice, 1 oz	90	4	1.5

Corned Beef:
Average, full fat, 1 oz	70	5	1.5
Healthy Choice, Hillshire Farm,1oz	30	1	0.5
Hebrew National, 4 slices, 2 oz	90	4.5	0
Loaf, jellied, 1 oz	45	2	0
Hash, canned, average, 1 oz	50	3	2
Dutch Brand Loaf, average, 1 oz	70	5	1.5

Continued Next Page

Ham, Luncheon:	C	F	Cb
Baked/Boiled, sliced, 1 oz	30	1	0.5
Chopped: *Eckrich* (97% FF), 1 oz	25	1	1
Armour, canned, 1 oz	35	1.5	0.5
97% Fat Free, 1 oz	25	1	1.5
Healthy Choice Deli Traditions:			
Baked, 6 sl., 2 oz	60	1.5	4
Larger Slice, 1 slice, 1 oz	30	1	1
Hormel (Black Label), 1 oz	70	6	0
Oscar Mayer, 1 oz slice	60	3	1
Honey, average, 1 oz	30	1	0.5
Healthy Choice Deli Traditions:			
6 slices, 2 oz	60	1.5	3
Prosciutto, average, 1 oz	70	5	1
Ham & Cheese Loaf, aver., 1 oz	70	5	1
Head Cheese *(Osc. Mayer),* 1 oz sl.	50	4	0
Honey Loaf *(Osc. Mayer),* 1 oz sl.	35	1	2
Italian Sausage, 2.6 oz	270	21	1
Kielbasa (Polish Sausage), 1 oz	85	7	0.5
Scott Petersen, 3.4 oz link	320	27	4
Beef, 2.8 oz link	290	25	4
Boar's Head, 1 oz	60	5	0
Kippered Beefsteak:			
(Hickory Farms), 3 slices, 0.75 oz	50	1	1
Knackwurst, 1 oz	90	8	0.5
Liverwurst, 1 oz	95	8	0.5
Liver Pate, fresh, average, 1 oz	110	10	3.5
Luncheon Loaf *(Foods Co),* 1 oz	80	7	2
Mortadella, 1 oz	90	7	0.5
Olive Loaf, average, 1 oz	70	5	3
Oscar Mayer, 1 oz slice	70	6	2
Pastrami (Beef), average, 1 oz	40	2	0.5
Healthy Deli, 1 oz	34	1	1
Hillshire (DeliSelect), 6 sl., 2 oz	60	1	1
Turkey Pastrami, 1 slice, 1 oz	30	1	1
Peppered Beef, 1 oz slice	40	2	1
Pepperoni: 5 slices, 1 oz	135	12	0
Pickle Loaf, average, 1 oz	80	6	1
Pickle & Pimiento Loaf			
(Oscar Mayer), 1 oz	80	6	3
Polish Sausage: See Kielbasa			
Proscuitti, average, 1 oz	70	5	0
Hormel, 1 oz	90	7	0
Roast Beef, lean, 1 oz	40	1	0.5

Salami:	C	F	Cb
Beef: average, 1 oz	80	7	1
Beer: average, 1 oz	70	6	0.5
Cotto: *Oscar Mayer,* 1 slice, 1 oz	70	5	1
Dry: Hard, aver. 3 slices, 1 oz	110	10	0.5
Oscar Mayer, 2 slices, 1.6 oz	120	10	1
Genoa: average, 1 oz	110	10	0
Stick *(Best's Kosher),* 2, 1.75 oz	180	15	2
Italian: *(Bridgeford),* 1 oz	120	11	0
Turkey: average, 1 oz	55	4	1
Spam: Original, 2 Tbsp, 1 oz	70	6	0
Summer Sausage: *Bridgeford,* 1 oz	100	9	0
Oscar Mayer, 1 slice, 0.8 oz	70	7	0
Treet *(Armour),* canned, 1 oz	100	9	1.5
Turkey: *Oscar Mayer,* 1 oz slice	30	1	0.5
¾ oz slice	22	0.5	0.5
Turkey Breast:			
Butterball Fat Free, 6 sl, 2 oz	50	0	2
Deli Thin Smoked, 1 sl., 1 oz	25	0	2
Hillshire Deli Select, 6 sl., 2 oz	50	0.5	2
Louis Rich Carvery Board,			
3 slices, (52g), 1.8 oz	50	0.5	1
Free, 2 slices, 2 oz	50	0	2
Healthy Choice, 6 sl., 2 oz	60	1.5	3
Hearty Deli Rst'd, 3 sl., 2 oz	60	0.5	1
Honey Roasted, 6 sl., 2 oz	60	1.5	4
Turkey Ham, 1 slice, 1 oz	35	1.5	0.5
Turkey Pastrami, 1 oz	35	1.5	0.5
Turkey Roll, 1 oz	40	2	0.5
Turkey Loaf, 1 oz	30	1	0.5

Meat Spreads

Average All Brands
Per ¼ cup (2 oz)

Chicken	120	8	2
Ham, deviled	160	14	0
Liverwurst	170	14	3
Roast Beef	140	11	0
Sandwich Spread	140	10	8
Turkey	110	7	2

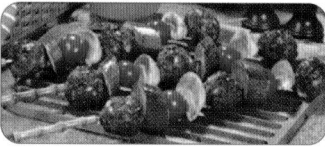

Paté | C | F | Cb

	C	F	Cb
Canned: *Average All Brands*			
Chicken Liver, 1 Tbsp, 1/2 oz	30	2	1
2 Tbsp, 1 oz	60	4	2
Foie Gras, goose liver, 1 oz	130	12	2
Sells, liverpate, 2 1/8 oz	190	16	3
Fresh (Refrigerated):			
Average all types, 1 oz	110	10	4
Marcel Henri, 2 oz serving	220	20	2
Pate de Campagne, 1 oz	105	9	1
Chicken Liver w. Port Wine, 1 oz	100	9	1
Duck Truffle w. Port Wine, 1 oz	120	12	1
Coeur de France:			
Smoked Salmon Pate, 1 oz	45	3.5	1
Spinach Pate w. Roquefort, 1 oz	50	4	1
Garden Fresh Vegetable Pate:			
Mushroom, Artichoke & Spinach in Puff Pastry, 2 oz	110	7	8

Lunch Packs | C | F | Cb

	C	F	Cb
Lunchables *(Oscar Mayer)*			
Per Package:			
Bologna/American Chse/Crackers	470	32	30
Bologna w. Cookies (4cpt)	480	33	31
w. Drink & M&M's	550	29	60
Deluxe Turkey/Chicken	390	22	26
Lean Ham	360	22	21
w. Drink & Jello	390	11	58
Lean Ham/Chedd./Crackers/Cookie	420	22	39
Lean Turkey/Amer. Chse/Cracker	360	19	33
Lean Turkey Brst./Chedd. Crackers	350	20	23
Red. Fat Turkey/Cheddar	250	9	24
Pancakes & Bac'n Bites	380	11	64
Pizza Dunks w. Drink	510	14	83
Pizza Swirls w. Drink	480	18	72
Turkey Breast:	370	20	33
w. Drink & Jello	350	9	53
Waffles & Sausage	350	12	54
Goosebumps (w. Capri Sun/Pudd.)			
Bologna/Amer. Chse/Crackers	550	29	60
Ham/Cheddar/Crackers	380	10	58
Turkey Brst/Cheddar/Crackers	350	9	53
Nachos: Cheese & Salsa	380	21	39
w. Capri Sun/Nestle Crunch	530	24	75
Pizza: Extra Cheesy, 3	300	12	30
w. Drink & Crunch Bar	460	15	62
Pepperoni Flavored Sausage, 3	310	14	30
Sandwiches: Ham, Turkey,Chedd.	470	22	47
Oven Rst. Turkey & Chse Sub	410	17	45
Smoked Ham & Cheddar Sub	380	14	44
Smoked Turkey & Chedd. Bagel	380	4	63
Tacos: Beef Taco & Cheese	310	11	34
w. Capri Sun/Butterfinger	470	13	67
Munch-A-Bunch *(Jewel):* Per 4 oz Package			
Bologna/Chse/Crackers/Cookies	430	29	27
Other varieties, average	350	19	29
Tastefuls! *(Jimmy Dean):* Per Package			
Real Pizza: 3 Cheese w. Hi-C	440	10	74
Pepperoni w. Chee-tos & M&M's	590	28	67
Combo w. Reeces P'nut Cup, Hi-C	470	16	66
Sandwiches: Rst. Chicken & Cheese			
w. M&M's, Doritos Tortilla Chips	520	20	63
Oven Rst Turkey & Cheese			
w. Reeces P'nut Cup, Pot. Chips	510	23	53
Ham & Turkey w. Kit Kat/ Chips	500	23	54

Quick Guide
Chicken

From 3lb ready-to-cook chicken

Breast/Wing Quarter	C	F	Cb
Roasted: With skin	300	15	0
Without skin	190	5	0
Fried, batter dipped	480	26	18
Leg Quarter: Thigh & Drumstick			
Roasted: With skin	265	15	0
Without skin	180	8	0
Fried, batter dipped	430	26	16

KFC ~ See Fast-Foods Section.

Average - All Meats

Average of Light & Dark Meats
Per 4 oz Serving (no bone)

	C	F	Cb
Roasted: With skin	270	15	0
Without skin	215	8	0
Stewed: With skin	250	14	0
Without skin	200	8	0
Fried: Batter-dipped	330	20	11
Flour coated	305	17	3.5

Chicken Parts

Broilers or Fryers: Edible Weights (no bone)
Breast: *Per 1/2 Breast*

	C	F	Cb
Raw: With skin, 5 oz	245	13	0
Without skin, 4 1/4 oz	130	2	0
Roasted: With skin, 3 1/2 oz	195	8	0
Without, 3 oz	140	3	0
Stewed: With skin, 4 oz	210	8	0
Without skin, 3 1/4 oz	140	3	0
Fried: Batter-dipped, 5 oz	370	19	12
Flour coated, w. skin, 3 1/2 oz	220	9	7

Drumstick: *Per Drumstick*

	C	F	Cb
Roasted: With skin, 2 oz	125	6	0
Without skin, 1 1/2 oz	75	2	0
Fried: Batter-dipped, 2 1/2 oz	195	11	7
Flour coated, 1 3/4 oz	120	7	1
Stewed: With skin, 2 oz	115	6	0
Without skin, 1 1/2 oz	80	3	0

Thigh Portion: Edible Wt. (no bone)

	C	F	Cb
Raw: With skin, 3.3 oz			
(4 1/4 oz with bone)	200	14	0
Without skin, 2.4 oz	80	3	0
Roasted: With skin, 2 1/4 oz	155	10	0
Without skin, 2 oz	110	6	0

Thigh Portion (Cont)

	C	F	Cb
Stewed: With skin, 2 1/2 oz	160	10	0
Without skin, 2 oz	105	5	0
Fried: Batter-dipped, 3 oz	240	14	8
Flour coated, 2 1/4 oz	165	9	2

Wing: *Per Wing*
Raw Weight 3.2 oz (with bone)

	C	F	Cb
Raw: With skin	110	8	0
Without skin	35	1	0
Roasted: With skin	105	7	0
Without skin	45	2	0
Fried: Batter-dipped	160	11	5
Flour coated	105	7	1
Stewed: With skin, 4 oz	100	7	0
Neck: Simmered, with skin	95	7	0
Without skin	30	2	0

Skin Only: *Skin from 1/2 Chicken*

	C	F	Cb
Raw skin, 2 3/4 oz	275	26	0
Roasted skin, 2 oz	255	22	0
Stewed skin, 2 1/2 oz	260	24	0
Fried, Flour coated, 2 oz	280	24	5
Fried, Batter-dipped, 6 3/4 oz	750	55	45

Roasters

Average of Light & Dark Meat:

	C	F	Cb
Roasted: With skin, 4 oz	250	15	0
Without skin, 4 oz	190	8	0
Light Meat: Without skin, rst.	175	5	0
Dark Meat: Without skin, rst.	206	10	0

Stewing Chicken

Stewed: *Per 4 oz Serving*
Average of Light & Dark Meat:

	C	F	Cb
With skin	325	21	0
Without skin	270	14	0
Light Meat: Without skin	240	9	0
Dark Meat: Without skin	295	17	0

Capon Chicken

	C	F	Cb
Roasted: With skin, 4 oz	260	13	0
1/2 Chicken, with skin	1460	74	0

Chicken Offal & Stuffing

	C	F	Cb
Giblets, simmered, 1 cup	230	7	1.5
Fried, flour-coated, 1 cup	400	20	6
Gizzard, simmered, 1 cup	220	5	1.5
Heart, simmered, 1 cup	270	12	0.5
Liver: Raw, 4 oz	140	5	3.5
Simmered, 1 cup	220	8	1
Liver Pate Fresh, 1 Tbsp, 1/2 oz	60	8	2
Stuffing: Average, 1/2 cup	200	2	22

Chicken Products

	C	F	Cb
Tyson			
Chicken Chunks: Regular, (6)	280	20	19
Breast, (6)	220	19	11
Southern Fried, (6)	260	19	11
Breast Patties: Regular, each	190	12	11
Chick 'n Quick/Chedd., 74g ea.	220	14	12
Crispy Baked, each	80	0	9
Thick 'n Crispy, each	200	19	10
Southern Fried, each	180	12	8
Nuggets: Breaded White Meat, (6)	250	18	12
Wings: Flavored, average, (3)	170	10	1
BBQ Style, (3)	200	13	2
Stir Fry Kit: Chicken, 2¾ c. froz.	430	4.5	73
Wraps: Southwest Black. 1½	560	12	82
Mandarin Sesame, 1½ wraps	560	12	82
M/wave S/wiches: Breast, 119g	320	15	33
Stove Top: *Per Serving*			
Chicken Stuffing Mix: 1 oz	110	1	20
½ cup prep.	170	9	20

Duck, Goose, Quail

	C	F	Cb
Duck: roasted, with skin, 3 oz	285	24	0
Without skin, 3 oz	170	10	0
½ whole duck, with skin	1300	108	0
Goose: roast, with skin, 3 oz	260	19	0
Without skin, 3 oz	200	11	0
Pheasant: ½ bird, raw	720	37	0
Quail: 1 whole, raw	210	13	0

Turkey

Fryer-Roasters

	C	F	Cb
Roasted: *Per 3 oz Serving*			
Light Meat: With skin	140	4	0
Without skin	120	1	0
Dark Meat: With skin	155	6	0
Without skin	140	4	0
¼ of Whole Turkey: (Approx. 3¼ lbs raw wt. w/out neck and giblets; 2 lb 6 oz cooked wt.)			
Roasted: With skin	1400	46	0
Without skin	1030	18	0
Ground Turkey, Raw: (4oz raw wt. = 3oz ckd wt.)			
Regular (85% lean), 4 oz	180	10	0
Lean (90% lean), 4 oz	160	8	0
Breast, no skin, 4 oz	115	1	0

Turkey Parts

	C	F	Cb
Roasted, Edible Weights (no bone)			
Breast (¼): (from 17¼ raw wt. w/bone)			
With skin, 12 oz (no bone)	525	11	0
Without skin, 10¾ oz	415	2	0
Back (½): With skin, 4½ oz	265	13	0
Without skin, 3½ oz	165	5	0
Leg (Thigh & Drumstick):			
(from 1 lb raw wt. w/bone)			
With skin, 8½ oz (no bone)	420	13	0
Without skin, 7¾ oz	355	8	0
Wing: (from 7¼ oz raw wt. w/bone)			
With skin, 3 oz (no bone)	185	9	0
Without skin, 2 oz	100	2	0
Neck: Simmered, 1 neck			
(9 oz w. bone)	275	11	0
Giblets, simm., 1 cup, 5 oz	240	7	3

Young Hens (Roasted)

	C	F	Cb
Light Meat: With skin, 3 oz	175	8	0
Without skin, 3 oz	135	3	0
Dark Meat: With skin, 3 oz	200	11	0
Without skin, 3 oz	165	7	0
Young Toms — Similar to Young Hens			

Turkey Products

	C	F	Cb
Banquet ~ Frozen Meals, Page 55			
Circle L: Boneless Turk Bacon,3 oz	120	9	1
Louis Rich			
Fat Free Breast of Turkey			
Rotiss'd/Smoked/Rstd, 2 oz	60	0	1
Turkey Ham & Chunks, cooked:			
Breast & White Turkey, 2 oz	60	1	2
Turkey Ham/Pastrami, 2 oz	70	3	1
Turkey Salami, 2 oz	100	8	0
Luncheon Slices — See Cold Meats, Page 48			
Franks: Medium, 1½ oz	80	6	2
Large, 2 oz	110	8	3
Smoked Sausage/Kielbasa, 1 oz	45	2	1
Turkey Nuggets, cooked, each	65	4	4
Turkey Patties, cooked, each	220	13	13
Turkey Sticks, cooked, each	75	5	4
Swanson ~ Frozen Meals, Page 59			
Turkey Store			
Gobble Stix: Honey, each	25	0	1
Lean Burger Patties, 1 patty	180	8	5
Lean Italian Sausage, 1 link	190	8	2

Quick Guide ⓒ Ⓕ ⓒᵇ

Fresh Fish

Low Oil (Less than 2.5% fat)
White/pale colored flesh. Examples:
Cod, Flounder, Haddock, Halibut, Monkfish
Perch, Pike, Pollock, Snapper, Sole, Whiting.

Per 4 oz Edible Portion

	C	F	Cb
Raw, 4 oz (no bones)	90	1	0
Steamed, Broiled, Baked	130	1	0
Fried: Lightly Floured	210	8	3.5
Breaded	260	12	8
In Batter	320	16	27

Medium Oil (2.5-5% fat)
Pale colored flesh. Examples:
Bluefin Tuna, Catfish, Kingfish, Salmon (Pink),
Swordfish, Rainbow Trout, Yellowtail.

	C	F	Cb
Raw, 4 oz (no bones)	140	5	0
Baked, Broiled, 4 oz	175	6	0
Fried, 4 oz	230	11	8

High Oil (Over 5% fat)
Darker colored flesh. Examples:
Albacore Tuna, Bluefish, Herring, Mackerel,
Orange Roughy, Salmon (Atl./Chinook/Sockeye),
Sardines, Trout, Whitefish.

	C	F	Cb
Raw, 4 oz (no bones)	230	16	0

Cooking Yields (Fin Fish):
4 oz Raw wt. = 3^1/$_2$ oz Cooked wt.
4 oz Cooked wt. = 5 oz Raw wt.

Calorie & Fat Variations
The amount of fat/oil in fish varies with the species, season and locality. Within the same fish, fat/oil content is generally higher towards the head.

Fish & Shellfish ⓒ Ⓕ ⓒᵇ

Edible Weights: (no bones/shell)

	C	F	Cb
Abalone: Raw, 4 oz	120	1	7
Anchovy: Paste, 1 Tbsp, ^{1}/$_4$ oz	15	1	0.5
Cnd. in oil, drnd., 5 only, ^{3}/$_4$ oz	40	2	0
Pickled, 1 oz	50	3	0
Barracuda (Pacific), raw, 4 oz	130	3	0
Bass: Black, raw, 4 oz	105	1	0
Striped, raw, 1 fillet, 5^1/$_2$ oz	150	4	0
Blue Fish, raw, 1 fillet, 5^1/$_4$ oz	185	6	0
Butterfish, raw, 4 oz	165	9	0
Calamari, breaded/fried, 1 serve	360	21	0
Carp, raw, 4 oz	145	6	0
Catfish: Raw, 4 oz	130	5	0
Fried, bread., 1 fillet, 3 oz	200	12	7
Caviar: black/red, 1 Tbsp, 16g	40	3	0.5
Clams: Raw, 3 oz (4 lge/9 sm)	65	1	2
Fried, breaded, 3 oz	170	10	9
Canned, 3 oz	125	2	4
Minced, ^{1}/$_4$ cup, 2 oz	25	0	0.5
Cod, Atl./Pacific, raw, 4 oz	95	1	0
Baked/Broil., 1 fill., 6^1/$_4$ oz	135	2	0
Canned, 3 oz	90	1	0
Minced, ^{1}/$_4$ cup, 2 oz	25	0	0
Crab: Alaska King, raw, 4 oz	95	1	0
1 leg, cooked, 4^3/$_4$ oz	130	2	0
Blue, raw, 1 crab			
(^{1}/$_3$ lb whole crab, ^{3}/$_4$ oz flesh)	18	<1	0
Canned, ^{1}/$_2$ cup, 2^1/$_2$ oz	65	<1	0
Dungeness, 1 crab, 5^3/$_4$ oz edible			
(from 1^1/$_2$ lb whole crab)	140	2	2
Imitation Crab Legs/Stix, 3oz	80	1	8.5
Crayfish, raw, 4 oz (edible)	100	1	0
Croaker, raw, 4 oz	120	3	0
Cuttlefish, raw, 4 oz	90	1	1
Dolphinfish, raw, 4 oz	95	1	0
Eel: Raw, 4 oz	210	13	0
Smoked, 2 oz	190	16	0
Flounder/Sole, raw, 4 oz	120	<1	0
Gefilte Fish: See Kosher Foods ~ Page 157			
Grouper, raw, 4 oz	105	1	0
Haddock: Raw, 4 oz	100	<1	0
Broiled, 1 fillet, 5^1/$_4$ oz	170	1	0
Smoked, 2 oz	22	<1	0
Halibut, raw, 4 oz	125	3	0
Herring: Atlantic, raw, 4 oz	180	10	0
Pickled, 2 pieces, 1 oz	60	4	2

Herring (Cont): Pickled	C	F	Cb
In Sour Cream, 1 oz	50	5	1
Party Snacks, 1/4 cup, dr., 2 oz	120	5	0
Rollmops, 1 1/2 oz	110	8	6
Canned: Plain w. liq., 4 oz	235	15	0
in Tomato Sauce, 4 oz	200	12	1
Smoked, kippered, 4 oz	245	14	0
Jellyfish: Raw, 4 oz	30	<1	0
Salted, 4 oz	40	<1	0
Kingfish, raw, 4 oz	120	3.5	0
Ling, raw, 4 oz	100	<1	0
Lobster, Northern: Raw, 4 oz	105	1	0.5
1 Lobster, 6 1/4 oz (from 1 1/2 lb whole lobster)	135	1.5	0.5
Cooked, 1 cup, 5 oz	140	1	2
Lobster Newberg, 3/4 cup	360	20	9
Lobster Thermidor, 1 serv.	370	22	15
Lobster Salads, 1/2 cup	220	13	5
Lox, Regular/Nova, 2 oz	65	2	0
Mackerel: Atlantic, raw, 4 oz	235	16	0
Jack, can., 1/2 cup, 3 1/3 oz	150	6	0
King, raw, 4 oz	120	2	0
Pacific/Jack, raw, 4 oz	180	9	0
Spanish, raw, 4 oz	160	7	0
Mahi-Mahi, raw, 4 oz	140	5	0
Monkfish, raw, 4 oz	75	1	0
Mullet, striped, raw	135	4	0
Mussels: Raw, 4 oz (edible)	100	2	4
1 cup, 5 1/4 oz (edible)	130	3	5
Cooked, moist heat, 3 oz	150	4	6
Ocean Perch, raw, 4 oz	90	1.5	0
Octopus, common, raw, 4 oz	95	1	0
Orange Roughy, raw, 4 oz	145	9	0

(Cals may be much lower. Over 90% of total fat is waxester which may not be metabolized)

	C	F	Cb
Oysters: Common, raw, 3 oz	70	1	3.5
Eastern raw:			
6 medium, 3 oz	60	2	3
1 cup, 8 3/4 oz	170	6	8.5
Fried/bread., 6 medium, 3 oz	170	11	10
Pacific, raw, 1 med., 1 3/4 oz	40	1	2
Oysters Rockefeller, 3 oysters	220	13	12
Perch, average, raw, 4 oz	105	2	0
Pollock, raw, 4 oz	100	1	0
Pompano, Florida, raw, 4 oz	190	10	0
Porgy/Scup, raw, 4 oz	130	4	0
Rockfish, Pacific, raw, 4 oz	110	2	0
Roe, raw, 1 oz	40	2	0.5

Salmon:	C	F	Cb
Raw: Chinook, 4 oz	205	7	0
Atlantic; Coho/Silver, 4 oz	160	7	0
Chum; Pink, 4 oz	135	4	0
Red/Sockeye, 4 oz	190	10	0
Smoked Salmon: Average, 2 oz	65	1	0
Pacific Supreme, 2 oz	100	4	0
Canned Salmon: Average All Brands			
Pink: 1 oz	40	2	0
1/4 cup, 63g (2.2 oz)	90	5	0
3 3/4 oz can, whole	155	8.5	0
7 1/2 oz can, whole	300	17	0
Skinless/boneless, 1/4 c., 2 oz	70	2	0
Red Sockeye: 1 oz	50	3	0
1/4 cup, 63g (2.2 oz)	110	7	0
3 3/4 oz can, whole	190	12	0
Atlantic, 1/2 cup, 3 1/2 oz	230	14	0
Chinook/King, 1/2 cup	210	14	0
Chum, 1/2 cup, 3 1/2 oz	140	5	0
Coho/Silver, 1/2 cup	155	5	0
Atlantic Steaks: Small, 8 oz	320	14	0
Medium, 12 oz	480	21	0
Large, 16 oz	640	28	0
Salmon Cake, take-out, 3 oz	240	15	6
Sardines: Canned: Average All Brands			
In Oil, undrained, 1 oz	85	7	0
Drained of oil, 1 oz	60	3	0
3 3/4 oz can, drained, (3 1/4 oz)	190	11	0
1 lrg/2 med. 3"/5 small, 0.8 oz	50	3	0
In Tom./ Mustard Sce, 1 oz	45	3	0
3 3/4 oz can (8 sardines)	170	11	0
Scallop: Raw, 6 lg./14 sm., 3 oz	75	<1	2.5
Breaded/fried, 6 lge, 3 oz	200	10	9
Shark: Raw, 4 oz	150	6	0
Batter-dipped, fried, 4 oz	260	16	7
Shrimps: Raw, in shell, 1/2 lb	140	2	1.5
Raw, shelled, 3 oz (12 lge)	90	1.5	0.5
Bread./fried, 3 oz (11 lge)	210	11	10
Canned, 2 oz	60	1	0.5
Smelt, Rainbow, raw, 4 oz	115	3	0
Snapper, raw, 4 oz	115	1	0
Sole, Lemon, raw, 4 oz	90	1	0
Squid, raw, 4 oz	105	1	3.5
Surimi, Imt. Crablegs/Shrimp, 4 oz	110	1	7.5
Swordfish, raw, 4 oz	140	5	0
Trout, Rainbow, raw, 4 oz	135	4	0
Smoked, 2 oz	110	6	0

Fish - Fresh/Canned/Frozen

Fish (Cont)

	C	F	Cs
Tuna:			
Raw, Bluefin, 4 oz	165	6	0
Skipjack, Yellowfin	120	1	0
Canned: *Average All Brands*			
In Water, drained:			
Chunk/Solid, 2 oz can	60	0.5	0
3 oz can	90	1	0
6 oz can	150	1.5	0
In Oil, drained:			
Chunk Light, 2 oz	110	5.5	0
6 oz can, drained	275	14	0
Solid White, 2 oz	90	2.5	0
6 oz can, drained	225	6.5	0
Tuna Salad: Deli Style, 1/2 c., 4oz	300	24	15
Whitefish, raw, 4 oz	155	7	0
Whiting, raw, 4 oz	100	1.5	0

Frozen Fish Products

	C	F	Cs
Fisher Boy			
Quik Stix: 6 sticks, 3 oz	200	11	16
Quik Bake Crunchy Fish Portions:			
2 portions, 3.2 oz	200	10	19
Fish Rings, 7 rings, 3.2 oz	230	12	20
Salmon Fillet, 1 pce, 3.8 oz	100	2.5	1
Gorton's			
Fish Sticks: Breaded, 6, 3 oz	210	12	17
Crunchy Fish Fillets: Breaded *(Per Fillet)*			
Lemon Pepper	135	9	9
Garlic & Herb; Hot & Spicy	125	7	10
Grilled: It. Herb; Lemon Pepper	130	6	2
Cajun Blackened; Lemon Butter	120	6	1
Battered: Parmesan	130	7.5	8
Plain, 1 fillet	120	6.5	10
Garlic & Herb, 1 fillet	125	6.5	11
Lemon Pepper, 1 fillet	135	9	9
Homestyle Baked:			
Au Gratin, 1 fillet, 4.6 oz	230	12	14
Primavera, 1 fillet, 4.6 oz	120	5	4
Fish Portions: 1 portion, 2^1/2 oz	170	11	12
Popcorn Shrimp: 20 shrimp, 2 oz	240	13	22
Tenders: 3^1/2 oz piece	250	14	20
Kroger Fish Portions: *Per 2 Pieces, 4 oz*			
Batter Dipt, 2 pces, 4 oz	260	14	22
Crispy Crunchy, 2 pces, 4 oz	270	18	18
Louis Kemp: Crab Delights,			
Surimi, 1/2 cup, 2.5 oz	80	0	10

Frozen Fish Products (Cont)

	C	F	Cs
Mrs Paul's			
Battered: Fish Sticks, 6	240	11	13
Fish Portions, 2	280	17	22
Batter Dipped: Fish Sticks, 2	330	17	28
Crispy Crunchy: Fish Sticks, 5	200	14	20
Fish Fillets, 2	250	13	11
Breaded Fish Portions, 2	240	12	20
Crunchy Batter: Fish Fillets, 2	280	13	23
Flounder Fillets, 2	260	14	24
Haddock Fillets, 2	250	12	25
Healthy Treasures:			
Fish Sticks, breaded, 4 sticks	140	6	14
Fish Cakes, 2 cakes, 4 oz	190	7	24
Light Seafood Entrees: Fish Dijon	200	5	17
Fish Florentine	220	8	10
Fish Mornay	230	10	12
Sea-Pak			
Crunchy Clam Strips, 1 pkt, 5 oz	410	2.5	41
Oven Crunchy Butterfly Shrimp,			
4 shrimp, 3 oz	200	9	20
Popcorn Fish, 7 pces, 3 oz	240	11	23
Popcorn Shrimp, 15 pces, 3 oz	210	12	18
Van De Kamp's			
Fish Sticks: Breaded, 6 stix, 4 oz	290	17	23
Battered Fillets: 2.6 oz Fillet	180	11	12
Crisp & Healthy: Breaded,			
1 fillet, 1.8 oz	85	1.5	14
Grilled: Italian Herb, 1, 4 oz	130	6	2
Breaded Butterfly Shrimp, 7, 4 oz	300	14	32
Lemon Pepper, 1, 3.6 oz	130	6	0
Salmon, Creamy Dill, 1	90	2.5	1
Tuna, Barbecue, 1, 1.8 oz	100	0.5	5
Tuna, Sesame Teriyaki, 1	110	1.5	4

"You're eating too much fish!"

Frozen Entrees & Meals

Banquet

	C	F	Cb
Meals: Per Meal			
Beef Enchilada	380	12	54
Boneless Pork Rib	400	19	39
Chicken Fingers & BBQ Sce, 9 oz	340	16	36
Chicken Fried Beef Steak	400	20	39
Chicken Nugget	410	21	42
Chicken Parmigiana	290	15	27
Fish Stick Meal, 6.6 oz	300	13	33
Meat Loaf	280	16	23
Mexican Style Enchilada Combo	360	11	55
Our Original Fried Chicken	470	27	35
Pork Cutlet	410	24	39
Roasted Honey Turkey	270	12	29
Salisbury Steak Meal, 9.5 oz	340	19	28
Turkey Mostly White Meat	290	10	34
White Meat Fried Chicken	470	28	40
Yankee Pot Roast, 9.4 oz	230	10	20
The Hearty One: Per Meal			
Beef Enchilada, 15.65 oz	520	16	73
Boneless Pork Rib Dinner, 15.25 oz	720	38	62
Chicken Fried Beef Steak, 16 oz	820	50	63
Fried Chicken Dinner, 14.7 oz	910	55	70
Salisbury Steak Dinner, 16.5 oz	780	54	47
Turkey Dinner, 17 oz	630	10	57
Pot Pies, each: Beef	330	15	38
Chicken	350	18	36
Turkey	370	20	38

Budget Gourmet

	C	F	Cb
Dinner: Per Meal			
Angel Hair Pasta w. Tom. Meat Sce, 8 oz	230	5	38
Beef Cheddar Melt w. Pot. Wedges, 9 oz	350	21	24
Italian Style Meatballs & Vege.	280	12	28
Low Fat Beef Salisbury Steak	240	7	27
Low Fat Fettucine Primavera	260	6	36
Low Fat Pasta in Wine & Mushr.	270	7	39
Mandarin Chicken	240	6	35
Potatoes Mozzarella in Sce	300	16	33
Regular Entrees			
Linguini w. Bay Shrimp & Clam	270	9	42
Pepper Steak w. Rice	290	8	37
Roast Beef Supreme	300	13	35
Swedish Meatballs	550	34	42
Three Cheese Lasagna	390	16	36

Budget Gourmet (Cont)

	C	F	Cb
Light Entrees			
Beef Stroganoff	290	7	30
Chicken Oriental & Vege.	300	5	43
Orange Glazed Chicken	300	2	51
Special Selections			
Escalloped Noodles & Turkey	430	21	32
Fettucini Alfredo w. Four Cheeses	480	22	40
Italian Style Vege. & Chicken	240	6	40
Lasagna Mozzarella	360	11	40
Macaroni & Chse w. Cheddar	310	7	45
Penne Pasta w. Italian Sausage	290	8	46
Rigatoni in Cream Sce & Chicken	230	5	37
Value Classics			
Chinese Style Vege & Chicken	250	6	39
Lasagna Alfredo w. Broccoli, 8 oz	310	11	41
Spaghetti Marinara	290	6	43
Spicy Szechuan Vege & Chicken	290	9	41
Stir Fry Rice & Vegetables	410	18	44
Wild Rice Pilaf w. Vegetables	400	16	50
Ziti Parmesano	350	10	40

Chef Boyardee

	C	F	Cb
Overstuffed Beef Ravioli, 1 cup, 9 oz (260g)	280	5	46

Don Miguel

Same Figures as El Charito

Empire Kosher

	C	F	Cb
Express Meal			
Chicken Fajita, 1	130	2.5	15
Chicken w. Pasta, 1 cup	140	2	17
Chicken Stir-Fry, 1 cup	160	2.5	20
Pierogies: Potato Cheese, 5.3 oz	250	4	44
Potato Onion, 5.3 oz	245	4	47
Pies: Chicken Pie, 8 oz	440	21	41
Turkey Pie, 8 oz	470	23	45
Blintzes: Cheese, 2	200	6	29
Blueberry, 2	190	4	36
Potato Pancakes: mini, 12, 3 oz	150	7	19

Continued Next Page

Frozen Entrees & Meals (Cont)

El Charrito

	C	F	Cb
Regular Dinners: Per 12 oz			
Beef Enchilada Dinner	490	15	65
Cheese Enchilada	470	15	70
Chicken Enchilada	390	7	65
Mexican Style (13.25 oz)	610	30	67
Queso Beef Dinner	460	14	69
Queso Dinner	420	10	72
Saltillo Dinner	450	13	69
Lean Ole Dinners: Beef Enchilada	380	7	60
Cheese Enchilada	360	4.5	66
Combo Enchilada	380	7	66
Grande Dinners: Saltillo, 20.75 oz	750	26	105
Beef Enchilada, 21 oz	830	35	99
Mexican Style Dinner, 20 oz	840	42	89
Entrees: Per 8 oz (227g)			
Beef Enchilada	270	9	38
Cheese Enchilada	250	7	38
Chicken Enchilada	250	9	38

Foster Farms

	C	F	Cb
Chicken Alfredo, 10 oz	390	6	42
Chicken & Homestyle Gravy, 10 oz	410	17	40

Healthy Choice

	C	F	Cb
Entrees: Beef Macaroni	220	4	34
Breaded Chicken Brst Strips, 8 oz	270	5	34
Chicken & Vegetable Marsala	230	1.5	32
Chicken Cantonese	280	6	34
Chicken Enchiladas Suiza	270	4	43
Chicken Glazed & Fettuccine Alfredo	260	1.5	35
Country Glazed Chick./Rst. Turkey	220	3	30
Grilled Chicken Sonoma	230	4	30
Grilled Chicken w. Mashed Pot.	170	3.5	18
Herb Breaded Pork Patty, 8 oz	280	6	38
Homestyle Chicken & Pasta, 9 oz	270	6	32
Honey Mustard Chicken	260	2	38
Macaroni & Cheese	320	7	50
Sesame Chicken	240	3	40
Stuffed Pasta Shells	370	6	60
Tuna Casserole, 9 oz	240	5	38
Hearty Handfuls:			
Ham & Cheese	320	5	50
Garlic Chick.; Italian Steak Meatball	320	5	51
Philly Beef Steak	290	5	47

Healthy Choice (Cont)

	C	F	Cb
Bowl Creations: Per Bowl			
Cheese & Chicken Tortellini	250	5	40
Chili & Cornbread	340	7	49
Colonial Chicken Pie	310	7	40
Country Chicken Bake	230	8	22
Fiesta Chicken	220	2	34
Garlic Lemon Chicken w. Rice	300	4	48
Roasted Potatoes w. Ham	210	4	26
Southern Style Chicken & Pasta	320	4	39
Turkey Divan, 9.5 oz	250	6	31
Meals: Beef Stroganoff	310	6	44
Charbroiled Beef Patty	280	6	41
Chicken Enchilada Supreme	270	4	46
Chicken Parmigiana	300	4	47
Chicken Picante	260	6	30
Chicken Teriyaki	230	3	37
Country Breaded Chicken	360	9	51
Country Herb Chicken	320	6	49
Country Inn Roast Turkey	250	4	28
Grilled Glazed Pork Patty	280	4	48
Herb Baked/Lemon Pepper Fish	340	7	54
Mesquite Beef w. BBQ Sauce	310	8	38
Roasted Chicken	220	5	25
Shrimp & Vegetables in Pasta	270	6	39
Traditional Beef Tips	260	6	32
Traditional Breast of Turkey	290	4.5	40
Traditional Meatloaf	320	5	52
Traditional Salisbury Steak	330	7	48
Yankee Pot Roast	290	7	38

Kid Cuisine

	C	F	Cb
Circus Show Corn Dog, 8.8 oz	490	20	30
Cosmic Chicken Nuggets	440	16	50
Fantastic Fish Sticks, 7 oz	370	14	48
Game Time Taco Roll, 7.35 oz	420	18	55
High Flying Fried Chicken	440	19	48
Magical Macaroni & Cheese	410	13	63
Parachuting Pork Ribettes, 7.55 oz	380	15	43

King Kold

	C	F	Cb
Potato Blintzees, 2.5 oz	110	3	18
Cheese Blintzees, 2.5 oz	110	1.5	14
Crepes, lowfat, w strwb. fill., 2.5 oz	110	1	19

La Choy *See Egg Rolls ~ Page 41*

Lean Cuisine

	C	F	Cb
American Favorites			
Baked Chicken	230	4	31
Beef Pot Roast	210	6	25
Beef Tips Barbecue	290	6	42
Country Veges. & Beef	210	4	33
Honey Roasted Chicken, 8.5 oz	290	6	46
Meatloaf w. Whipped Potatoes	250	6	30
Oven Rst Beef w. Veg. Rice, 9.24 oz	260	8	28
Roasted Turkey Breast	270	3	49
Shrimp & Angel Hair Pasta, 10 oz	290	6	42
Entrees			
Alfredo Pasta Primavera	290	7	46
Angel Hair Pasta	220	3	41
Cheese Cannelloni	230	4	28
Cheese Ravioli	270	7	40
Chicken a l'Orange	250	2	40
Chicken & Vegetables	250	6	31
Chicken Chow Mein w. Rice	220	5	33
Chicken Enchilada Suiza w. Rice	280	5	48
Chicken Fettucini	280	6	36
Chicken Lasagna	270	8	30
Fettucini Alfredo	300	7	47
Fettucini Primavera	270	7	38
Lasagna w. Meat Sauce	290	6	37
Macaroni & Cheese	290	7	43
Oriental Style Dumplings	300	6	51
Penne Pasta w. Tomato Basil Sce	270	6	39
Roast Potato w. Broc./Ched. Sce	260	6	39
Spaghetti w. Meat Sauce	300	4	50
Spaghetti w. Meat Balls	280	6	40
Stuffed Cabbage w. Whipped Pot.	180	5	24
Swedish Meatballs w. Pasta	280	7	33
Teriyaki Stir-Fry	290	4	48
Three Bean Chilli w. Rice	250	6	38
Vegetable Egg Roll, 9 oz	340	6	64
Vegetable Lasagna	260	7	35
Hearty Portions			
Cheese & Spinach Manicotti	340	6	52
Chicken & BBQ Sauce	380	8	54
Grilled Chick. & Penne Pasta	380	6	52
Rigatoni w. Meatballs	440	9	62
Roast Chicken w. Mushroom	290	5	40
Roast Turkey Breast Dinner	380	6	57
Salisbury Steak Dinner	340	7	40

Lean Cuisine (Cont)

	C	F	Cb
Cafe Classics			
Baked Fish	270	6	36
Beef Peppercorn, 8.75 oz	220	7	23
Beef Portabello, 9 oz	220	7	24
Cheese Lasagna w. Chicken	290	8	33
Chicken Breast in Wine Sauce	210	6	23
Chicken Carbonara	280	8	33
Chicken in Peanut Sce	290	6	35
Chicken Parmesan	220	5	27
Chicken Piccata	270	6	41
Chicken w. Basil Cream Sce	270	7	35
Fiesta Chicken	270	5	36
Glazed Chicken w. Veg. Rice	240	6	25
Glazed Turkey	240	5	37
Grill. Chick. w. Pasta, 9 3/8 oz	260	8	28
Herb Roasted Chicken	210	5	27
Honey Mustard Chicken	250	5	39
Honey Roasted Pork, 9.5 oz	250	6	32
Oriental Beef, Vege & Rice	240	3.5	35
Salisbury Steak	280	8	29

Lady Lee (Lucky Stores)

	C	F	Cb
Chicken Tenderloins w. Pasta	380	13	40
Cheddar Pasta w. Beef & Tomato	500	24	44
Pot Pies: Average, 7 oz	400	23	40

Marie Callender's

	C	F	Cb
Café Creations:			
Chicken Teriyaki, 13 oz	510	13	71
Glazed Chicken w. Rice, 13 oz	490	25	40
Complete Skillet Meals			
Per 1/2 Container Unless Indicated			
Beef Pot Roast w. Noodles	290	9	33
Beef Stroganoff	310	11	31
Chicken Alfredo w. Gdn Vegies	490	29	32
Chicken & Rice w. Broccoli	440	14	47
Chicken Teriyaki	340	1	61
Garlic Mashed Potatoes, 2/3 cup	220	12	24
Herb Chicken w. White Wild Rice	290	4	42
Penne Pasta w. Meatballs	600	31	53
Roast Chicken & Vegies	260	6	30
Rst Pot. w. Cheddar & Broc., 3/4 c.	160	7	20
Pot Pies: Chicken; Yankee, 10 oz	680	44	58
Turkey, 10 oz	710	46	56
Chicken & Broccoli, 10 oz	780	48	88
Chicken Au Gratin, 10 oz	720	48	53

Marie Callender's (Cont)

Meals & Dinners	C	F	Cb
Breaded Fish w. Mac. Cheese	550	28	53
Cheese Ravioli in Marinara Sauce w. Spirals & Garlic bread, 1 c. + 1 oz brd	370	14	57
Chicken & Dumplings, 1 cup	260	12	23
Chicken Cordon Bleu, 1 dinner	590	25	58
Chicken Fried Beef Steak & Gravy	650	31	69
Chicken Marsala, 1 dinner	450	17	42
Chicken Parmigiana	620	28	63
Chicken Pasta Fiesta	640	40	44
Chili/Cornbread, 1 c. + 1 1/2 oz br.	350	13	45
Chunky Chicken & Noodle, 1 meal	520	30	42
Country Fried Chick. & Gvy, 1 din.	610	27	63
Country Fried Pork Chop, 1 dinner	550	27	50
Escalloped Noodles/Chicken, 1 c.	270	16	38
Extra Cheese Lasagna, 1 cup	330	16	30
Fettucine Alfredo & Garlic Brd, 1 cup + 1 oz bread	460	27	71
Fettucine Alfredo Supreme	450	27	35
Fettucine Primavera w. Tortellini,1 c.	310	19	35
Fettucine w. Broccoli & Chick.,1 c.	410	24	32
Grilled Chick. Breast w. Rice Pilaf	360	14	38
Grilled Chick. in Mushroom Sce	480	15	54
Ham Steak w. Macar. & Chse, 1 din.	450	9	63
Herb Rst. Chicken w. Mashed Pot.	670	31	32
Homestyle Tuna & Noodles, 1 meal	960	35	143
Lasagna w. Meat Sauce, 1 cup	370	18	34
Linguini & Italian Sausage, 1 meal	710	36	70
Meatloaf & Gvy w. Mashed Pot.	540	30	42
Old Fash. Pot Roast & Gravy, 1 c.	250	6	31
Salisbury Steak & Gravy, 1 dinner	550	25	51
Spagh. & Meat Sce,1 c. + 1 oz brd	260	10	51
Stuffed Pasta Trio	380	18	40
Swedish Meatballs	520	26	44
Sweet & Sour Chicken, 1 dinner	530	9	56
Turkey with Gvy/dress., 1 dinner	530	17	52
Per Packet			
Beef Tips & Mush. Sce, 13.6 oz	430	19	39
Bow Tie Pasta Marinara, 13 oz	430	19	46
Breaded Fish w. Mac. Chse, 12 oz	550	28	53
Cheesy Rice Chick. Broccoli, 12 oz	390	13	44
Chicken Pasta Fiesta, 12.5 oz	640	40	44
Chunky Tuna & Noodles, 12 oz	960	35	143
Fettucini Alfredo Supreme, 13 oz	450	27	35
Grilled Turkey Breast Strips w. Rice Pilaf, 11.75 oz	310	10	34
Macaroni Chse w. Brocc., 13.5 oz	510	18	65

Michelina's

Per Serving	C	F	Cb
Black Bean Chili w. Rice, 8 oz	300	4	58
Chili-Mac, 8 oz	280	9	36
Fettucine Alfredo w. Broc., 8.5 oz	310	10	37
Four Cheese Lasagna, 8 oz	290	7	42
Lasagna w. Meat Sce, 9 oz	290	7	40
Linguini w. Clams & Sauce	310	4.5	55
Macaroni Cheese	360	14	40
Meatloaf, Gravy, Mash. Potato	290	16	22
Noodles Stroganoff w. Beef, 8 oz	350	15	39
Noodles w. Chicken, 8 oz	300	10	40
Pepper Steak & Rice	260	4.5	46
Salisbury Steak Mashed Potato	300	13	33
Spaghetti Marinara, 8 oz	250	2.5	47
Wheels & Cheese	290	8	40
Signature Entrees:			
Beef Burgundy, 9 oz	320	16	23
Beef Pot Roast, 10.5 oz	300	6	40
Breaded Chick. Parmigiana,10 oz	420	14	46
Cheddar Broccoli Pot., 10.5 oz	420	20	41
Chicken Marsala, 9 oz	310	17	23
Chicken Piccata, 9 oz	380	17	41
Jumbo Chse Ravioli w. Sce, 11 oz	410	13	54
Lasagna w. Meat Sce, 10 oz	400	16	40
Shrimp Alfredo, 9 oz	370	15	36
Sirloin Beef Peppercorn, 9 oz	280	12	33

Nancy's

	C	F	Cb
Mushroom Turnovers, 5 oz	450	30	39
Quiche: Florentine, 6 oz	440	26	35
Lorraine; Monterey, 6 oz	490	29	34
Petite Quiche, 4.5 oz	390	23	31
Seafood Crab Cakes, 6 oz	350	20	28

Poppers

	C	F	Cb
Mozzarella Cheese Sticks, 30g ea.	100	6	7
Stuffed Jalapenos Crm Chse, 25g	70	3.5	6

President's Choice

	C	F	Cb
3 Bean Beef Chili, 1 cup, 225g	240	8	22
5 Cheese Cannelloni, 1 pce, 189g	220	7	26
Beef Shepherd's Pie, 1 cup, 225g	460	32	25
Macaroni & Cheese, 1 cup, 230g	390	20	35
Pizza Lasagne, 1 cup, 227g	380	17	33
Seafood Lasagne, 1 cup, 216g	360	23	20
Vegetable Lasagne, 1 cup, 230g	350	18	27

Frozen Entrees & Meals (Cont)

Stouffer's	C	F	Cb
Entrees: Beef Pie	450	26	36
Beef Stroganoff	390	20	30
Cheddar Pasta w. Beef & Tom.	450	19	45
Cheese Ravioli	380	13	51
Chicken a la King	350	13	41
Chicken Pie, 10 oz	540	33	38
Chili w. Beans	270	10	30
Creamed Chicken	260	19	8
Creamed Chipped Beef	160	11	6
Escalloped Chick. & Noodles, 10 oz	430	27	30
Fettucini Alfredo	520	28	50
Five Cheese Lasagna	360	13	40
Fish Fillets w. Mac. Cheese, 9 oz	430	21	37
Green Pepper Steak	330	9	43
Lasagna Bake	370	12	47
Lasagna w. Meat Sauce, 10$^{1}/_2$ oz	370	14	40
Macaroni & Beef	420	20	40
Macaroni Cheese, 1 cup	380	17	40
Macaroni & Chse, w. Broccoli	350	16	36
Meat Lasagna, 1 cup	270	10	28
Noodles Romanoff	490	25	48
Pasta Shells & American Cheese	260	10	36
Salisbury Steak & Macaroni Chse	410	19	34
Spaghetti w. Meatballs	440	15	56
Spaghetti w. Meat Sauce	350	12	46
Stuffed Pepper, 10 oz	200	5	27
Swedish Meatballs	480	24	43
Tuna Noodle Casserole	320	10	37
Turkey Pie	530	33	36
Turkey Tetrazzini	360	17	33
Side Dishes: Corn Souffle	170	7	21
Creamed Spinach	160	12	8
Escalloped Apples	180	3	38
Potatoes au Gratin	130	6	15
Scalloped Potatoes	140	5	18
Spinach Souffle	150	10	10
Welsh Rarebit	120	9	5
Hearty Portions			
Beef Pot Roast, 16 oz	370	11	44
Chicken Fettuccini, 16$^{3}/_4$ oz	640	24	67
Country Fried Beef Steak, 16 oz	560	25	61
Fried Chicken Breast, 15$^{1}/_8$ oz	520	16	66
Meatloaf w. Potatoes, 17 oz	480	23	46
Pork w. Roast Potatoes, 15$^{3}/_8$ oz	570	15	75
Roast Turkey Breast	490	20	52
Salisbury Steak, 16 oz	570	24	47
Veal Parmagiana	630	26	68

Stouffer's (Cont)	C	F	Cb
Skillet Sensations: Per $^{1}/_2$ pkg			
Cheddar Beef	600	29	58
Chicken Alfredo	490	16	63
Homestyle Beef	360	11	34
Homestyle Chicken	390	13	47
Teriyaki Chicken	340	3	59
Homestyle: Beef Pot Roast	250	8	30
Baked Chicken in Gravy/Potato	260	11	18
Breaded Pork Cutlet	420	23	27
Chick. Breast w. Mushr. Gravy	360	15	32
Fried Chicken & Mashed Potato	400	17	38
Meatloaf & Whip. Potato	360	21	28
Salisbury Steak in Gravy/Onions	350	16	27

Swanson	C	F	Cb
Microwave Pies: Beef, 7 oz	415	23	41
Chicken; Turkey, 7 oz	400	21	43
Pot Pies: Beef, 14 oz	415	23	41
Chicken, 14 oz	650	35	22
Turkey, 14 oz	650	34	65
Hungry Man Dinners:			
Boneless Pork Rib	770	38	78
Boneless White Meat Fried Chick.	430	16	49
Classic Fried Chicken, 16$^{1}/_2$ oz	790	45	75
Country Fried Beef Steak	660	33	66
Fisherman's Platter, 13 oz	640	25	80
Fried Chicken Dinner, 11 oz	430	16	50
Fried Chicken Dinner, 13.75 oz	460	26	73
Fried Chicken, mostly white meat	800	39	79
Mexican Style	690	27	87
Salisbury Steak	610	33	46
Sirloin Beef Tips	440	15	53
Traditional Pot Roast	360	6	48
Turkey, mostly white meat	510	15	64
4 Compartment Meals			
Boneless Pork Rib, 10.5 oz	470	19	58
Classic Fried Chicken, 11$^{1}/_2$ oz	600	31	58
Country Fried Beef Steak w. Gravy	460	22	47
Chicken Nuggets	590	25	71
Fish 'N Chips	490	20	59
Herb Roasted Chicken	310	7	44
Mexican Style Comb., 13.25 oz	470	18	59
Salisbury Steak	340	15	35
Turkey Most. White Meat, 11.34 oz	320	8	42
Veal Parmigiana, 11$^{1}/_4$ oz	390	18	40
Yankee Pot Roast	250	4.5	39

Frozen Entrees & Meals (Cont)

Thai Chef
C F Cb

Per Meal

	C	F	Cb
Peanut Satay Chicken, 12 oz	400	14	50
Lemon Basil Chicken, 12 oz	390	10	55
Thai Sweet & Sour Veges, 12 oz	340	5	70
Vegetarian Mussaman, 12 oz	390	9	71

Taj

Per Meal

	C	F	Cb
Asparagus Subzi/Dal Baahar	385	13	58
Bean Masala/Chunna Bahji	330	6	60
Chicken Masala/Korma	330	9	35
Eggplant Bhartha	300	7	55
Mushroom/Green Pea Masala	390	13	61
Palak Paneer	320	7	25
Raj Mah	340	5	62
Shahi Paneer	410	24	42
Vegetable Korma	340	12	54

Topps

	C	F	Cb
Chicken Nuggets, 4, 2.5 oz	200	12	12
Hamburger: 100% Pure Ground Beef			
Grilled or Panfried, 2.7 oz	230	17	1
Kabobs:			
Beef, 1 kabob, 1.5 oz	170	7	2
Chicken, 1 kabob	120	1.5	0

Tyson

See Page 51

Wolfgang Puck's

Per Meal

	C	F	Cb
Breaded Chick. Parmagiana, 12 oz	540	21	58
Chick. & Spinach Pasta Wrap	460	11	68
Chicken Bolognese & Spaghetti	480	22	48
Chicken Pappardelle	460	18	47
Eggplant Parmesan	370	28	14
4 Cheese Lasagna; Meat Lasagna	490	22	51
4 Cheese Macaroni	610	33	51
Italian Sausage Pasta Wrap	700	29	67
Meatloaf in Wine Sauce	560	32	36
Mushroom & Spinach Ravioli	260	18	54
Mushroom Lasagna/Tortellini	440	17	53
Penne Pasta w. Beef & Vege	410	18	38
Radiatore Pasta Primavera	310	10	41
Spicy Chicken Tortellini	490	24	51

Weight Watchers
C F Cb

Smart Ones: Per Meal

	C	F	Cb
Angel Hair Pasta	180	2	32
Broccoli & Chse Baked Pot., 10 oz	250	6	39
Chick. Chow Mein; Fiesta Chicken	205	2	34
Chicken Enchiladas Suiza, 9 oz	270	9	33
Fettucini Alfredo w. Broc., 9.25 oz	270	6	39
Fiesta Chicken, 8.5 oz	210	2	35
Grilled Salisbury Steak	260	10	24
Honey Mustard Chicken, 8.5 oz	210	3.5	33
Lasagna Florentine, 10.5 oz	290	8	36
Lasagna w. Meat Sauce, 9 oz	240	2	43
Lemon Herb Chicken Piccata	210	2	31
Mac. & Chse; Ravioli Florentine	220	2	43
Pasta & Spinach Romano	240	8	35
Penne Pasta w. Sundr. Tom., 10 oz	300	8	43
Ravioli Florentine, 8.5 oz	220	2	43
Roast Turkey Medallions, 9 oz	200	2	33
Santa Fe Style Rice & Beans, 10 oz	300	8	49
Spaghetti & Meat Sce, 11.5 oz	280	5	43
Spaghetti Marinara, 9 oz	280	7	46
Spicy Penne & Ricotta; Rigatoni	280	6	45
Spicy Szechuan Veg. & Chicken	220	2	39
Swedish Meatballs, 9 oz	290	9	34
Tuna Noodle Casserole	280	7	38
Ziti Mozzarella, 9 oz	290	7	47

Main Street Bistro Selections: Per Meal

	C	F	Cb
Basil Chicken, 9 oz	280	7	35
Chicken Carbonara, 9.5 oz	300	6	36
Fajita Chicken Supreme, 9.25 oz	280	7	33
Fire-Grilled Chick. & Vegies, 10 oz	280	5	40
Golden Baked Garlic Chick., 10 oz	280	6	40
Oven Roast Veg. Primavera, 10 oz	300	8	46
Slow Roast Turkey Breast, 10 oz	220	2	20
Pizza: 5.5 oz each	390	12	50

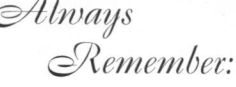

Always Remember:

In the end, we are not measured in inches or pounds, but rather by the size of our heart and soul.

Pockets

	C	**F**	**Cb**
Per Serving			
Big Stuffs: Ham & Cheese	420	16	50
Cheese & Steak; Pepperoni	440	20	48
Croissant Pockets			
Supreme Pizza	390	20	40
Pepperoni Pizza	360	16	41
Philly Steak & Cheese	350	16	37
Ham & Cheddar	320	12	40
Egg, Sausage & Cheese	340	15	40
Chick. Broccoli & Chse; Turk./Ham	290	4	37
Delistuffs			
Ham & Cheese	340	13	41
Cheese Steak; Pepperoni Pizza	350	14	40
Hot Pockets			
Beef & Cheddar	350	16	36
Pepperoni Pizza	350	15	41
Sausage Pizza; Beef Fajita	340	6.5	38
Ham & Cheese	320	12	40
Meatballs w. Mozzarella	320	11	39
Other flavors	300	6	38
Pizza Minis: Pepperoni	250	11	31
Sausage & Pepperoni	230	8	31
Double Cheese	240	10	32
Toaster Breaks: *Per Piece, 2.1 oz*			
Pizza: Pepperoni; Dble Cheese	190	9	22
Sausage & Pepperoni	180	8	22
Melts: Grilled Cheese	210	10	24
Ham & Cheese	180	8	22
Philly Steak & Cheese	190	10	20
Lean Pockets			
Chicken Parmesan	280	7	41
Philly Steak & Chse; Turkey/Broc.	260	7	35
Other flavors	270	7	40
Taj Samosa Pockets: *Per 9 oz*			
Aloo (potato)	170	8	26
Gobi (mixed vegetable)	150	5	22
Subzi (cabbage/potato)	150	5	22

Pizza & Egg Rolls

	C	**F**	**Cb**
Totino's: Pizza Rolls, 6 rolls, 3 oz			
Sausage	210	10	20
Pepperoni	230	12	20
Chun King: Munchers (Mini Egg Roll), 6 rolls, 3 oz	210	9	15

Burritos & Waffles

	C	**F**	**Cb**
Per Serving			
Belgar Chef			
Waffles	180	2	34
El Monterey: King Size, 8 oz			
Beef & Bean/Green Chili	580	27	30
Old El Paso			
Burrito: Bean & Cheese	300	9	44
Beef & Bean	320	10	47
Pizza, all types	250	9	30
Chimichanga, all types	350	18	38
Tina's Burrito			
Bean & Cheese, 8.5 oz	420	15	5
Microwaveable Pouch, 5 oz			
Chicken Burrito	240	4	15
Red Hot Beef	370	15	10
Beef & Bean	380	15	15
w. Green Chili	370	15	10

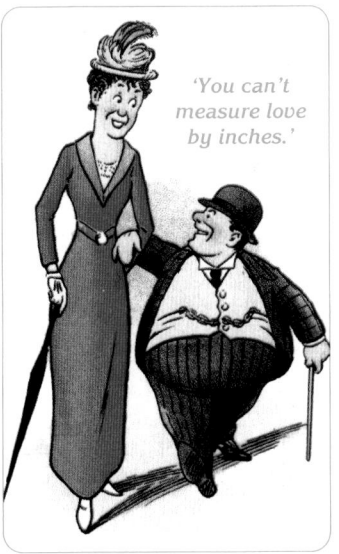

'You can't measure love by inches.'

Frozen Pizza

	C	F	Cb
Amy's			
Cheese; Spinach, 13 oz	320	11	40
Roasted Vegetable, 12 oz	270	8	43
Pizza Pockets: Regular, 4$\frac{1}{2}$ oz	290	9	38
Veggie Pepperoni, 4$\frac{1}{2}$ oz	220	7	28
Celeste			
Large Pizza: Per $\frac{1}{4}$ Pizza			
Cheese	320	16	32
Deluxe; Pepperoni	350	20	34
Suprema, $\frac{1}{5}$ pizza	290	16	27
Large Premium Pizza: Per $\frac{1}{4}$ Pizza			
Cheese	350	18	33
Deluxe; Pepperoni	390	22	34
Sausage/Pepperoni	380	22	33
Pizza For One: Per Pizza			
Cheese; Vegetable	420	21	45
4-Cheese Orig.; Pepperoni	475	27	41
Deluxe; 4-Cheese Zesty	470	25	45
Sausage	530	27	52
Suprema	500	27	49
Rising Crust: Per $\frac{1}{6}$ Pizza			
4-Cheese	320	11	39
Pepperoni	380	16	43
Suprema; Three Meat	385	17	40
Connie's Pizza (Chicago Deep Dish)			
Cheese, $\frac{1}{4}$ pizza, 4.5 oz	300	12	34
Sausage, $\frac{1}{4}$ pizza, 4.6 oz	300	11	39
Spinach Mushroom, $\frac{1}{4}$ pizza, 5 oz	310	12	30
Di Giorno			
Rising Crust Pizza			
Large: Per $\frac{1}{6}$ Pizza			
Four Cheese	320	11	39
Pepperoni; Three Meat	390	17	41
Supreme	400	17	41
Small (Individual) Size:			
Pepperoni, 12.75 oz	300	13	34
Supreme, 14.3 oz	300	14	34
Vegetable, 13.8 oz	900	39	90
Dominick's			
Per $\frac{1}{6}$ Pizza			
Four-Cheese, 5 oz	290	9	38
Italian Sausage/Supreme, 5 oz	320	13	38
Empire Kosher			
Bagel Cheese Pizza, 1	140	1.5	24
Cheese Pizza (11oz), $\frac{1}{4}$, 2.8 oz	170	3.5	27
English Muffin Cheese, 1	120	2.5	18

	C	F	Cb
Healthy Choice			
French Bread Pizza			
Cheese; Pepperoni, 6 oz	340	5	50
Supreme, 6.35 oz	330	5	51
Vegetable, 6 oz	280	4	44
Home Run Inn: *Per $\frac{1}{4}$ Pizza*			
Cheese, 4.5 oz	390	30	34
Sausage, 5 oz	400	22	32
Sausage & Mushroom, 5.5 oz	390	23	29
Jack's Pizza			
Original 12": Per $\frac{1}{4}$ Pizza			
Canadian Style Bacon	280	10	31
Cheese, $\frac{1}{3}$ pizza	360	13	41
Hamburger; Saus.; Spicy Italian, $\frac{1}{4}$	300	14	28
Pepperoni	330	15	31
Original 9": Per $\frac{1}{2}$ Pizza			
Pepperoni; Sausage, average	380	18	37
Great Combinations (12"): Per $\frac{1}{4}$ Pizza			
Bacon Cheeseburger; Dble Cheese	380	19	32
Pepperoni; Sausage, average	400	19	41
Sausage & Mushroom	310	15	29
Other types, average	350	18	30
Great Combinations (9"): Per $\frac{1}{2}$ Pizza			
Double Cheese	430	21	38
Pepperoni & Sausage	380	18	36
Naturally Rising (12"): Per $\frac{1}{6}$ Pizza			
Canadian Style Bacon; Cheese	290	10	35
Other types, average	340	16	34
Naturally Rising (9")			
Cheese, $\frac{1}{3}$ pizza	300	10	38
Comb. w/Saus. & Pepperoni, $\frac{1}{4}$	300	14	29
Pepperoni; Sausage, $\frac{1}{3}$ pizza	360	16	38
The Works, $\frac{1}{4}$ pizza	280	12	29
Pizza Bursts: All types, 6 pieces	250	13	26
Jeno's			
Crisp 'n Tasty: Per Pizza			
Canadian Style Bacon	440	19	17
Cheese	460	19	17
Combination; Sausage; Supreme	520	28	17
Hamburger; Three Meat	500	25	16
Pepperoni	510	27	17
Lean Cuisine			
French Bread Pizza:			
Deluxe, 6$\frac{1}{8}$ oz	300	6	46
Pepperoni, 5$\frac{1}{4}$ oz	310	7	46
Sundried Tomato, 6 oz	340	8	48

62

Frozen Pizza (Cont)

	C	F	Cb
Pepperidge Farm			
Croissant & Pastry Pizza:			
Cheese	390	20	39
Deluxe	450	27	40
Pepperoni	420	23	39
Pillsbury			
Microwave: Cheese, 1/2 pizza	240	10	28
Pepperoni, Combination, 1/2 pizza	310	15	29
Sausage, 1/2 pizza	280	13	29
French Bread Pizza: Cheese (1)	370	13	41
Pepperoni, 1 pizza	430	19	46
Sausage, 1 pizza	410	16	48
Sausage & Pepperoni	450	21	47
Porretta Pizza			
Four Cheese, 1/6 pizza, 4.6 oz	310	9	48
Supreme, 1/8 pizza, 4.4 oz	220	9	29
Power Dogz Pizza For Kids			
Gonzo's Cheeseburger Max, each	460	20	44
KT's Poppin' Pepperoni, each	500	24	46
Shaggy's Cheezy Cheese, each	420	14	46
Red Baron			
Large: 4 Cheese, 1/4 pizza	430	21	45
Pepperoni, 1/4 pizza, 154g	450	23	41
Special Deluxe, 1/5 pizza	340	17	34
Supreme, 1/5 pizza	350	18	38
Deep Dish Singles: Pepperoni	540	31	47
Supreme, 1/5 pizza	490	27	46
Reggio's: Cheese, 1/4, 4.5 oz	330	12	41
Deluxe/Sausage, 1/4, 5 oz	380	16	41
Stouffer's: *French Bread Pizzas,* 1/2 Pkg			
Bacon Cheddar/Deluxe Pizza	430	21	45
Cheese; Vegetable Deluxe	370	16	47
Cheeseburger; Pepperoni	430	21	45
Extra Cheese	400	16	50
Pepperoni & Mushr./Sausage	440	21	50
Sausage & Pepperoni/White Pizza	460	23	45
Three Meat	460	21	48
Tombstone			
Original 12" Pizza: Per Serving			
Canadian; Extra Cheese, 1/4	350	14	36
Pepperoni, 1/4 pizza	400	21	35
Other varieties, average, 1/5	320	15	29
12" Special Order: Per 1/5 Pizza			
Four Cheese	400	19	37
Other varieties, average	360	18	32

	C	F	Cb
Tombstone (Cont)			
Original 9" Pizza (Cont):			
Deluxe; Hamburger; Saus., 1/3	280	13	27
Extra Cheese, 1/2 pizza	380	16	40
Pepperoni & Sausage, 1/3 pizza	300	15	27
Pepperoni Supreme, 1/3 pizza	310	16	27
Double Top:			
Two Cheese, 1/5 pizza	380	19	29
Other varieties, average, 1/6	330	18	25
Oven Rising: Per 1/6 Pizza			
All types, average	330	15	34
Thin Crust: 3 Cheese; Italian, 1/4	370	22	26
4 Meat Combo, 1/4 pizza	380	23	26
Pepperoni, 1/4	400	25	25
Supreme; Supreme Taco, 1/4	370	23	27
For One: Pepperoni; Supreme	550	32	42
Extra Cheese	520	28	41
For One (1/2 Less Fat): Cheese	360	10	43
Vegetable, 1 pizza	360	9	48
Tony's Pizza			
Italian Style: Pepperoni, 1/3, 146g	450	26	37
Pastry Crust, Cheese, 1/3, 140g	400	21	37
Super Rise: Supreme, 1/5, 129g	300	12	35
Four Cheese, 1/4, 138g	330	12	42
Pepperoni, 1/4, 147g	370	16	42
Totino's			
Party Pizza: Per 1/2 Pizza			
Cheese; Can Bacon; Vegetable	320	14	34
Combination; Zesty Italiano	390	21	35
Hamburger	380	20	34
Sausage & Mushr.; Three Meat	380	19	34
Sausage; Bacon; Pepperoni	380	21	34
Supreme	380	20	35
Pizza Family Size			
Cheese, 1/3 pizza	360	16	39
Combination, 1/4 pizza	310	17	29
Pepperoni, 1/3 pizza	410	22	38
Sausage, 1/4 pizza	300	16	29
Pizza Rolls: Per 6 Rolls			
Combination	230	12	23
Pepperoni	240	12	24
Sausage	230	11	24
Supreme; Cheese	210	10	25
Three Meat	220	10	24
M'wave Pizza For One: Cheese	240	11	26
Pepperoni; Sausage	290	16	26
Supreme	300	17	26

Canned & Packaged Meals

	C	F	Cb
Austex			
15 oz Can: Beef Stew, 1 cup	340	26	14
B & M			
Baked Beans: *Per 1/2 Cup (4 1/2 oz)*			
Bacon & Onion w. Brown Sugar	190	2	36
Baked Beans w. Pork	180	2	33
Barbeque; Vegetarian	170	1	33
w. Natural Honey; Red Kidney	170	2	30
Yellow Eye Baked Beans	180	3	30
Betty Crocker			
Chicken Helper: *Per 1 Cup Made Up*			
Chicken & Herb Rice	260	7	26
Average other flavors	300	9	28
Potato Buds: Plain, *1/3 cup mix*	80	0	18
As prepared, *1/2 cup*	160	8	19
Campbell's: *Per 1/2 Cup, 4 1/2 oz*			
Barbecue; Old Fashioned Beans	170	2.5	29
Brown Sugar & Bacon Beans	170	3	29
Chili Beans	130	3	21
New England Beans	180	3	32
Pork & Beans in Tomato Sauce	130	2	24
Chef Boyardee			
Microwave Cup Meals: *Per Bowl*			
Beef Ravioli	190	3.5	28
Lasagna	220	6	30
Pasta w. Meatballs	230	8	30
Pasta w. Chicken & Veges.	220	6	34
Rice w. Beef & Veges.	250	7	38
Spaghetti & Meatballs	210	7	28
Pull Ring 7 oz Can: Beef Ravioli	170	4	27
Spaghetti w. Meatballs	210	8	27
Homestyle 15 oz Can: *Per Cup, 9 oz*			
Cannelloni; Rigatoni	250	10	31
Ravioli Primavera	240	5	38
Pull Ring 16 oz Can: *Per Cup*			
Beef/Cheese Ravioli	220	5	38
99% Fat Free Beef Ravioli	210	1	41
Spaghetti w. Meatballs	270	10	32
Lasagna Dinner Kit: *Per Serving*			
(add your own cheeses)	290	7	44
Cheese Pizza Kit: *Per Serving*	300	5	51
Chef Jr: Micro Ravioli, 8 3/4 oz	210	5	33
Flying Saucers & Aliens, 9 oz	240	1.5	47
Other varieties, 1 cup, 9 oz	200	0.5	43
Cup A Ramen: Average, 1 ctn	310	17	36

	C	F	Cb
Dennison's Chili			
15 oz Can: Per 1 CupServing			
Chili Con Carne With Beans:			
Original; Hot, 1 cup	350	15	36
Chunky; Hot & Chunky	320	12	32
Beef Chili w. Beans (99% Fat Free)	220	2	27
Mild Green w. Beans	370	17	32
Vegetarian w. Beans (99% FF)	180	1	35
No Bean Chili Con Carne	330	18	21
Dinty Moore (*Hormel Foods*)			
1 1/2 lb Can: Beef Stew, 1 cup	230	14	16
7 1/2 oz Can: Beef Stew	190	10	15
Noodles & Chicken	200	9	21
American Classics: *Per 10 oz Microwave Bowl*			
Beef Pot Roast	200	3	19
Chicken & Noodles	270	8	28
Chicken Breast & Gravy w. Pot.	240	4	25
Hearty Lasagna	340	16	28
Roast Beef & Gravy w. Potato	240	5	24
Salisbury Steak w. Potato	300	13	24
Turkey & Dressing w. Gravy	290	8	32
Dr. McDougall's: *Per Cup*			
Pasta w. Beans, Mediterranean	180	1	29
Pinto Beans & Rice, Sthwestern	190	2	38
Ramen Noodles; Chicken; Beef	140	1	39
Rice & Pasta Pilaf	210	1	36
Eden: *Per 1/2 Cup, 4 1/2 oz*			
Baked Beans w. Sorghum, Mustard	150	0	27
Black Soy Beans	90	1.5	9
Chili Beans w. Jalapeno & Peppers	130	0	21
Ginger Blacks w. Ginger, Lemon	120	0	21
Lentils w. Onion, Bay Leaf	90	0	13
Fantastic			
Cup Meals: *Per Packet*			
Bombay Curry Rice & Beans	250	1.5	53
Cajun Rice & Beans	230	3	46
Cha-cha Chili	220	1	37
Chili Ole, average	260	2.5	48
Ready, Set, Pasta!, average	230	3.5	41
Spanish Rice & Beans	210	1.5	49
Tex Mex Rice & Pinto Beans	240	2.5	48
Vegetarian Chili	160	1	27
Noodles: Average	140	1	27
Couscous: Black Bean Salsa	240	1.5	46
Creole Vegetable	220	1.5	41
Nacho Cheddar	120	2	21
Sweet Corn	180	1	36

Franco-American
Per 1 Cup Serving

	C	F	Cb
Life w. Louise Pasta	190	2	36
Spaghetti in. Tom Sce w. Cheese	210	2	41
Spaghettios: in Tomato & Cheese	190	2	36
w. Sliced Franks/Meatballs	260	11	32
Beef Ravioli	230	3.5	42

Hamburger Helper
Prepared as Directed: Per Cup

Beef Pasta	270	10	26
Beef Stew	250	10	24
Cheeseburger Macaroni	360	15	33
Cheesy Hashbrowns; Chili; Pizza	290	10	31
Cheddar Cheese Melt	310	12	31
4-Cheese Lasagna; Stroganoff	330	14	31
Lasagna; Ravioli	280	10	32
Southwestern Beef	300	10	32
3-Cheese	340	15	38

Hormel: *Per Cup*

Kid's Kitchen: Beans 'N Wieners	310	13	37
Beefy Macaroni	190	6	23
Cheesy Macaroni 'N Beef	260	7	33
Cheezy Mac 'N Cheese	260	11	30
Mini Beef Ravioli	240	7	34
Noodle Rings & Chicken	150	5	16
Spaghetti Rings w. Meatballs	230	7	35
Microwave Cup: Beef Stew	190	10	15
Chicken & Noodles	200	9	16
Low Calorie	110	2.5	16
Chili w. Beans	220	6	27
Chili no Beans	190	8	15
Lasagna w. Meat Sauce	210	6	29
Scalloped Potatoes & Ham	240	14	20
Spaghetti w. Meat Sce	220	7	31
Chili, 15 oz Can: Per Cup			
With Beans: Reg./Hot/Chunky	270	7	34
Homestyle Chili	330	19	24
Turkey (99% Fat Free)	200	3	26
Vegetarian (99% Fat Free)	200	1	38
No Beans, 1 cup	210	9	17

Hungry Jack Potatoes

Casseroles: Per 1/2 cup, average	150	5	24
Idaho Mashed: Per 1/2 cup, aver.	155	5	21
Inst. Potato Flakes: Per 1/3 cup	80	0	18
1/2 cup, prepared	160	8	19
Mashed: Aver. all types, 1/3 cup	150	7	19
Pot. Pancake Mix, 2 T., Made Up	90	1.5	16

Hy Top: *Per Serving*

	C	F	Cb
Deluxe Shells & Ched. Chse Dinner	410	16	51
Refried Beans, 1/2 Cup	150	2.5	24
Cans: Per 1 Cup			
Spagh. Rings & Tom. Meatballs	410	16	51
Spagh. Rings in Tomato Sce	190	0.5	40
Spaghetti w. Tom. Sce & Chse	180	0	39
11/2lb Can: Beef Stew, 247g	190	7	18
15oz Can: Corned Beef Hash	430	28	28
Chili w. Beans, 270g	510	32	34

Kraft Pasta Dinners
Prepared as Directed: Per Cup

Deluxe: Four Cheese	320	10	44
Sharp Cheddar	270	4	38
Macaroni & Cheese:	320	10	44
Light	290	4.5	48
Child's/Cartoon Pack	410	19	47
Light (Only 1 T. fat + skim milk)	290	6	47
Velveeta: Creamy Herb & Garlic	360	13	46
Shells/Radiatore & Cheese	360	13	46

Lipton Packet Meals
Prepared as Directed: Per 1 Cup Serving

Rice & Sauce: Spanish	270	7.5	47
Cheddar Broccoli; Chicken	280	9	46
If no fat used in prep'n, deduct 55 Cals and 6g Fat			
Noodles & Sauce: Butter/& Herb	310	14	42
Chicken Flavor; Chick. Broccoli	300	11	42
If no fat used in prep'n, deduct 55 Cals and 6g Fat			
Pasta & Sauce: Creamy Garlic	350	13	47
Crmy Mushr./Tom.; Zesty Ched.	310	11	43
Mild Ched. Chse; Rst Garlic Chick.	290	10	40
Roasted Garlic Olive Oil w. Tom.	270	8.5	42
Other varieties, average	290	9	40
If no fat used in prep'n, deduct 55 Cals and 6g Fat			
Recipe Secrets: Golden Onion	50	1	9
Onion	20	0	4
Onion & Mushroom; Savory Herb	30	0.5	6
Vegetable	30	0	9

Lunch Basket: *Per Serving*

Microwave: Dumplings 'n Chicken	140	5	21
Hearty Beef Stew	170	9	17
Lasagna w. Meat Sauce	160	3	29
Pasta 'n Chick. w. Veg	150	5	22

Manischewitz: Taco Dinner

Taco Dinner	290	12	38
Vegetarian Chili, 3/4 cup	145	1.5	31

Maruchan: *Per Pkt*

	C	F	Cb
Instant Noodles: all flavors, aver.	280	13	35
Instant Wonton, all flavors	200	12	19
Oriental Noodle, all flavors	290	12	38
Ramen flavors, 1/2 pkt, 1 1/2 oz	180	7	26
Wonton flavors, 1/3 pkt	90	5	9

Near East: *Prepared as Directed, Per Cup*

	C	F	Cb
Couscous: Original Plain	230	2	46
Chicken & Herbs	270	6	51
Toasted Pine Nut	230	6	40
Creamy Parmesan	280	7	48
Roasted Garlic	220	5	41
Roasted Pecan & Garlic	240	9	37
Broccoli	210	3	42
Rice Pilaf	190	0.5	42

Nile Spice: *Per Cup*

	C	F	Cb
Couscous: Lentil Curry	200	1.5	36
Minestrone	180	1.5	34
Parmesan	200	3	34

Old El Paso: *Per Serving*

	C	F	Cb
Refried Beans, 1/2 cup: Reg, Black	110	2	18
Vegetable; w. Green Chilies	100	1	17
w. Cheese	130	3.5	18
w. Sausage	200	13	14
Fat Free varieties	100	0	18
Mexe/Pinto Beans, 1/2 cup	110	0.5	19
Black/Garbanzo Beans, 1/2 cup	110	1.5	17
One Skillet Mexican (Prepared):			
Nacho Cheese, (2)	490	19	56
Salsa; Taco, average, (2)	450	16	56
Dinner Kits (Prep'd): Soft Taco	400	20	57
Burrito; Fajita	300	13	34
Taco Dinner	330	20	40
Side Dishes: Per Serving			
Canned: Chili with Beans, 1 cup	240	11	19
Spanish Rice, 1 cup	130	1	28
Tamales in Chili Gravy (3)	320	19	31
Boxed: Cheesy Mexican Rice (1/3)	290	6	55
Spanish Rice, 1/3 pkt	280	5	55

Pasta-Roni
Prepared as Directed: Per Cup

	C	F	Cb
Broccoli	340	15	41
Broccoli Au Gratin	280	10	41
Chicken; Shells & White Cheddar	310	13	41
Chicken & Broccoli	370	16	49
Chicken & Garlic (Lowfat)	210	3	39
Creamy Garlic	420	25	41

Pasta-Roni (Cont): *Per Cup*

	C	F	Cb
Fettucini Alfredo: Reduced Fat	310	8	50
Garlic & Olive Oil w. Vermicelli	360	16	48
Homestyle Chicken	230	6	39
Parmesano	390	17	49
White Cheddar & Broccoli	400	19	48

Pritikin

	C	F	Cb
Vegetarian Chili, 1 cup	160	1	27

Progresso: Beef Rav., 1 c., 9 oz

	C	F	Cb
Progresso: Beef Rav., 1 c., 9 oz	260	5	45
Cheese Ravioli, 1 cup, 9 oz	220	2	43
Italian Style Zucchini, 1/2 c., 4.2 oz	50	2	7

Ramen Noodles: *Per Serving*

	C	F	Cb
Beef/Chicken Flavor, 3 oz	190	8	27
Baked Noodle: 1/2 Block, 1 1/2 oz	140	1	30
Noodles: Fat Fried Shrimp, 1 1/2 oz	170	6	26
Other Flavors, 1 1/2 oz	160	6	26
Fried Cup: Beef, 1 packet, 2.2 oz	290	11	41
Lowfat: Average, 2 oz	215	1.5	45

Rice-A-Roni
Prepared as Directed: Per Cup

	C	F	Cb
Beef; Herb & Butter	310	9	52
Broccoli Au Gratin	370	17	47
1/3 Less Salt	320	11	50
Chicken	310	9	52
1/3 Less Salt	280	5	53
Lowfat	210	3	41
Chicken & Broccoli	230	6	41
Chicken & Garlic	260	9	41
Chicken & Mushroom	360	14	52
Fried Rice	320	11	51
Long Grain & Wild Rice	240	6	43
Red Beans & Rice	290	7	51
Rice Pilaf; Risotto	310	9	51
Savory Chicken Vegetable	210	3	41
Spanish Rice	270	8	46
White Cheddar & Herbs	340	13	48

(Reduced Fat Recipe: If only 1 Tbsp fat is used instead of 2 Tbsp, deduct 35 calories and 4g fat.)

Stagg Chili
15 oz Can: Per 1 Cup

	C	F	Cb
Chili w. Beans: Classic/Dynamite	330	17	28
Country Brand/Laredo	320	16	29
Rancho House Chicken	290	9	32
No Beans: Steakhouse/Double	330	21	16
99% Fat Free: 4-Bean Chili	200	1	37
Turkey Ranchers/Silverado Beef	240	3	31

Sweet Sue	C	F	Cb
Chicken & Dumplings, 1 cup	240	7	31
Canned Whole Chicken:			
w/out giblets, 2 oz	80	5	0

Trader Joe's			
Quiche: Broccoli & Cheddar, 6 oz	490	33	33
Mexicaine, 6 oz	510	36	29
Spinach & Mushroom, 6 oz	470	30	32

Tuna Helper (Betty Crocker)			
Prepared as Directed: Per Cup			
Cheesy Pasta	310	14	32
Creamy Pasta	300	13	31
Tuna Melt; Creamy Broccoli	310	12	34

Uncle Ben's			
Rice Bowls: Per Bowl, 12 oz (340g)			
Barbeque Beef	430	4.5	85
Chicken & Vegetable	340	5	56
Teriyaki Chicken	430	5	78
Teriyaki Stir Fry Vegetable	340	3	70

Wolf			
Chili w. Beans: 227g Can	300	16	27
15 oz Can, 1 cup, 254g	330	18	30
Chili No Beans: 227g Can	390	27	18
15 oz Can, 1 cup, 248g	420	30	20
Chunky Beef w. Beans:			
15 oz Can, 1 cup, 254g	300	15	28
No Beans, 1 cup, 246g	330	22	18

"Take two of these and call me in the morning."

Soybean Products

	C	F	Cb
Cheeses (Soy): See Page 38			
Miso, 1/2 cup, 5 oz	280	8	39
Cold Mountain: Red, 1 T., 0.5 oz	25	1	3
Mellow White, 1 Tbsp, 0.5 oz	35	0.5	6
Natto, 1/2 cup, 3 oz	190	10	13
Tempeh, 1 piece, 3 oz	170	6	14
Fried, 3 oz	250	14	14
SoyBoy, White Wave ~ See Page 70			
Soybean Protein (TVP), 1 oz	90	0	7
Soy Drinks ~ See Page 24			

Tofu

	C	F	Cb
Azumaya Tofu:			
Soft (Silken), 3 oz	45	2	4
Firm, 3 oz	60	2.5	3
Extra Firm, 3 oz	75	3.5	10
Age (Tofu Puff),1/2 oz	40	1.5	2
Nama-Age (Fried Tofu), 3 oz	130	5	8
Calco: Tasty Tofu, 3 oz	50	3	2
Hinoichu Tofu:			
Soft, 3 oz, 1" slice	45	2.5	5
Reg. (Japanese), 3 oz, 1" slice	60	3	6
Firm (Chinese), 3 oz, 1" slice	60	3	6
Extra Firm, 3 oz	90	5	10
Mori-Nu Tofu (Silken):			
Soft, 4 oz	60	3	3
Firm, 4 oz	70	3	3
Extra Firm, 4 oz	70	2	3
Nasoya Tofu:			
Soft, 3 oz	60	3	2
Silken, 3 oz	50	2	2
Firm, 3 oz	80	4	2
Extra Firm, 3 oz	90	5	1
Chinese 5 Spice Tofu, 3 oz	80	4	2
Pulmuone Tofu:			
Soft, 3 oz	45	2	5.5
Silken, 3 oz	45	2	5.5
Firm, 3 oz	55	2.5	6
SoyBoy:			
Firm Organic, 3 oz	100	5	2
X-Firm Organic, 3 oz	120	6	2
X-Firm LowFu, 3 oz	90	2	5
TofuLin, 2 oz	100	5	4
Baked, Seasoned, Smoked, 2 oz	100	5	3
Carribean Tofu, 2 oz	100	5	3
Tofu Stir Fried, 4 oz	120	8	3

Vegetarian Meals & Products

	C	F	Cb
Amy's (Frozen): Per Serving			
Pot Pies: Country Vege, 7 1/2 oz	370	16	47
Broccoli, 7 1/2 oz	430	22	46
Mexican Tamale, 8oz	220	3	41
Non-Dairy Vegetable, 7 1/2 oz	320	9	50
Shepherd's Pie, 8 oz	160	4	27
Vegetable, 7 1/2 oz	360	18	44
Entrees: Chse Enchilada, 4.75 oz	210	12	13
Blk Bean Vege. Enchilada, 4.75 oz	130	4	20
Cheese Lasagna, 10.25 oz	310	11	37
Macaroni & Cheese, 9 oz	390	14	50
Macaroni & Soy Cheeze, 9 oz	360	14	42
Pasta Primavera, 9 1/2 oz	320	12	39
Ravioli w. Sauce, 8 oz	340	12	44
Vege./Tofu Lasagne w. Chse, 9 1/2 oz	300	10	39
Burritos: Bean & Rice, 6 oz	250	5	44
Bean & Cheese, 6 oz	280	8	43
Black Bean Vegetable, 6 oz	320	8	54
Breakfast, 6 oz	230	5	38
Asian Meals: Asian Noodle Stir Fry	240	4.5	41
Whole Meals: Cannelloni, 9 oz	330	12	34
Black Bean Enchilada, 10 oz	250	8	41
Country Dinner, 11 oz	380	12	60
Cheese. Enchilada, 9 oz	330	14	38
Chili & Cornbread, 10.5 oz	320	6	59
Veggie Loaf, 10 oz	260	5	47
Pocket Sandwich: Broccoli & Chse	270	10	37
Cheese Pizza, 4 1/2 oz	290	9	38
Mediterranean Vegetable, 4 1/2 oz	220	7	33
Roasted Vegetable, 4 1/2 oz	220	8	35
Spinach Feta, 4 1/2 oz	200	7	27
Tamale, 4 1/2 oz	250	7	39
Vegetable Pie, 5 oz	230	6	37
Veggie Pizza, 4 1/2 oz	240	6	35
Pizza: Cheese; Spinach	320	11	40
Peasto w. Tomato & Broccoli	300	11	39
Roasted Vegetable, 4 oz	270	8	43
Soy Cheese, 4.3 oz	280	11	37
Boca Burger: Breakfast Patties, 1	70	3	4
Chef Max's Favorite, 2.5 oz patty	110	2	10
Hint of Garlic, 2.5 oz patty	100	1	9
Vegan Original, 1 patty	80	0	8
Celentano (Frozen)			
Eggplant: Rollettes, 10 oz Tray	220	12	19
Parmagiana, 1/2 Tray, 7oz	320	21	22
Lasagna Primavera, 10 oz Tray	230	4	37
Spinach & Broccoli: Manicotti	230	4	36
Stuffed Shells, 10 oz Tray	210	4	31

	C	F	Cb
Dr McDougall's/Eden			
See Page 64			
Gardenburger: (Wholesome & Healthy Foods Inc.)			
Gardenburger: Per 2 1/2 oz Patty			
Classic Greek	120	3	17
Fat Free	100	0	7
Five Roasted Vegetable	110	2.5	16
Original	130	3	18
Santa Fe	130	2.5	20
Savory Mushroom	120	3	18
Sautéed Onion	100	0	8
Tayburn Smoked Cheddar	140	3	23
Veggie Medley, 2 1/2 oz	100	0	17
Zesty Bean, 2 1/2 oz	120	2.5	19
GardenDog: 2 oz	120	2.5	4
GardenSausage: 2 1/2 oz patty	130	3	18
Lifeburger: 3 oz patty	100	1	9
Harvest Burger (Green Giant)			
Original, each	140	4	8
Southwestern, each	140	4	9
Health Valley			
Fat-Free Beans & Chili:			
Honey Baked Beans, 1/2 cup	110	0	25
Chili in a Cup, all types, 3/4 cup	120	1	21
Mild/Spicy Vegetarian Chili:			
all flavors, 1/2 cup	80	1	15
Chili Burrito/Enchilada, 1/2 cup	80	1	15
Chili, Fajito flavored, 1/2 cup	80	1	15
Ken & Robert's			
Veggie Burger, 2.5 oz	130	1	26
Veggie Pockets, average, 4.5 oz	250	8	39
Litelife (Frozen)			
Smart Deli Slices, 3 slices, 1 1/2 oz	50	0	2
Smart Dogs, 1 link, 1 1/2 oz	45	0	1
Tofu Pups, 1 link, 1 1/2 oz	60	2.5	2
Wonderdogs, 1 1/2 oz	55	1	1
Loma Linda			
Frozen: Corn Dogs, 1 corn dog	150	4	22
Chik Nuggets, 5 pieces, 3 oz	240	16	13
Canned & Dry Products			
Big Franks, 1 link	110	7	2
Lowfat, 1 link	80	3	3
Chicken Supreme Mix, 1/3 cup mix	90	1	6
Dinner Cuts, 2 slices, 3 1/4 oz	90	1.5	3
Fried Chik'n/Gravy, 2 pcs, 3 oz	160	10	3

Vegetarian Meals & Products

Loma Linda (Cont)	C	F	Cb
Canned & Dry Products Cont:			
Gravy Quik: Aver.,1 Tbsp mix	20	0	4
Linketts, 1 link	70	4.5	1
Little Links, 2 links	90	6	2
Nuteena, 3/8" slice, 2 oz	160	13	6
Ocean Platter, 1/3 cup dry mix	90	1	8
Patty Mix, 1/3 cup dry mix, 1 oz	90	1	7
RediBurger, 5/8" slice, 3 oz	120	2.5	7
Sandwich Spread, 1/4 cup, 2 oz	80	4.5	7
Savory Dinner Loaf, 1/3 cup, drain.	90	1.5	7
Soyagen, all varieties. 1/4 c. drain.	130	6	12
Swiss Stake, 1 piece, 3 1/4 oz	120	6	8
Tender Bits, 6 pieces, 3 oz	110	4.5	7
Tender Rounds, 6 pieces, 2 3/4 oz	120	5	5
Vege Burger, 1/4 cup, 2 oz	70	1.5	2
Vita Burger Chunks, 1/4 cup	70	1	7
Vita Burger Granules, 3 Tbsp	70	1	6
Morningstar Farms			
American Orig. Veggie Dog, each	80	0.5	6
Better'n Burger, 1 pattie	70	0	7
Better'n Eggs, 1/4 cup, 2 oz	20	0	0
Breakfast Links, 2 links	60	2.5	2
Breakfast Patties, 1 pattie	70	3	2
Breakfast Strips, 2 strips	60	4.5	2
Chik Nuggets, 4 pieces	160	4	17
Chik Patties, 1 pattie	150	6	15
Corn Dog, 1 link	150	4	22
Garden Grille, 1 pattie, 3 oz	120	2.5	18
Garden Vege patties, 1 pattie	100	2.5	9
Grillers, 1 pattie, 2 1/4 oz	140	6	5
Ground Meatless, 1/2 cup, 2 oz	60	0	4
Homestyle Noodles, 1/2 cup, 2 oz	160	4	33
Prime Patties, 1 pattie, 2 3/4 oz	140	2	5
Recipe Crumbles, 2/3 cup, 2 oz	90	3	5
Roasted SoyButter, 2 Tbsp, 1 oz	170	11	10
Scramblers, 1/4 cup, 2 oz	35	0	1
Spicy Bl. Bean Burger, 1 pattie	110	1	16
Breakfast Scramblers: Per Sandwich			
Bagel/Scramblers/Pattie/Cheese	320	4.5	40
Engl.Muf./Scramblers/Pattie/Chse	280	3	35
English Muffin/Scramblers/Pattie	240	2.5	32
Dry Products			
Garden Vegie Burger Kit, 1/4 pkg	80	0	6
Sth.West.Veggie Burger, 1/4 pkg	90	0	9

Midland Harvest	C	F	Cb
Fat Free & Lowfat Dry Mix:			
Taco Filling & Dip, 2.7 oz	50	0	7
Chili Fixin's, 8 oz	70	1	10
Sloppy Joe Fixin's, 3.6 oz	60	0	11
Burger Loaf Dry Mix: Per 3.2 oz	120	4	8
Frozen Patties: Sausage, 2 oz	80	4	5
Other varieties, 3.2 oz	120	4	8
Natural Touch			
Frozen Products			
Dinner Entree, 1 pattie, 3 oz	220	15	2
Garden Vege pattie, 1 pattie	110	2.5	8
Lentil Rice Loaf, 1" slice, 3 oz	170	9	14
Nine Bean Loaf, 1" slice, 3 oz	160	8	13
Okara Pattie, 1 pattie, 2 1/4 oz	110	5	4
Spicy Bl.Bean Burger, 1 pattie	100	1	15
Vegan Burger, 1 pattie, 2 3/4 oz	70	0	6
Vegan Burger Crumbles, 1/2 cup	60	0	4
Vegan Saus.Crumbles, 1/2 cup	60	0	4
Vege Frank, 1 link	100	6	2
Canned & Dry Products			
Kaffree Roma, 1 rounded tsp, 2g	10	0	2
Roma Cappuccino, 3 Tbsp, 10g	50	3	5
Loaf Mix, 4 Tbsp dry mix, 1 oz	100	0.5	10
Original Veggie Burger, 1/4 pkg	80	0	6
Sthwestern Veggie Burger, 1/4 pkg	90	0	9
Roasted Soy Butter, 2 Tbsp	170	11	10
Stroganoff Mix, 4 Tbsp dry mix	90	3.5	10
Taco Mix, 3 Tbsp dry mix, 0.6 oz	60	1	7
Vegetarian Chili, 1 cup, 8 oz	170	1	21
New Menu (Vitasoy)			
VegiBurgers, 3 oz	110	1	12
VegiDogs, 1 link, 1.5 oz	45	0	1
Tofumate (Seasoning Mixes):			
Average all varieties, 1/4 cup	25	0	4
SoyBoy			
Breakfast Links, 1 link, 1 oz	65	2.5	6
5-Grain Tempeh	135	6	9
Leaner Weiners, 1 weiner, 1.5 oz	55	0	2
Not Dogs, 1 link, 1.5 oz	95	3	10
Ravioli Rosa/Verde, 1 cup, 3.5 oz	180	3	29
Soysage, 2 oz	120	5	12
Soy Tempeh, 3 oz	150	6	9
Tofu Ravioli, 1 cup, 3.5 oz	180	3	31

Tofu & Tempeh Products
~ See Page 67 ~

Vegetarian Meals & Products (Cont)

White Wave	C	F	Cb
Stir Fry: Chick'n & Herbs, 3 oz	110	4	7
Italian Style, 4 1/2 oz	150	6	14
Mexican Fajita, 3 oz	180	3.5	6
Thai Peanut, 4 oz	230	6	12
Seitan: Chicken w. Broth, 5 oz	130	0	12
Traditional, 4 oz	140	0	4
Tempeh: Five Grain, 1/3 pkg	140	4	15
Original, 1/3 pkg	150	6	10
Sea Veggie, 1/3 pkg	120	3	11
Wild/Soy Rice, 1/3 pkg	140	5	13
Tofu: Baked: All variet., 2 oz pce	120	6	3
Organic: Soft/Firm, 1/5 pkg, 3.2 oz	90	6	1
Fat-Reduced, 1/5 pkg, 3.2 oz	90	4	4
Extra Firm, 1/4 pkg, 3 oz	80	5	1

Worthington	C	F	Cb
Frozen Products			
Beef Style Meatless, 3/8" slice	110	7	4
Bolono, 3 slices, 2 oz	80	3.5	2
Chic-Ketts, 2 slices (3/8"), 2 oz	120	7	2
Chick., Sliced or Roll, 2 sl., 2 oz	80	4.5	1
ChikStiks, 1 piece, 1 1/2 oz	110	7	3
Corned Beef Meatless, 4 sl., 2 oz	140	9	5
Crispy Chic Patties, 1 pattie	170	9	15
Dinner Roast, 3/4" slice, 3 oz	180	12	5
Fillets, 2 pieces, 3 oz	180	10	8
FriPats, 1 pattie	130	6	4
Golden Croquettes, 4 pieces	210	10	14
Leanies, 1 link	100	7	2
Prosage Links, 2 links	60	2.5	2
Prosage Patties, 1 pattie	100	3	4
Prosage Roll, 5/8" slice, 2 oz	140	10	2
Salami, Meatless, 3 slices, 2 oz	130	8	2
Smkd Beef, Meatless, 6 sl., 2 oz	120	6	6
Smkd Turkey., Meatless, 3 sl, 2 oz	140	10	3
Stakelets, 1 piece, 2 1/2 oz	140	8	6
Stripples, 2 strips, 1/2 oz	60	4.5	2
Tuno, 1/2 cup (drained), 2 oz	80	6	2
Veelets, 1 pattie, 2 1/2 oz	180	9	10
Veggie Dog, 1 link	80	0.5	6
Vegetarian Egg Rolls, 1 roll	180	8	20
Wham, 2 slices, 1 1/2 oz	80	5	2
Canned & Dry Products			
Chili, 1 cup, 8 oz	290	15	21
Low Fat Chili, 1 cup, 8 oz	170	1	21
Choplets, 2 slices, 3 1/4 oz	90	2	3
Country Stew, 1 cup, 8 1/2 oz	210	9	20
Cutlets, 1 slice, 2 1/4 oz	70	1	2

Worthington (Cont)	C	F	Cb
Canned & Dry Products (Cont)			
Diced Chik, 1/4 cup, 2oz	40	0	1
FriChik, 2 pieces, 3 oz	120	8	1
Low Fat FriChik, 2 pcs, 3 oz	80	3	2
GranBurger, 3 Tbsp, 0.6 oz	60	0.5	3
Multigrain Cutlets, 2 sl., 3 1/4 oz	100	2	5
Numete, 3/8" slices, 2 oz	130	10	5
Prime Stakes, 1 piece, 3 1/4 oz	120	7	4
Protose, 3/8" Slice, 2 oz	130	7	5
Saucettes, 1 link	90	6	1
Savorex, 1 tsp	10	0	1
Savory Slices, 3 slices, 3 oz	150	9	6
Sliced Chik, 3 slices, 3 oz	70	0.5	2
Super Links, 1 link	110	8	2
Turkee Slices, 3 slices, 3 1/4 oz	190	14	3
Vegetable Skallops, 1/2 c., 3 oz	90	1.5	3
Vegetable Steaks, 2 pieces	80	1.5	3
Vegetarian Burger, 1/4 c., 2 oz	60	2	2
Veja Links, 1 link, 1 oz	50	3	1
Low Fat Veja Links, 1 link	40	1.5	1

Yves	C	F	Cb
Jumbo Veggie Dogs, 2.6 oz each	90	0	5
Veggie Weiners/Chili Dogs, 1.6 oz	55	0	3
Tofu Weiners, 1.3 oz each	45	0.5	2
Veggie Ground Round:			
Original & Italian, 1/3 cup	60	0	3
Deli Slices, 3.5 slices, 1.8 oz	60	0	2
Burger Burgers, 1 patty, 3 oz	70	0	7
Pepperoni, 3.5 slices, 1.8 oz	70	0	4
Garden Vegetable Patties, 1, 3 oz	70	0	12
Canadian Veggie Bacon, 3 sl., 2 oz	80	0	2
Veggie Breakfast Links, 2, 1.8 oz	65	0	4
Veggie Pizza Pep'roni, 16 sl., 1.7 oz	70	0	5

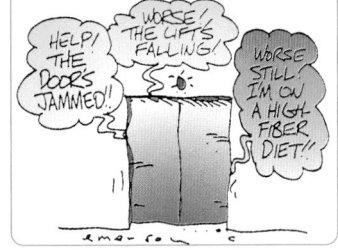

Homemade & Restaurant

	C	F	Cb
Restaurant & Take-Out			
Per 8 fl.oz			
Bean Medley	200	3	34
Beef Consomme	30	0	2
Borscht (w. Cream)	130	8	14
Bouillabaisse	400	15	10
Chicken & Corn	290	14	20
Chicken & Wild Rice	80	4	9
Chicken Consomme	50	0	2
Chicken Curry	180	8	18
Chicken Jambalaya	160	7	8
Chicken Noodle	80	2	12
w. Chicken	160	4	12
Chicken Soup	80	2	6
Chili with Beans	250	12	25
Clam Chowder	240	15	17
Corn & Crab	120	3	18
Corn Chowder	150	8	16
Cream of Broccoli	200	12	20
Cream of Potato	220	12	25
Cream of Mushroom	290	21	20
Creamy Pumpkin	210	10	26
Fish Chowder	220	15	6
French Onion	420	15	25
Gazpacho	60	0	13
Lentil Soup	250	9	28
Lobster Bisque	320	15	14
Matzo Ball (w.1 large ball)	180	7	24
Minestrone	140	2	14
Mulligatawny	300	15	8
Pea & Ham	240	10	25
Potato & Bacon	170	7	19
Shark Fin Soup	220	6	4
Split Pea Soup	150	6	18
Vegetable (Fat Free)	75	0	18
Vegetable Beef	80	2	10
Vichyssoise	200	9	15
Watercress	90	4	13

● Ethnic & Restaurant Section: Pages 155-159
● Fast Foods/Restaurant Section: Pages 161-247
(*Arby's, Au Bon Pain, Boston Market, Dunkin' Donuts, Denny's, Schlotzsky's, Sizzler, Souplantation, Sweet Tomatoes*)

Homemade Soups:
Calculate calories, fat and carbohydrates from ingredients.

Bouillon Cubes & Powders

	C	F	Cb
Bouillon Cubes: Aver. all types			
Regular, 1 cube	8	0	1
Low Sodium (LiteLine)	12	0	1
Powders: Average, 1 tsp	8	0	1
Herb-Ox:			
Instant Broth & Seasoning			
Beef, 1 envelope	10	0	2
Chicken, vegetarian	10	0	2
Herbs, Spices: 1 tsp	5	0	1
Soup Oyster Crackers			
40 small/20 large, 1/2 oz	60	2	8

Arrowhead Mills

Soup Mixes: Per 1/4 Cup	170	0	35
Cans: Per 1 Cup Serving			
Chicken Broth	60	1	12
Chicken Vegetable	100	3	10
Creamy Onion	100	1.5	21
4-Bean	130	2	23
Minestrone	110	2	19
Mushroom Barley	70	1	13
Mushroom Broth	10	0	1
Red Lentil	100	1.5	17
Smoky Bean	140	1	25
Tomato Vegetable	90	2	17
Vegetable Broth	15	0	3

Barnum & Bagel

Frozen Soup: Per 1 Cup Serving			
Chicken Noodle	100	1.5	17
Chicken Matzo Ball	100	5	11
Minestrone	140	2	24
Mushroom Barley; Vegetable	130	1	26
Sweet & Sour Cabbage	160	1	36

Bean Cuisine

Made as Directed: Per 1 Cup Serving			
Florentine/Country Bean; Barcelona	210	1.5	29
Basque Beans; Italian Market Bean	195	1.5	30
13 Bean Bouillabaisse	240	0	18

Campbell's

Red & White Label
Per 1 Cup Prepared (from ¹/₂ Cup Condensed)

	C	F	Cb
Bean & Bacon	180	5	25
Beef Broth	15	0	1
Beef w. Vegetable & Barley	80	2	11
Broccoli Cheese	110	7	9
Californian Veg.; Chicken Gumbo	60	1	10
Cheddar Cheese	130	8	11
Chicken Broth	30	2	1
Chicken Noodle/w. Stars	70	2	9
Chicken Vegetable	80	2	12
Clam Chowder Manhattan	60	0.5	12
Clam Chowder New England	100	2.5	15
Cream of Asparagus; Celery	110	7	9
Cream of Broccoli; Shrimp	100	6	9
Cream of Chicken & Broccoli	120	8	11
Cream of Mushroom	110	7	9
Double Noodle in Chicken Broth	100	2.5	14
French Onion	70	2.5	10
Golden Mushroom	80	3	10
Minestrone	100	2	16
Split Pea w. Ham; Green Pea	180	3.5	28
Tomato	80	0	18
Tomato Bisque	130	3	24
Tomato Rice (Old Fashioned)	120	2	23
Vegetable	90	1	16
Vegetable & Beef; Turkey Noodle	80	2	10
Won Ton	45	1	5

Healthy Request (Blue Label), 10³/₄ oz Can:
	C	F	Cb
Average all varieties	80	2	10

16 oz Can: *Per ¹/₂ Can Serving*
	C	F	Cb
Hearty Chicken & Rice	110	2.5	16
Hearty Chicken Noodle	100	3	14
New England Clam Chowder	120	3	17
Split Pea & Ham	170	1.5	29

98% Fat Free (Green Label): *Per 10³/₄ oz Can*
	C	F	Cb
Cream of Broccoli/Cheese	80	3	12
Cream of Celery/Mushroom	70	3	9
Cream of Chicken	80	3	10

Home Cookin' (White 19 oz Can): *Per ¹/₂ Can*
	C	F	Cb
Chicken Rice	110	1.5	17
Chicken Vegetable	130	3.5	20
Chicken w. Egg Noodle	90	2	13
Country Mushroom & Rice	80	0.5	16
Creamy Potato	180	9	21
Fiesta; Tomato Garden	130	2.5	24
New England Clam Chowder	200	13	16

Campbell's (Cont)

Chunky (Red Can):
19 oz Can: *Per ¹/₂ Can Serving*

	C	F	Cb
Cheese Tortellini	110	2	18
Chicken Broccoli Cheese	200	12	14
Chicken Chowder Mushroom	210	12	18
Chicken Corn Chowder	250	15	18
Classic Chicken Noodle	130	3	16
Hearty Chicken & Vegetable	90	2	12
New England Clam Chowder	300	18	26
Potato Ham Chowder	220	14	16
Savory Chicken & Rice	140	3	18
Sirloin Burger	180	7	20
Vegetable	160	4	15
Vegetable Beef	150	5	17

Microwave Soups:
Per Container

	C	F	Cb
Bean with Bacon 'n Ham	280	6	40
Chicken Noodle	130	4	18
Chicken Rice, 10¹/₂ oz	120	2.5	20
Vegetable Beef	140	0.5	26

Soup & Recipe Mixes (Dry):
Per 1 Tbsp

	C	F	Cb
Chicken Noodle/w. Broth	30	0.5	5
Onion	20	0	5

Soup Jar (24 oz Jar):
Per 1 Cup Serving

	C	F	Cb
Chicken & Pasta	90	10	14
Garden Vegetable & Pasta	110	0.5	21
Hearty Chick. Noodle w. Wh. Meat	80	1	12
Minestrone	110	1.5	21
Vegetable Beef w. Pasta	110	1.5	17

Campbell's Restaurant Soup (Frozen):
Per 1 Cup Serving (Prepared)

	C	F	Cb
Baked Potato w. Cheddar	160	8	18
Chicken Noodle	100	2.5	11
New England Clam Chowder	140	4.5	19

College Inn

Per 1 Cup Serving

	C	F	Cb
Beef/No Fat Broth	20	0	0
Chicken Broth/Lower Sodium	25	1.5	1

Cup-A-Ramen

Per 1 Cup Serving

	C	F	Cb
Beef; Cajun Chicken	310	16	36
Chicken ; Shrimp	320	17	36

Dominick's   **C** **F** **Cb**

Canned:

	C	F	Cb
Tomato, condensed, 1/2 cup	80	0.5	18
Chicken Broth: Regular, 1 cup	15	0.5	0
Reduced Salt, 1 cup	15	0	0

Dr McDougall's

Cup Mix:

	C	F	Cb
Minestrone & Pasta, 1 cup	180	1	31
Ramen Noodles, 1 container, 43g	150	0.5	29
Split Pea w. Barley, 1 cup	200	2	36
Tamale Pie w. Baked Chips, 1 cup	200	1.5	39
Tortilla Soup w. Baked Chips, 1 c.	190	1.5	37

Fantastic Cup Soups

Per 1 Cup

	C	F	Cb
Country Lentil	230	1	41
Creamy Soups: Average	150	2.5	27
5 Bean	230	1	43
Jumpin' Black Bean	210	1	39
Minestrone	150	1	29
Split Pea	190	1	35
Vegetable Barley	150	0.5	29

Goodman's

Soup Mixes (Prep.): Per 1 Cup

	C	F	Cb
Alphabet Vegetable	45	0	9
Noodle Soup: Regular	45	0.5	9
Salt Free	50	0.5	9
w. Vegetables	45	0	9
Onion Soup	30	1	5

Hain

Canned: Per 1 Cup

	C	F	Cb
Homestyle Naturals:			
Chicken Broth	25	2	3
Chicken Noodle	150	3	24
Chunky Tomato	80	0.5	18
Minestrone	110	2	20
Healthy Naturals:			
Black Bean	90	0	18
Mushroom Barley	130	1.5	26
Vegetable Broth	30	0	8
Vegetarian Lentil	120	1	20
Vegetarian Split Pea	170	1	30
Wild Rice	80	1.5	15

Healthy Choice   **C** **F** **Cb**

	C	F	Cb
Baked Potato, 1 cup	140	2	25
Bean and Ham, 1 cup	160	1.5	29
Chicken Corn Chowder, 1 cup	160	2.5	26
Chicken with Rice, 1 cup	100	2	13
Chili Beef, 1 cup	170	1.5	29
Country Vegetable, 1 cup	100	0.5	22
Garden Vegetable, 1 cup	120	1	24
Lentil, 1 cup	150	1	29
New England Clam Chowder, 1 c.	120	1	22
Old Fashioned Chick. Noodle, 1 c.	150	2.5	23
Split Pea & Ham, 1 cup	160	0.5	29
Turkey w. White & Wild Rice, 1 c.	90	2	14
Zesty Gumbo, 1 cup	90	1.5	15

Health Valley

	C	F	Cb
Bean Vegetable, 1 cup	140	0	32
Beef Broth, 1 cup	20	0	0
Chicken Broth, 1 cup	45	1.5	0
Garden/Tomato Vegetable, 1 cup	80	0	17
Real Minestrone; Italian Plus, 1 c.	80	0	20
Split Pea & Carrots, 1 cup	110	0	17
Country Corn & Vegetable, 1 cup	70	0	17
Carotene varieties, average, 1 cup	70	0	17
Lentil & Carrots, 1 cup	90	0	25
Pasta Soups: Pasta Fagioli, 1 cup	120	0	25
Other varieties, 1 cup	110	0	23
Organic: Black Bean; Split Pea	110	0	25
Mushroom Barley; Potato Leek	60	0	15
Lentil; Tomato; Minestrone, 1 c.	90	0	20
Vegetable, 1 cup	80	0	18
Dry Soups: Per 1/3 cup, average	120	0	24

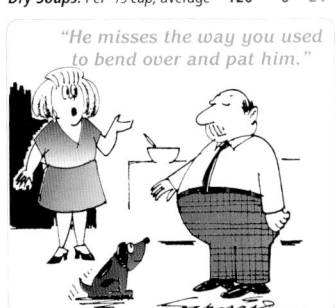

"He misses the way you used to bend over and pat him."

Hormel **C** **F** **Cb**

Microwave Cup Hearty Soup: *1 cup, 7 1/2 oz*

Chicken w. Vegetable & Rice	110	2	17
Beef Vegetable	90	1	15
Beef & Ham	190	4	29
Chicken Noodle	110	2.5	13
Chicken w. Vegetable & Rice	110	2	17
Beef Vegetable	90	1	15
Beef & Ham	190	4	29
Chicken Noodle	110	2.5	13

Hy-Top Soups

Condensed *(10 1/2 oz Can): Per 1/2 Cup*

Chicken w. Rice	70	1.5	11
Chicken Noodle	60	2	8
Cream of Chicken	100	5	10
Cream of Mushroom	110	7	10
Tomato	70	0	16
Vegetable	80	2	12

Knorr's Soup

Soup & Recipe Mixes: *Per Serving (1/3 Pkg)*

Chicken Flavor Noodle	90	1.5	16
Cream of Broccoli/Spinach	70	2.5	10
Creamy Chicken w. Rice	100	3.5	13
Fine Herb	100	5	13
French Onion	45	1	8
Hot & Sour	50	1.5	8
Leek	70	2.5	9
Oxtail	60	2	9
Roasted Garlic & Herb	80	1.5	13
Spring Vegetable	25	0	5
Tomato Basil	80	2.5	13
Vegetable, 1/4 Pkg	30	0.5	6

Lipton

Cup-a-Soup: *Per Envelope*

Broccoli & Cheese	70	3	9
Cream of Chicken	70	2	12
Creamy Chicken Vegetable	80	4.5	10
Chicken Noodle	50	1	8

Recipe Secrets Mixes: *Per Serving*

Golden Onion	50	1	9
Onion Mushroom	30	0.5	5
Savory Herb w. Garlic; Vegetable	30	0	7
Noodle	60	2	9

Manischewitz **C** **F** **Cb**

Condensed:
Per 1/3 Cup (Unprepared)

Chicken	15	0.5	2
w. 3 Matzo Balls	80	4	9
Four Bean	70	1	13
Lentil	140	2	24
Minestrone	90	1.5	16

Per 8 fl.oz Serving (Prepared)

Borscht w. Beets	90	0	21
Borscht Low Calorie	25	0	6

Instant Cup (Mrs Manischewitz): *Per Cup*

Black Bean	200	1	37
Chicken Noodle	140	2	26
Chicken Rice	130	1	28
Hearty Lentil	140	1	26
Minestrone	210	1.5	39
Potato Leek	100	1	39

Near East

Per Serving

Black Bean; Split Pea	195	1.5	34
Chicken; Sweet Corn	120	2.5	20
Chili & Corn	160	3	25
Country Mushroom	140	2.5	26
Italian Tomato	140	4	21
Lentil; Mediterranean Pasta	180	2	34
Minestrone; Parmesan Pasta	160	3	32
Potato Leek; Tomato & Rice	130	3	21
Primavera Pasta	190	2.5	36
Red Beans & Rice	190	2.5	36

Nile Spice

Per Cup

Chicken Flavored Vegetable	110	1.5	21
Lentil	180	1.5	31
Minestrone	140	1	30
Potato Leek	110	3	19
Red Beans & Rice	170	1	36
Split Pea	200	1	35
Tomato & Rice	140	2.5	27

Pacific Foods

Ready To Eat: *Per Cup (8 fl.oz)*

All Natural Chicken Broth	15	0	2
Organic Vegetable Broth	0	0	0

Progresso

Per 1/2 Can Serving (9 1/2 oz)

	C	**F**	**Cb**
19 oz Can:			
Bean & Ham	160	2	25
Beef Barley	130	4	13
Beef Minestrone/Noodle	140	3	16
Beef Vegetable & Rotini	130	2.5	14
Chickarina	130	5	12
Chicken & Wild Rice	100	1.5	11
Chicken Barley	110	1.5	16
Chicken Broth	20	1.5	1
Chicken Minestrone	110	1.5	15
Chicken Noodle	80	1.5	7
Chicken Rice w. Vegetable	90	2	13
Chicken Vegetable	90	1.5	13
Clam & Rotini Chowder	190	9	21
Escarole in Chicken Broth	25	1	2
Green Split Pea	170	3	25
Hearty Black Bean	170	1.5	30
Hearty Chicken & Rotini	90	1.5	15
Hearty Penne in Chicken Broth	80	1	14
Hearty Tomato	100	2	19
Home Style Chicken w. Veges	90	1.5	11
Lentil, 10.5 oz	170	8.5	27
Macaroni & Bean, 9.5 oz	160	4	23
Manhattan Clam Chowder	110	2	11
Meatballs & Pasta Pearls	140	7	13
Minestrone	120	2	21
Minestrone Parmesan	100	2.5	16
New England Clam Chowder	190	10	20
Potato Broccoli/Ham & Cheese	165	6.5	21
Rotisserie Seasoned Chicken	100	1.5	15
Spicy Chicken & Penne	110	1.5	14
Split Pea w. Ham	150	4	20
Tomato; Tomato Basil	100	2	19
Tomato Vegetable	90	2	15
Tortellini in Chicken Broth	70	2	10
Turkey Noodle	90	1.5	11
Turkey Rice w. Vegetable	110	1.5	18
Vegetable	90	2	15
Pasta Soups:			
Basil Rotini Tomato	120	1.5	22
Cheese & Herb Tortellini Tomato	140	3	23
Italian Herb Shells Minestrone	120	1.5	22
Oregano Penne Italian Style Vege.	90	2	15
Peppercorn Penne Vegetable	100	1	20
Roasted Garlic Pasta Lentil	120	1.5	20

Progresso (Cont)

	C	**F**	**Cb**
99% Fat Free:			
Beef Barley	140	2	20
Beef Vegetable	160	2	24
Chicken Noodle	90	1.5	13
Chicken Rice w. Veges	110	2	16
Creamy Mushroom Chicken	90	2	12
Lentil; Minestrone	130	1.5	21
New England Clam Chowder	130	2	22
Split Pea	170	1.5	28
Tomato Garden Vegetable	100	1.5	19
Vegetable	70	1	13
White Cheddar Potato	140	2.5	26

Pritikin

Per Cup

	C	**F**	**Cb**
Black Bean w. Rice	200	1	37
Chicken Flavored Vegetable	160	1	27
Minestrone	130	0.5	25
Potato Broccoli	110	0	22

Ralph's

	C	**F**	**Cb**
Chicken Broth, 1 cup	30	1	3
Fat Free/Reduced Salt, 1 cup	20	0	2

Ramen Noodles

See Page 66

Rokeach

15 oz Can (Ready to Serve):
Per Serving

	C	**F**	**Cb**
Barley & Mushroom	110	1	23
Chicken Consomme	50	4	0
Cream of Mushroom	120	7	13
Minestrone	170	1	32
Potato	100	1	20
Seven Bean	130	1	24
Split Pea & Egg Barley	190	1.5	35
Vegetable	110	1.5	22

Enjoy nutritious soup as part of a meal or as a snack. Soup is an excellent filler for dieters - especially to beat the 4.30pm snack syndrome. Choose low fat varieties.

Soups (Cont)

Shari's

	C	F	Cb
Cream of Tomato, 1 cup	80	0	17
Great Plains Split Pea, 1 cup	150	0	26
Indian Black Bean & Rice, 1 cup	150	1	30
Italian White Bean, 1 cup	170	1	32
Spicy French Green Lentil, 1 cup	130	0	22
Spicy Mexican Bean, 1 cup	210	1	38
Tomato w. Red Bell Pepper, 1 cup	100	0	19
Vegetarian French Onion, 1 cup	60	0	9

Shelton's

Canned: Per Cup

	C	F	Cb
Black Bean & Chicken	170	4	22
Turkey Meatball; Chicken Noodle	90	3	11
Chicken Tortilla	110	1.5	16
Chicken Broth	35	2.5	0

Streit's

Instant Soups: Per Serving

	C	F	Cb
Chicken Flavor; Mushr. & Barley	70	0.5	11
Garden Vegetable	70	0.5	13
Mild Chili; Split Pea	60	0	14
Tomato Minestrone; Veg. Chicken	80	0.5	18

Swanson

Canned: Per Cup

	C	F	Cb
Beef Broth	20	1	1
Chicken Broth	30	2	1
100% Fat Free	15	0	1
Vegetable Broth	20	1	3

Tabatchnick

Frozen: Per Serving (1 bag, 7^1/2 oz)

	C	F	Cb
Barley Mushroom	70	0	13
Cream of Broccoli/ Spinach	90	4	11
Old Fashioned Potato	70	0	16
Pea	180	2	31
Vegetable	110	1	20
Yankee Bean	160	2	27

Uncle Ben's

Hearty Soup Mix: Per Serving (^{1}/3 pkg)

	C	F	Cb
Black/Red Bean & Rice	150	2	28
Southwest Vegetable	90	1	19
White Bean & Pasta	100	1.5	18

Weight Watchers

	C	F	Cb
Chicken Noodle, 10^1/2 oz	150	2	25
Chicken & Rice, 10^1/2 oz	110	1.5	17
Minestrone, 10^1/2 oz	130	2	23
Vegetable, 10^1/2 oz	130	1	27
Instant Beef/Chicken Broth, 1 pkg	10	0	2

Westbrae

Canned:
Per Cup Unless Indicated

	C	F	Cb
Alabama Black Bean Gumbo	80	0	23
Calif. Unchicken Broth, ^{3}/4 cup	15	0.5	2
Chattanooga Corn Chowder	110	1	23
French Country Onion, ^{3}/4 cup	60	0	12
Great Plains Savory Bean	70	0	20
Irish Isle Potato Leek	110	1	22
Monte Carlo Cr. Mushroom, ^{3}/4 c.	70	3	10
Natural Wellington Unbeef	60	0	13
Rocky Mount. Crmy. Unchick., ^{3}/4 c.	70	3	10
Santa Fe Vegetable	120	0	23
Savanna Unchicken Rice	60	0.5	11
Spicy Southwest Vegetable	90	0	23
Tuscany Tomato	60	0	9
Versailles Garden Vegetable	70	0	15

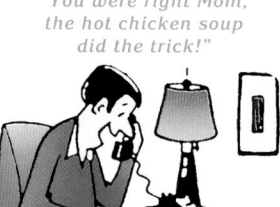

"You were right Mom, the hot chicken soup did the trick!"

ENGLEMAN

Herbs & Spices ◆ Condiments

Herbs & Spices

Per 1 Teaspoon

	C	**F**	**Cb**
Average all types: 1 tsp	5	0	1
Allspice, ground	5	0	1
Chili Powder	8	0	1
Cinnamon, ground	6	0	2
Curry Powder	6	0	1
Garlic Powder	9	0	2
Nutmeg, ground	12	0	1
Onion Powder	7	0	2
Parsley, dried	4	0	1
Pepper, black/red/white, aver.	6	0	1
Saffron	2	0	1
Tumeric, ground	8	0	1
Seeds: Fenugreek	12	1	2
Mustard,Poppyseed	15	1	1
Other types, average	7	0	2
Parsley Patch, Sesame, 1 tsp	16	1	1
Salt-free blends, average	10	0	2
All-purpose, 1 tsp	6	0	1

Seasonings & Flavorings

	C	**F**	**Cb**
Accent Flavor Enhancer, 1 tsp	10	0	0
Angostura Bitters, 1 tsp	12	0	3
Bacon Bits, average, 1 Tbsp	30	1	0
Bacon Chips (*Durkee*), 1 Tbsp	45	1	2
Best O'Butter, 1 tsp	10	<1	2
Braggs Liquid Aminos, 1 tsp	5	0	0
Butter Buds, 1 tsp	8	<1	2
Garlic Bread Sprinkle, 1 tsp	8	<1	2
Garlic Salt, 1 tsp	2	0	0
Italian Seasoning, 1 tsp	4	0	1
Lemon Pepper Season., 1 tsp	7	0	1
Meat Tenderizer, aver., 1 tsp	7	0	1
Molly McButter, 1 tsp	5	0	2
Mrs Dash Blends, 1 tsp	0	0	2
Perc Salt-free Seasoning, 1 tsp	8	0	2
Salad Sprinkles (*Lawry's*), 1 tsp	16	<1	2
Salad Supreme (*McCormick*), 1 tsp	10	<1	1
Salt: Regular, Sea Salt, Lite Salt	0	0	0
Seasoning Mixes, aver., ¼ pkg	70	1	1
Taco Seasoning, aver., ¼ pkg	30	<1	4
Old El Paso:			
Chili Season. Mix, 1 T.	25	0.5	4
Taco/Burrito Seasoning Mix, 2 tsp	15	0	3
Enchilada Seasoning Mix, 2 tsp	10	0	2
Fajita Seasoning Mix, 1 Tbsp	30	0	6
Vegit Seasoning Mix, 1 tsp	5	0	1

Condiments, Sauces

Average of Brands & Homemade

	C	**F**	**Cb**
Apple Sauce:			
Sweetened., ¼ cup, 2¼ oz	45	0	11
Unsweetened, ¼ cup, 2 oz	27	0	12
Eden; Tree of Life, ½ cup	50	0	15
Barbecue: Average, 1 Tbsp	25	0	6
Average, 2 Tbsp	50	0	12
Bearnaise Sce, ¼ cup, 2½ oz	190	19	5
Braggs Liquid Aminos, 1 tsp	5	0	0
Catsup (Ketchup): Reg., 1 Tbsp	15	0	4
Cheese, h/made, ¼ cup, 2½ oz	150	10	12
Chili Sauce: *Heinz,* 1 Tbsp	15	0	4
Del Monte, 1 Tbsp	20	0	5
Wolf Hot Dog, 1 Tbsp	15	1	2
Cocktail Sce: ¼ cup	110	0	15
Cranberry, jellied, ¼ cup, 2½ oz	110	0	27
Escoffier Sauces, 1 Tbsp	20	0	4
Honey Mustard (*French's*): 1 tsp	5	0	1
Horseradish: 1 Tbsp	2	0	0
Sauce: *Sauceworks,* 1 Tbsp	20	2	0
Ketchup: Regular, 1 Tbsp	16	0	4
Heinz Lite, 1 Tbsp	8	0	2
Mayonnaise: See Page 82			
Mushroom Sauce, ½ cup, 2 oz	50	2	5
Mustard, average, 1 tsp	0	0	0
Pizza Sauce, cnd., ¼ cup, 2 oz	25	0	5
Seafood Cocktail Sce, ¼ cup	60	0	14
Soy Sauce, all types, av., 1 Tbsp	10	0	0
Sour Cream Sce, ½ cup	250	15	22
Spaghetti Sce, ½ cup, 4½ oz	135	6	19
Steak Sauce: *Heinz/A.1..,* 1 Tbsp	15	0	3
Lea & Perrins, 1 Tbsp	25	0	6
Str'berry Puree Sce: Unsweet., 2 T.	9	0	2
Sweet & Sour Sauce:			
Contadina, 2 Tbsp	40	1	8
Kikkoman Lite Soy, 2 Tbsp	10	0	1
La Choy, 2 Tbsp, 34g	60	0	14
Tabasco Sauce, 1 Tbsp	2	0	0
Taco Sauce, average, 2 Tbsp	10	0	1
Tartar Sauce: *Heinz,* 2 Tbsp, 30g	140	14	4
America's Choice, 2 Tbsp, 27g	160	17	1
Hellman's: Regular, 2 Tbsp, 30g	80	7	3
Lowfat, 2 Tbsp, 30g	40	1.5	7
Teriyaki Sauce: *Kikkoman,* 1 Tbsp	15	0	2
Vinegar: White or wine, 1 fl.oz	4	0	1
White Sauce, ½ cup, 5 oz	130	7	12
Worcestershire Sauce, 1 tsp	5	0	1

Pickles ◆ Gravy ◆ Sloppy Joe

Pickles & Relish | C | F | ●

Average All Brands

	C	F	
Bread & Butter Pickles, 4 sl.,1 oz	20	0	5
Chutney, 2 Tbsp, 1¼ oz	40	0	12
Dill Pickle:			
Slices, 4 slices, 1 oz	3	0	0.5
1 large, (3¾"x 1¼" diam.), 2¼ oz	12	0	3
Extra lrg (4"x 1¾" diam.), 5 oz	30	0	6
Halves: Small, 1 oz	3	0	0.5
Large, 2½ oz	8	0	2
Sweet, small, ½ oz	22	0	6
Gherkins, sweet, 1 med., 1 oz	15	0	7
Green Chilies, chopped, 2 Tbsp	5	0	1
Horseradish, 1 Tbsp	10	0	2
Jalapenos, pickled, 2 whole	5	0	1
Jalapeno Relish, 1 Tbsp, ½ oz	5	0	1
Mustard, aver. all brands, 1 tsp	5	0	0.5
Peppers: Hot/Mild, 1 oz	8	0	2
Pickled: Beets, ½ cup, 4 oz	75	0	19
Onions, 1 medium, ¾ oz	10	0	2
Cocktail Onion, 1 onion	2	0	0
Red Cabbage, ½ cup, 3 oz	60	0	13
Pickles:			
Sweet, 2 Tbsp, 1 oz	35	0	0
Large (3" x ¾ diam.), 1¼ oz	40	0	10
Pickle in a Pouch, 1 large	12	0	3
Relishes: Sandwich Spread, 1 tsp	20	1	5
Cranberry-Orange, 1 Tbsp	30	0	7
Hot Dog (*Heinz*), 1 Tbsp	17	0	28
Sweet Pickle, 1 Tbsp	20	0	5
Sauerkraut, ½ cup, 3½ oz	25	0	5
Sweet Cauliflower	35	0	8

Salsa

Average all types

	C	F	
Regular, no oil, 2 Tbsp	15	0	3.5
w. Oil, homemade, 2 Tbsp	40	3	8
Chef's Kitchen, 2 Tbsp	10	0	2
Del Monte, all flavors, 2 Tbsp	10	0	2
Kaukauma, 2 Tbsp	15	0	3

Pasta Sauces: *See Page 79*

Pasta Sauces: See Page 79

Gravy | C | F | Cb

	C	F	Cb
Homemade Gravy:			
Thin, little fat, 2 Tbsp, 1 oz	20	1	3
Thick, 2 Tbsp, 1¼ oz	50	2	9
¼ cup, 2½ oz	100	4	18
Franco-American (Canned)			
Au Jus Gravy, ¼ cup, 2 oz	10	0	2
Beef/Mushrm; Turkey Gravy, 2 oz	25	1	3
Chicken Gravy, 2 oz	40	4	3
Golden Pork Gravy, 2 oz	45	4	3
Fat Free, Average, 2 oz	25	0	4
Pillsbury (Gravy Mixes)			
Brown; Homestyle, ¼ cup	15	0	3
Chicken, as prep., ¼ cup	20	0	4

Sloppy Joe Sauce

Per Serving

	C	F	
Del Monte: ¼ cup, 67g	50	0	11
Heinz: ½ cup, 125g	70	0.5	14
Hunt's Manwich: ¼ cup, 64g	30	0	6
Libby's: ⅓ cup, 78g	45	0	10

Tomato Products

Whole/Chopped/Crushed/Diced

	C	F	
1 cup, 8½ oz	50	0	10
In Aspic, ½ cup	50	0	12
w. Green Chili, 1 cup, 8½ oz	45	<1	11
Stewed, ½ cup	40	2.5	9
Wedges in Tom Juice, 1 cup	70	0.5	15
Salsa, average, 1 Tbsp	15	0	3.5
Tomato Ketchup, regular, 1 Tbsp	16	0	4
Tomato Paste, 2 Tbsp	25	0	5
Regular, 6 oz, ¾ cup	150	0	34
Tomato Puree, ½ cup	50	0	10
Tomato Sauce:			
Regular, ½ cup	40	0	9
Spanish Style, ½ cup	40	0	9
w. Mushrooms, ½ cup	40	0	9
w. Onions, ½ cup	50	0	11
Tomato Seasoning, 3 tsp	20	0	4
Sundried Tomatoes:			
Natural, 5-6 pces, 0.4 oz	22	0	5
In Oil, drained, 6 pces, ½ oz	60	4	5

Sauce Mixes

	C	F	Cb
Knorr (Mix)			
Made As Directed: *Per 1/4 Cup, 2 oz*			
Au Jus	8	0.2	1
Bearnaise	170	17	5
Classic Brown Gravy	25	1	5
Demi-Glace	30	1	4
Hollandaise	170	18	5
Hunter; Lyonnaise	25	0.3	4
Mushroom Sauce	60	3	5
Napoli Sauce	100	3	17
Pepper Sauce	20	1	3
McCormick			
Grillmates:			
Marinade, aver. all flavors, 2 tsp	15	0	2
Sauce Blend Seasoning Mixes:			
Lemon Herb Chicken, 1 Tbsp	30	0	5
Chicken Fried Rice, 1 Tbsp	35	0	6
Stir Fry Chicken, 1 Tbsp	20	0	4
Chicken Teriyaki, 1 1/3 Tbsp	40	1	5

Pizza & Enchilada Sauce

Per 1/4 Cup	C	F	Cb
Pizza Squeeze *(Contadina)*	35	1.5	6
Progresso Pizza Sauce	10	0	2
Ragu: Pizza Sauce	30	1	4
Pizza Quick; average all types	40	1.5	6
Enchilada Sauce *(Old El Paso)*	10	0	2

"Well, I did swallow some melon seeds about five months ago. . ."

Brands

	C	F	Cb
Barilla: *Per 1/2 Cup*			
Arrabbiata; Siciliana	80	3.5	9
Marinara; Ortolana	80	4	10
Mushr. & Garlic; Pepperonata	70	2	12
Puttanesea	80	2.5	13
Classico: *Per 1/2 Cup*			
Florentine Spinach & Cheese	80	4.5	8
Italian Sausage & Fennel	90	5	7
Mushroom & Olive	50	1	8
Roasted Peppers & Onions/Garlic	60	2	9
Spicy Red Pepper	60	2.5	6
Sun Dried Tomato; 4 Cheese	80	4	8
Tomato & Basil	50	1	9
Contadina: *Per 1/2 Cup*			
Alfredo Sauce	360	32	10
Lite	160	10	10
Garden Vegetable Sauce	40	0	9
Marinara Sauce	80	4	9
Mushroom Alfredo	200	14	12
Mushroom Marinara Sauce	70	2.5	11
Pesto with Basil, Red. Fat	460	26	22
Pesto w. Sundried Tomato	380	30	20
Roasted Garlic Marinara	60	2	10
Del Monte: *Per 1/2 Cup*			
Chunky: Average all varieties	60	1.5	11
D'Italia Pasta: Four Cheese	60	2	8
Other varieties	50	1.5	9
Spaghetti Sauce: Traditional	60	0.5	15
Garlic & Onion	60	1.5	11
w. Mushroom/Meat	70	1.5	14
Dominick's: *Per 1/2 Cup*			
All Natural: Garlic & Onion	80	4	10
Marinara	80	4	10
Mushr. & Olive; Tomato & Basil	80	1	8
Italian Classics: Four Cheese	80	2.5	12
Portabella Mushroom	60	2	8
Puttanesea	70	3	8
Spicy Roasted Garlic	70	2	10
Sun Ripened Tomatoes	80	4	8
Tomato Basil	50	1	8
Estee: Spaghetti Sce, 1/4 cup, 4 oz	60	2	13
Frank Sinatra: *Per 1/4 Cup*			
Alfredo	160	14	4
Pesto	160	14	3

Brands (Cont)

Five Brothers: Per 1/2 Cup	C	F	Cb
Alfredo w. Mushrooms	160	12	6
Creamy Alfredo/Pesto	200	18	4
Fresh/Summer Tomato Basil	60	1.5	11
Grilled Summer Vegetable	80	5	12
Marinara w. Burgundy Wine	80	3	12
Mushroom & Garlic	90	3	13
Oven Roasted Garlic & Onion	70	1.5	10
Imported Romano & Garlic	90	4	10

Garden Valley: Per 1/2 Cup	C	F	Cb
Chunky Vege. Primavera	35	0.5	12
Four Cheese	35	1	8
Millina's Finest; Roasted Garlic	50	0	12
Sundried Tomato; Tom. Mushroom	50	0	11
Sweet Tomato Basil	60	0	13

Hagerty Foods: Per 4 oz	C	F	Cb
Asparagus Garlic	95	7	9
Caponata	60	3.5	8

Healthy Choice: Per 1/2 Cup	C	F	Cb
Garlic & Herbs	50	0	10
Marinara w. Burgundy	50	5	11
Roasted Garlic & Romano	60	1	11
Sundried Tomato & Herb	60	0.5	12

Hy Top: Per 1/2 Cup, 125g	C	F	Cb
Spaghetti Sauce: All flavors	90	4	11

Mama Coco's: Per 1/2 Cup	C	F	Cb
Basil & Garlic	70	4	9
Marinara	100	7	8
Mushroom	110	8	8

Newman's Own: Per 1/2 Cup	C	F	Cb
Bombolina	100	5	12
Other flavors	60	2	9

Prego: Per 1/2 Cup	C	F	Cb
Extra Chunky: Garden Comb.	90	2	16
Garlic Supreme	120	3	23
Mushroom & Green Pepper	120	4.5	18
Mushroom Supreme	120	4.5	21
Zesty Mushroom	120	4	20
Tomato, Onion & Garlic	110	3.5	19
Regular:			
Diced Onion & Garlic	110	3	19
Flavored w. Meat	140	6	21
Fresh Mushroom; Traditional	150	5	23
Hamburger	120	4	17
Italian Sausage & Garlic	120	5	16
Mushroom & Garlic	110	2	20
Mushroom/Tomato Parmesan	120	3.5	19
Pepperoni	120	4.5	18
Roast Red Pepper/Herb & Garlic	110	3.5	17
Roast Garlic Parmesan	120	1.5	23
Three Cheese	100	2	18

Progresso: Per 1/2 Cup, 4 1/4 oz	C	F	Cb
Pasta Sauces: Alfredo (Authentic)	200	15	7
Creamy Clam	110	6	8
Lobster	100	7	8
Marinara (Authentic)	100	4	12
Marinara, regular	85	4.5	8
Meat Flavor; Spaghetti	100	4.5	12
Red Clam	60	1	8
White Clam (Authentic)	150	10	5
White Clam, regular	140	10	5

Ragu: Per 1/2 Cup	C	F	Cb
Chunky Garden Style:			
Creamy Tomato Romano	120	5	14
Classic Alfredo	240	24	6
Four Cheese	240	22	4
Light Parmesan Alfredo	160	12	4
Mushroom Green Pepper	110	3.5	18
Roasted Garlic Parmesan	240	22	6
Tom. Garlic Onion; Super Mushr.	120	3.5	19

Rinaldi: Meat/Mushroom, 1/2 c.	C	F	Cb
	90	4	11

Seeds of Change: Per 1/2 Cup	C	F	Cb
Average all varieties	50	0.5	9

Sutter Home: Per 1/2 Cup	C	F	Cb
Italian Style Pasta Sauce	80	2	12
Sicilian Style; Spicy Mediterranean	80	2	12
Marinara Pasta Sauce	70	2	11

Brands (Cont)

	C	F	Cb
Taj: *Per 1/2 Cup*			
Bombay Curry Simmer Sauce	90	5	10
Calcutta Masala Simmer Sauce	100	5	13
Kashmir Tandoori Marinade Sce	50	3	5
Seasoning Mixes: *Per 2 tsp*			
Meat Loaf; Sloppy Joe's	30	0	4
Beef Stew	15	0	3
Chili	40	1	6
Chicken/Taco Seasoning	25	0	4
Spaghetti Sauce: Italian Style, 1 T.	25	0	5
Timpone's: *Per 1/2 Cup*			
Spaghetti Sauce: Classic	50	2.5	8
Mom's	70	3.5	8
Tomaso's: *Per 1/2 Cup*			
Basil & Fresh Garlic; Spicy Eggplant	60	3	7
Black Olive Fresh Basil	40	2	5
Extra Garlic	55	2	8
Fresh Mushroom & Artichoke	50	2	7
Sugo Rosa	105	7.5	8
Tree of Life: *Per 1/2 Cup*			
Pasta Sauce Plus: All varieties	45	0	9
Organic: Classic Tomato	40	0	8
Average other varieties	30	0	7

Other Sauces

	C	F	Cb
Bookbinders: *Per 1/2 Cup*			
White Clam Sauce	300	30	4
Bullseye: *Per 2 Tbsp*			
BBQ	50	0	13
Estee			
Barbecue Sauce, 1 Tbsp	18	<1	3
Steak Sauce, 1 Tbsp	14	<1	3
Heinz			
Per 1 Tbsp: Approx. 1/2 oz			
Barbecue Sauces: All flavors	35	0	9
Chili Sauce	15	0	4
Horseradish Sauce	70	7	13
Mustard: Pourable/Mild	8	<1	5
Spicy Brown	13	1	6
Seafood Cocktail Sauce	20	0	10
Steak Sauce 57	15	0	4
Tartar Sauce	70	7	2
Tomato Ketchup	16	0	26
Worcestershire Sauce	8	0	11

Other Sauces (Cont)

	C	F	Cb
Hunt's BBQ: *Per 2 Tbsp*			
Original, 36g	50	0	13
Hickory & Brown Sugar, 38g	70	0	18
Kraft			
Sauceworks: Cocktail, 2 Tbsp	30	0.3	6
Horseradish, 1 tsp	20	1.5	0
Sweet 'n Sour, 1 Tbsp	30	0	7
Tartar: 1 Tbsp	50	5	2
Lemon & Herb, 1 Tbsp	75	8	0
Barbecue Sauces:			
Average all types, 2 Tbsp	50	0.5	9
Other Sauces: *Per 1 Tbsp*			
Horseradish: Reg./Cream Style	10	0	0
Mustard	10	0	0
Sandwich Spread & Burger	50	4	3
Sweet 'n Sour	40	0.5	9
Nonfat Tartar	12	0	5
Las Palmas			
Red Chile Sauce, 1/4 cup, 2oz	15	0.5	2
Enchilada Sauces: Green Chile	25	1.5	3
Hot/Original, 1/4 cup, 2oz	15	0.5	3
Salsa: Mexicana. Mild, 2 Tbsp, 1oz	5	0	1
Mexicana Hot/Medium, 2 Tbsp	10	0	2
Old El Paso			
Salsa: Thick 'n Chunky, 2 T., 1 oz	10	0	2
Homestyle; Green Chili; Verde			
2 Tbsp, 1 oz	10	0	2
Taco Sce: All varieties, 2 Tbsp, 1 oz	10	0	1
Thick 'n Chunky Sauces: 2 T., 1 oz	10	0	2
Enchilada Sauces:			
All varieties, 1/4 cup, 2 oz	30	1.5	4
Grilling Sauces: All types, 2 Tbsp	60	0	14
Tomatoes & Green Chiles,			
1/4 cup, 2 oz	10	0	2
Tomatoes & Jalapenos, 1/4 c., 2 oz	10	0	2
Open Pit: *Per 2 Tbsp*			
Honey	40	0	10
Hickory	50	0.5	11
Original BBQ	50	0.5	11
Thick & Tangy	50	0	12
President's Choice: *Per 2 Tbsp*			
Honey Dijon	50	0.5	11
Hot & Spicy	55	0	13
Original BBQ	60	0	12

Salad Dressings

Quick Guide
C **F** **Cb**

Mayonnaise

	C	F	Cb
Regular			
Average All Brands, 1 Tbsp	100	11	0
(Bestfoods, Kraft), 1 Tbsp	100	11	0
1/2 cup, 4 oz	800	88	0
Light/Reduced Fat			
Kraft; Best Foods, 1 Tbsp	50	5	1
1/2 cup, 4 oz	400	40	8
Hain, 1 Tbsp	60	6	2
Hellman's; Estee, 1 Tbsp	50	5	1
Smart Beat, 1 Tbsp	40	4	1
Weight Watchers, 1 Tbsp	25	2	1
Fat Free			
Kraft; Weight Watchers, 1 Tbsp	10	0	3
1/2 cup, 4 oz	80	0	16

Mayonnaise Type Dressing

Per 1 Tbsp (Approx. 1/2 oz)

	C	F	Cb
BAMA Dressing, 1 Tbsp	50	4	3
Miracle Whip Salad Dressing:			
Regular, 0.5 oz	70	7	2
Light, 0.5 oz	40	3	3
Free, 0.5 oz	15	0	3
Nayonaise (Nasoya)			
(Tofu Base/Dairy Free/Eggless)			
Regular, 1 Tbsp, 0.5 oz	35	3	1
Fat-Free, 1 Tbsp, 0.5 oz	10	0	2

*Enjoy a healthy salad
but don't drown it
in high-fat salad dressings.*

Quick Guide
C **F** **Cb**

Salad Dressings

Average All Brands
Per 2 Tbsp (Approx 1 oz)

	C	F	Cb
Blue Cheese: Regular	150	16	2
Light/Reduced Fat	80	8	1
Caesar: Regular	140	14	2
Light/Reduced Fat	50	5	0.5
French: Regular	130	11	5
Light/Reduced Fat	50	3	4
Fat/Oil-Free	40	0	4
Italian: Regular	130	11	3
Light/Reduced Fat	70	7	2
Fat/Oil-Free	10	0	2
Ranch: Regular	180	18	3
Light/Reduced Fat	90	8	3
Fat-Free	50	0	2
Russian: Regular	130	10	3
Light/Reduced Fat	50	5	2
Fat-Free	30	0	2
Thousand Island: Regular	130	12	5
Light/Reduced Fat	50	4	3
Fat-Free	35	0	3

Brands ~ Salad Dressings

Per 2 Tbsp (Approx 1 oz)

C **F** **Cb**

	C	F	Cb
Benecol: *Per 2 Tbsp*			
Creamy Italian	100	10	3
French Style	130	11	6
Ranch	130	13	3
Thousand Island	130	12	5
Bernstein's			
Balsamic	110	11	2
Cheese: Garlic Italian; Fantastico	110	11	2
Creamy Caesar	120	13	1
Fat Free Cheese & Garlic Italian	10	0	2
French Herb Garden	130	11	2
Restaurant Recipe Italian	130	13	1
Best Foods			
Caesar, 2 Tbsp	100	9	6
Chardonnay Vinaigrette	50	4	4
Chunky Blue Cheese	140	15	1
Creamy Caesar	170	18	2
Creamy French	160	16	4

Per 2 Tbsp (Approx 1 oz)

	C	F	Cb
Best Foods (Cont)			
Creamy/Garlic/Spr. Onion Ranch	140	15	1
Creamy Thousand Island	130	13	4
Fat Free Caesar; Dijonnaise	30	0	7
Fat Free Ranch	45	0	4
Fat Free Italian	15	0	4
Rst. Tomato & Balsamic Vinegar	100	9	3
Brianna's			
Blush Vintage	100	6	12
Cardini's			
Caesar, 2 Tbsp	160	17	1
Herb Poppy Seed	35	1	7
Zesty Garlic	120	13	2
Summer Honey Mustard	150	14	5
Carolina's Swamp Stuffs'			
Per 2 Tbsp			
Blue Tick Dressing	220	16	6
Cedar Spray	40	3	2
Milk Weed	100	10	2
Pure Tar	60	5	2
Red Tide	30	3	2
Seaweed Splash	30	2	2
Swamp Sauce	20	0	6
Tadpole Tea	30	2	2
Girards: *Per 2 Tbsp*			
Caesar	150	16	1
Lite	80	7	2
Lite Champagne	60	5	2
Oriental	120	11	6
Original French	120	13	0
Spinach Salad	80	2	14
Fat Free: Caesar	40	0	9
Raspberry Vinaigrette	40	0	9
Red Wine Vinaigrette	40	0	2
Good Seasons (Mix)			
As Prepared, 2 Tbsp (Approx 1 oz)			
Blue Cheese, Cheese Garlic	145	16	2
Cheese Italian, Garlic & Herbs	145	16	2
Classic Dill, 1 pkg	28	0	5
Italian	145	16	2
Italian Lite	55	6	2
Lite Cheese Italian	55	6	2
Mild Italian; Zesty Italian	145	16	2
Ranch	115	12	2

Per 2 Tbsp (Approx 1 oz)

	C	F	Cb
Hain			
Regular Pourable: Per 2 Tbsp			
Canola: Garden Tomato	120	12	2
Italian; French Mustard	100	10	2
Creamy Caesar: French	120	12	2
Creamy Italian	160	16	0
Garlic & Sour Cream	140	14	0
Poppyseed Rancher's	120	14	0
Savory Herb (No Salt Added)	180	20	0
Thousand Island	100	10	5
Traditional Italian	160	16	0
(No Salt Added)	120	12	2
Mix: Made Up Per 2 Tbsp			
No Oil Range: Bleu Cheese	28	2	2
Buttermilk	22	0	2
Caesar	12	0	2
French	24	0	6
Italian	4	0	2
Healthy Sensation			
Blue Cheese, French, 2 Tbsp	40	2	8
Honey Dijon	50	2	10
Italian	15	0	2
Ranch	30	0	6
Thousand Island	40	0	8
Hidden Valley			
Fat Free: Caesar	30	0	6
Honey & Bacon French	50	0	11
Honey Dijon	35	0	7
Italian Herb & Cheese; Ranch	30	0	6
Italian Parmesan	20	0	4
Red Wine & Herb Vinaigrette	45	0	11
Roasted Garlic Italian	40	0	5
Honey & Bacon French	150	12	10
Original Ranch	140	14	1
Light Original Ranch	80	7	3
Original Ranch w. Bacon	140	14	1
Ranch Caesar Creamy	110	11	1
Ranch Cole Slaw	150	15	5
Ranch Garden Vegetable	130	13	3
Ranch Garlic & Spice	130	13	2
Hollywood			
Caesar; Creamy French	140	14	4
Italian; Creamy Italian	180	18	3
Italian Cheese	160	16	4
Poppy Seed Rancher's	150	16	2
Thousand Island	120	12	6

Salad Dressings (Cont)

Per 2 Tbsp (Approx 1 oz)

	C	F	Cb
Knott's Berry Farm			
Honey Dijon, 2 Tbsp	130	13	4
Raspberry Vinaigrette	30	2	8
Roasted Garlic Caesar	140	14	3
Sun Dried Tomato Vinaigrette	100	10	3
Kraft			
Regular Dressings: *Per 2 Tbsp*			
Bacon & Tomato	140	14	2
Buttermilk Ranch	150	16	2
Caesar; Salsa Ranch	130	13	2
Caesar Ranch; Pesto Italian	140	15	1
Catalina French/ with Honey	140	12	8
Chunky Blue Cheese	90	7	3
Coleslaw	150	12	8
Creamy Caesar; Cucumber Ranch	140	15	2
Creamy Garlic; Creamy Italian	110	11	3
French	120	12	4
Honey Dijon	150	15	4
House Italian	120	12	3
Peppercorn Ranch; Ranch	170	18	1
Free	50	0	11
Roka Brand Blue Cheese	90	7	5
Russian	130	10	10
Salsa Zesty Garden	70	6	3
Sour Cream & Onion Ranch	170	18	1
Thousand Island	110	10	5
Thousand Island w. Bacon	120	12	5
Zesty Italian	110	11	2
Kraft Deliciously Right			
(Red. Calorie Dressings):			
Bacon & Tomato; Caesar	60	5	3
Creamy Italian	50	5	3
Cucumber Ranch	60	5	2
French	50	3	6
Italian	70	7	1
Ranch	110	11	2
Thousand Island	70	4	8
Kraft Free (Fat Free):			
Blue Cheese, Catalina, French	50	0	12
Honey Dijon, Peppercorn/Ranch	50	0	11
Italian	10	0	2
Red Wine Vinegar	15	0	3
Thousand Island; Sr Cream & Onion	45	0	11
Light Done Right: Classic Caesar	70	6	3
Italian; Red Wine Vinaigrette	50	4.5	3
Raspberry Vinaigrette	60	4	6
Thousand Island	70	4	17

Per 2 Tbsp (Approx 1 oz)

	C	F	Cb
Kraft (Cont)			
Special Collection:			
Balsamic Vinaigrette	110	12	1
Creamy Cucumber Dill	120	12	4
Creamy Parmesan Romano	170	18	1
Creamy Roasted Garlic	160	17	2
Greek Vinaigrette	120	13	2
Savory Mayo:			
Roast Garlic/Onion	100	10	1
Tangy Tomato Bacon	130	11	8
Vinaigrette: Caesar Parmesan	60	5	1
Roast Garlic	50	4.5	2
LadyLee (Lucky Stores)			
Fat Free French	120	11	7
Fat Free Italian	10	0	2
Fat Free Ranch/Thousand Island	35	0	8
Lawrey's			
Caesar; Italian, 2 Tbsp	130	13	2
Creamy Caesar	130	14	8
Red Wine Vinaigrette	90	7	7
Manischewitz			
Garlic Ranch, 2 Tbsp	15	0	4
Maple Grove			
Fat Free: Caesar, 2 Tbsp	30	0	6
Honey Dijon	45	0	10
Marzetti			
Regular Dressings:			
Blue Cheese	160	17	0
Buttermilk: Bacon Ranch; Ranch	180	19	1
Blue Cheese	160	18	1
Caesar; Chunky Blue Cheese	150	16	1
California French; Celery Seed	160	13	11
Classic Caesar Ranch	190	20	2
Country French	150	13	7
Creamy Italian	150	16	1
Dijon Honey Mustard	140	13	6
Garden Ranch; Ranch	180	19	1
Honey French/Blue Cheese	160	13	11
Italian w. Olive Oil	120	13	1
Potato Salad Dressing	120	13	7
Red Wine Vinegar & Oil	130	14	2
Slaw	170	16	6
Southern Slaw	100	11	14
Thousand Island	150	15	5

Per 2 Tbsp (Approx 1 oz) — **C** **F** **Cb**

Marzetti (Cont)

	C	F	Cb
Fat Free Dressings: Italian	15	0	3
California French; Honey French	45	0	11
Honey Dijon	60	0	14
Ranch; Peppercorn Ranch	30	0	7
Slaw; Sweet & Sour	45	0	12
Thousand Island	35	0	9
Light Dressings: Blue Cheese	60	6	4
Buttermilk Ranch	90	9	4
California French	80	6	8
Chunky Blue Cheese	80	7	4
French	40	2	6
Honey French	80	4	12
Italian	60	5	3
Ranch	90	8	7
Red Wine Vinegar & Oil	20	1	3
Slaw	60	7	10
Sweet & Sour	100	6	11
Thousand Island	70	5	6

Newman's Own

	C	F	Cb
Caesar; Olive Oil & Vinegar, 2 T.	150	16	1
Italian Light	20	0	3
Ranch	180	18	2

Nasoya

Vegi-Dressing (Tofu Base/Dairy Free):

	C	F	Cb
Thousand Island	60	4	6
Other flavors	60	5	3
(Nayonaise - See Mayonnaise)			

Pfeiffer

	C	F	Cb
California French, 2 Tbsp	140	12	9
French	150	13	7
Honey Dijon	140	13	6
Lite Italian	50	5	3
Ranch	180	20	1
Savory Italian	110	12	3
Thousand Island	140	14	4

Pritikin

	C	F	Cb
Dijon Balsamic; Zesty Italian	30	0	6
Honey Dijon	45	0	11
Honey French Style	40	0	10
Raspberry	35	0	11

Ralph's Chef Express

	C	F	Cb
Blue Cheese, 2 Tbsp	170	18	1
Lite Ranch	90	8	3

Per 2 Tbsp (Approx 1 oz) — **C** **F** **Cb**

Red Wing

	C	F	Cb
Chunky Blue Cheese, 2 Tbsp	130	13	3
Creamy Ranch	150	15	2
French Tradit'nal; Spicy Sw. French	130	11	8
Italian Traditional	100	9	4
"K" Dressing	140	14	8
Thousand Island	110	9	8

San-J

	C	F	Cb
Fat Free: Honey Curry, 2 Tbsp	25	0	6
Tamari Mustard	25	0	5
Thai Peanut (lowfat)	50	2.5	4

S & W

	C	F	Cb
Light: Oriental Rice Wine, 2 Tbsp	30	0	7
Red Wine Vinegar Herb	40	0	10
Low Calorie Range: Blue Cheese	50	4	4
Creamy Cucumber; Thousand Island	50	4	4
Creamy Italian	20	2	2
French	35	0	6
Italian No-Oil	4	0	0
Russian	50	2	8

Seven Seas

	C	F	Cb
Regular Dressings: Chunky Blue	90	7	5
Creamy Caesar	140	15	1
Creamy Italian	110	12	2
Green Goddess	120	13	1
Herbs & Spices	120	12	1
Ranch	150	16	2
Red Wine Vin. & Oil; Viva Italian	110	11	2
Two Cheese Italian	70	7	3
Viva Caesar	120	12	2
Viva Russian	150	16	3
Free (Fat-Free): Italian	10	0	2
Ranch	50	0	12
Red Wine Vinegar	15	0	3
Reduced Calorie:			
Crmy Italian; Red Wine Vin. & Oil	60	5	2
Italian w./Olive Oil	50	5	2
Ranch	100	9	5
Viva Italian	45	4	2

Spike Splashes!

	C	F	Cb
Original, 2 Tbsp	100	11	1
Salt Free	100	10	2
Fat Free	10	0	2

Per 2 Tbsp (Approx 1 oz)

	C	F	Cb
Spectrum			
Fat Free: Creamy Dill	25	0	4
Creamy Garlic	20	0	4
Sweet Onion & Garlic; Tstd Sesame	15	0	3
Lowfat: Blue Cheese Style	35	2	3
Creamy Roasted Pepper	45	2	5
Honey Dijon	35	2	4
Mango Madness	50	2	7
Southwestern Caesar	40	2	3
Zesty Italian	30	2	1
The Spice Hunter			
Mix: ~ As Prepared, Per 2 Tbsp			
Caesar Salad, 2 Tbsp	150	13	1
Chinese Salad	140	12	1
Garlic & Herb	140	13	2
Tree of Life			
House Dressing: Cafe Venice	120	12	2
Maison Caesar	70	6	1
Shanghai Palace	80	7	3
Lowfat Free: Blue Cheese	15	1	2
Fat Free: Honey French	35	0	8
Italian Garlic	20	0	4
Oriental Ginger	15	0	3
Walden Farms			
Fat Free, Calorie Free Range			
Average All Types, 2 Tbsp	0	0	0
Weight Watchers			
Salad Celebrations Dressings			
Fat Free: Caesar (Single), 0.75 oz	5	0	1
Caesar, 2 Tbsp	10	0	1
Creamy Italian (8 oz), 2 Tbsp	30	0	7
French Style, 2 Tbsp	40	0	9
Honey Dijon, 2 Tbsp	45	0	11
Italian (8 oz), 2 Tbsp	10	0	2
Ranch Style, 2 Tbsp	35	0	7
Ranch (Single), 0.75 oz	25	0	6
Wishbone			
Chunky Blue Cheese: Regular	170	17	2
Lite	80	8	3
Caesar	110	10	2
Classic House Italian	140	14	2
Classic Lite Olive Oil	40	4	2
Creamy Caesar	180	18	1
Creamy Italian	110	12	4

Per 2 Tbsp (Approx 1 oz)

	C	F	Cb
Wishbone (Cont)			
Fat Free: Caesar	25	0	5
Honey Dijon	45	0	10
Italian	15	0	2
Parmesan - Onion	45	0	9
Ranch	40	0	9
Red Wine Vinaigrette	35	0	7
French: Lite	60	6	8
Fat-Free	12	0	2
Sweet 'N Spicy; Red French	140	12	6
Lite	35	0	7
Italian: Regular	80	8	3
Lite	15	0.5	2
Italian Cream Lite	50	4	4
Olive Oil Vinaigrette	60	5	4
Parmesan - Onion	110	10	5
Ranch: Regular	160	17	1
Lite	100	8	5
Robusto Italian	90	8	4
Russian: Regular	110	6	15
Thousand Island:			
Regular	130	12	7
Lite	80	5	8
Thousand Island	35	0	9
Vinaigrette: Berry	50	4.5	2
Roast Garlic	60	5	3
Sun-dried Tomato	50	5	2

STOP-SMOKING
NICOTINE PATCH

STOP-EATING
FOOD PATCH

Quick Guide
Cooked Cereals

	C	F	Cb
Buckwheat Groats, roasted:			
Dry, 1/2 cup, 3 oz	280	2	60
Cooked, 1 cup, 7 oz	180	1	39
Bulgar: Dry, 1/2 cup, 2 1/2 oz	240	1	53
Cooked, 1 cup, 6 1/2 oz	150	<1	34
Corn/Hominy Grits:			
Dry, 1/4 cup, 1.4 oz	145	<1	33
3 Tbsp, 1 oz	110	<1	25
Cooked, 3/4 cup, 6 1/2 oz	110	<1	25
Instant, 1 pkt, 0.8 oz	80	<1	18
w. Imitation Bacon Bits, 1 oz	100	<1	22
Cream of Rice, ckd, 3/4 c, 6 oz	90	0	20
Cream of Wheat:			
Regular, ckd, 3/4 cup, 6 oz	180	<1	37
Quick, ckd, 3/4 cup, 6 oz	95	<1	20
Instant, ckd, 3/4 cup, 6 oz	110	<1	23
Farina: Cooked, 3/4 cup, 6 oz	85	0	18
Millet, dry, 1/4 cup, 1 oz	100	0	20
Oat Bran:			
Raw, 1/3 cup, 1 oz	75	2	14
Cooked, 1/2 cup	45	<1	8
Oatmeal:			
Dry, 1/3 cup, 1 oz	110	0	19
Regular, ckd, 3/4 cup, 6 oz	110	2	19
1 cup, 8 oz	145	3	25
Instant: Regular, aver., 1 oz	100	2	18
Flavored, average	150	2	32
Quaker: *See Brands*			
Wheat Hearts, 1 oz dry, 3/4 c. ckd	110	1	21

Quick Guide
Cold Cereals
Average All Brands

	C	F	Cb
Bran (processed), 1/3 cup, 1 oz	70	<1	20
Bran Flakes, 3/4 cup, 1 oz	90	<1	23
Corn Flakes, 1 cup, 1 oz	110	<1	24
Granola, 1/4 cup, 1 oz	130	4	21
Oat Bran Cereal, 1/3 cup, 1 oz	110	1	23
Puffed Rice, 1 cup, 1/2 oz	55	0	12
Puffed Wheat, 1 cup, 1/2 oz	55	0	12
Raisin Bran, 1/2 cup, 1 oz	85	<1	22
Rice Crisps, 1 cup, 1 oz	110	1	25
Shredded Wheat, 1 bisc., 3/4 oz	80	<1	18
Sugar-frosted Flakes, 3/4 c, 1 oz	110	<1	26
Wheat Flakes, 1 cup, 1 oz	105	<1	23

Brans & Wheatgerm

	C	F	Cb
Bran: Wheat, unprocessed, 1 Tbsp, 3g	10	0	3
Rice Bran, raw, 1 Tbsp, 5g	16	1	2.5
1/3 cup, 1 oz	90	6	14
Oat Bran, 1 Tbsp, 5g	15	<1	3
1/3 cup, 1 oz	75	2	15
Wheat Germ, 1 Tbsp, 1/4 oz	25	1	3.5
1/4 cup, 1 oz	108	3	15

Cereal Add-ons

	C	F	Cb
Milk: *Per 1/2 Cup, 4 fl.oz*			
Whole, 1/2 cup	80	4.5	6
2%, 1/2 cup	60	2.3	6
1%, 1/2 cup	50	1	6
Nonfat, 1/2 cup	43	0	6
Yogurt: *Per 1/2 Cup, 4 fl.oz*			
Plain: Whole	90	4	7
Skim	60	0	8
Yogurt, fruit: Whole, 1/2 cup	125	2.6	23
Lowfat, 1/2 cup	120	2	23
Nonfat, 1/2 cup	60	0	13
Soy Drink: Regular, 1/2 cup	65	2	4
Lite, 1/2 cup, 4 fl.oz	50	1	3
Fruit: Dried, average, 1 oz	80	0	21
Banana, 1/2 medium	50	0	23
Prunes in Syrup, 5, 3 oz	90	0	24
Honey: 1 Tbsp, 3/4 oz	65	0	17
Lecithin Granules, 1 Tbsp, 10g	50	5	1
Nuts: Almonds, 6 (1/4 oz)	40	4	5
Pollen (Bee) Granules, 1 T., 8g	25	1	2
Psyllium Husks, 1 Tbsp, 5g	10	0	1
Seeds: Sunflower, 1 Tbsp	65	6	2
Soy Grits, 1 Tbsp, 8g	32	1.5	3
Sugar: 1 heaping tsp	25	0	7
1 Tbsp, 12g	46	0	12

*S*tart the day right
with a high fiber breakfast
of cereals, milk/soy and fruit.

*It will help prevent
high-calorie snacking.*

Breakfast Cereals (Cont)

Ready-To-Eat

	C	F	Cb
Arrowhead: Amaranth, 1 c., 1.2oz	130	2	25
Bran Flakes, 1 cup, 1 oz	100	1	22
Kamut Flakes, 1 cup, 1.1 oz	120	1	25
Maple Corns, 1 cup, 1.9 oz	190	3	43
Multi Grain Flakes, 1 cup, 1.2 oz	140	2	29
Nature O's, 1 cup, 1.1 oz	120	1	24
Oat Bran Flakes, 1 cup, 1.2 oz	110	2	24
Puffed Corn/Rice, aver., 1 c., 0.8 oz	80	0	18
Puffed Kamut, 1 cup, 0.6 oz	50	0	11
Puffed Millet/Wheat, 1 cup, 0.9 oz	90	1	19
Puffed Rice, 1 cup, 0.8 oz	90	0	19
Spelt Flakes, 1 cup, 1.1 oz	100	1	22
Barbara's Bakery			
Breakfast O's, 1 cup, 1 oz	120	2	22
Brown Rice Crisps, 1 cup, 1 oz	120	1	25
Cinnamon Puffins, 3/4, 1 oz	100	1	26
Corn Flakes, all types, 1 cup, 1 oz	110	0	26
Fruity Punch, 1 cup, 1 oz	110	0.5	26
Organic Ultra Minis, 3/4 cup, 2 oz	190	1	46
Shredded Oats, 1 1/4 cup, 2 oz	220	2.5	46
Shredded Puffins, 3/4 cup, 1 oz	90	1	23
Shredded Spoonfuls, 3/4 cup	120	1.5	23
Shredded Wheat, 2 bisc., 1.4 oz	140	1	31
Stars: Cocoa/Honey Crunch, 1 c., 1oz	110	0.5	24
Toasted O's, average, 3/4 cup	120	2	24
Betty Crocker: Scooby Doo! 25g	80	0	21
Breadshop: Granola, 1/2 c. 1.7 oz	220	9	31
Flakes 'n Frostin', 3/4 cup, 1 oz	100	0	24
Kamut 'n Honey, 1 cup, 1 oz	120	3	22
Puffs 'n Honey, 1 cup, 1 oz	120	3	21
Shapes 'n Honey, 1 cup, 1 oz	110	0.5	24
Cap'n Crunch: All types, 3/4 cup	110	2	22
Chex: Corn, 1 1/4 cup, 1 oz	110	0	26
Wheat, 3/4 cup, 1.8 oz	190	1	41
Country Inn			
Green Gables Inn, 1/2 cup, 1.8 oz	210	7	36
Greyfield Inn, 3/4 cup, 1.8 oz	210	5	39
Inn at Ormsby Hill, 1 cup, 2.1 oz	220	2.5	48
Dominick's: Corn Flakes, 1 1/4 cup	120	0	27
Crispy Corn & Rice, 1 1/4 cup, 1 oz	120	0	26
Crispy Rice, 1 cup, 1 oz	130	0	28
Frosted Flakes, 3/4 cup, 1 oz	120	0	28
Fruit Rings, 3/4 cup, 1 oz	100	1	23
Tasteeos, 1 1/4 cup, 1 oz	120	2	24

Dr McDougall's	C	F	Cb
Oatmeal & Wheat, 1 cup, 2.4 oz	220	2	57
Oatmeal & 4 Grains, 1 cup, 2.3 oz	210	1.5	52
Erewhon			
Aztec, 1 oz	100	0	24
Crispy Brown Rice, 1 cup	110	1	24
Fruit 'n Wheat, 1 oz	100	1	21
Raisin Bran; Super O's, 1 oz	100	0	24
Wheat Flakes, 1 oz	100	0	22
Estee			
Corn Flakes, 1 oz pkg	90	0	24
Raisin Bran, 1 oz pkg	90	1	21
Familia: Muesli, 1/2 cup, 2.1 oz	210	3	45
No Added Sugar, 1/2 cup	200	3	41
Glenny's			
Maple Frosted Corn, 1 oz	110	0	20
Oat/Rice Mini Puffs, 1 oz	110	0	24
General Mills			
Basic 4, 1 c., 2 oz	200	3	43
Body Buddies, 1 cup, 1 oz	120	1	26
Boo Berry, 1 cup, 1 oz	120	1	27
Cheerios: Regular, 1 cup, 1 oz	110	2	22
Apple Cinnamon, 3/4 c., 1 oz	120	2	25
Frosted; Team, 1 cup, 1 oz	120	1	25
Honey Nut, 1 cup, 1 oz	120	1.5	24
Multi-Grain, 1 cup, 1 oz	110	1	24
Chex: Corn, 1 cup, 1 oz	110	0	26
Honey Nut, 3/4 cup, 1 oz	120	0.5	26
Multi-Bran, 1 cup, 2 oz	200	1.5	49
Rice, 1 1/4 cup, 1 oz	120	0	27
Wheat, 1 cup, 2 oz	180	1	41
Cinnamon Grahams, 3/4 c., 1 oz	120	1	26
Cinnamon Tst Crunch, 3/4 c., 1 oz	130	3.5	24
Cocoa Puffs, 1 cup, 1 oz	120	1	27
Cookie Crisp; Count Choc, 1 c., 1 oz	120	1	26
Count Chocula, 1 cup, 1 oz	120	1	26
Country Corn Flakes, 1 c., 1 oz	120	0	26
Crispy Wheaties 'N Rais., 1 c., 2 oz	190	1	45
Fiber One, 1/2 cup, 1 oz	60	1	24
Frankenberry, 1 cup, 1 oz	120	1	27
French Toast Crunch, 3/4 c., 1 oz	120	1.5	26
Golden Grahams, 3/4 cup, 1 oz	120	1	26
Grand Slams, 1 cup, 1 oz	120	1	26
Honey Nut Clusters, 1 cup, 2 oz	210	2.5	46
Jurrasic Park Crunch, 1 cup, 1 oz	120	1	26
Kaboom, 1 1/4 cup, 1 oz	120	1.5	24

Ready-To-Eat (Cont)

General Mills (Cont)

	C	F	Cb
Kix, 1¹/3 cup, 1 oz	120	0.5	26
Berry Berry, 3/4 cup, 1 oz	120	1.5	26
Lucky Charms, 1 cup, 1 oz	120	1	25
NesQuik: Choc Puff, 1 cup, 1 oz	120	2	25
Oatmeal Crisp Almond, 1 c., 2 oz	220	5	41
Apple Cinn.; Raisin, 1 cup, 2 oz	210	2.5	45
Raisin Nut Bran, 1 cup, 2 oz	200	4	41
Reese's P'nut Butter Puffs, 3/4 cup	130	3	24
Sunrise, 3/4 cup, 1 oz	110	0.5	26
Total Corn Flakes, 1¹/3 cup, 1 oz	110	0	26
Total Raisin Bran, 1 cup, 2 oz	180	1	43
Total Whole Grain, 1 cup, 1 oz	110	1	24
Trix, 1 cup, 1 oz	120	1.5	26
USA Olympic Crunch, 1 cup, 1 oz	120	1	26
Wheaties, 1 cup, 1 oz	110	1	24
Honey Frosted, 3/4 cup, 1 oz	110	0	27

Grist Mill

	C	F	Cb
Apple Cinn. Nat., 1/2 c., 1.9 oz	260	10	36
Bran, 1/2 cup, 1.9 oz	250	8	37
Oat & Honey Nat., 1/2 c., 1.9 oz	270	12	34
Oat Honey & Rais., 1/2 c., 1.9 oz	260	10	35

Healthy Choice

	C	F	Cb
M/grain Rais. & Almd, 3/4 c., 1 oz	100	1	22
Flakes, 1 cup, 1.1 oz	100	0	26

Heartland

	C	F	Cb
Granola: Lowfat, 1/2 cup, 2 oz	210	3	40
Original; Raisin, 1/2 cup, 2¹/4 oz	300	11	41

Health Valley

	C	F	Cb
Amaranth Flakes, 3/4 cup	100	0	24
Bran Cereal (w. Fruit), 3/4 cup	160	0	40
Corn Bran Flakes, 3/4 cup	100	0	24
Fiber 7 Flakes (100% Orig.), 3/4 c.	100	0	24
Golden Flax, 1/4 cup	190	3	38
Granola O's, all types, 3/4 cup	120	0	26
Healthy Crunches & Flakes, 3/4 c.	130	0	31
Healthy Fiber Flakes, 3/4 cup	100	0	23
Hot Cups: Maple; Banana, 1 pkt	240	2.5	46
Apple; 10 Grain, 1 pkt	220	2.5	42
98% Fat Free Granola 2/3 cup	180	1	43
Oat Bran Flakes, all types, 3/4 c.	105	0	26
Oat Bran/10 Bran O's, 3/4 cup	100	0	23
Puffed: Honey Sweetened, 1 cup	110	0	28
Raisin Bran Flakes, 1¹/4 cup	190	0	47
Real Oat Bran, 1/2 cup	200	3	34

Kashi

	C	F	Cb
Breakfast Pilaf, 1/2 c., ckd, 5 oz	170	3	30
Honey Puffed Kashi, 1 oz	120	1	25
Kashi Go, 1/2 cup, 5 oz	270	3	59
Kashi Good Friends, 3/4 cup, 1 oz	90	1	24
Kashi Medley, 1/2 cup, 1 oz	100	1	20
Kashi Pillows, 3/4 cup, 2 oz	200	1	45
Puffed Kashi, 1 cup, 0.9 oz	70	0.5	13

Kellogg's

	C	F	Cb
All-Bran, 1/2 cup, 1 oz	80	1	23
with Extra Fiber, 1/2 cup, 1 oz	50	0.5	20
Apple Cinn. Rice Krispies, 3/4 c.	110	0	26
Apple Cinn. Squares, 3/4 c., 2 oz	180	1	44
Apple Jacks, 1 cup, 1 oz	120	0	30
Apple Raisin Crisp, 1/2 cup, 1 oz	90	0	23
Blueberry Squares, 3/4 cup, 2 oz	180	1	43
Bran Buds, 1/3 cup, 1 oz	80	0.5	24
Cinnamon Mini Buns, 3/4 cup	120	0.5	27
Complete Bran Flakes, 3/4 cup	90	0.5	24
Cocoa Krispies, 3/4 cup	120	1	27
Common Sense O/Bran, 3/4 cup	110	1	23
Corn Flakes, 1 cup, 1 oz	110	0	24
Honey Crunch, 3/4 cup, 1 oz	120	1	26
Corn Pops, 1 cup, 1 oz	120	0	28
Cracklin' Oat Bran, 3/4 c., 2 oz	190	6	36
Crispix, 1 cup, 1 oz	110	0	25
Double Dip Crunch, 3³/4 cup	110	0	25
Froot Loops, 1 cup	120	1	28
Marshmallow Blasted, 1 c., 1 oz	120	0.5	27
w. Jungleberry Swirls, 1 c., 1.1 oz	120	1	28
Frosted: Bran, 3/4 cup, 1 oz	100	0	26
Flakes, 3/4 cup, 1 oz	120	0	28
Krispies, 3/4 cup, 1 oz	100	0	24
Mini-Wheats, 1/2 cup, 1 oz	85	0.7	19
Bite Size, 1 cup, 1 oz	200	1	48
Fruity Marshmallow Krispies, 3/4 c.	110	0	25
Healthy Choice:			
Almond Crunch 1/4 cup	210	2	50
Golden Multi-Grn Flakes, 3/4 c.	110	0	26
Tst Brown Sugar Sq., 1 cup	190	1	44
Just Right, all varieties, 1 cup, 2 oz	210	1.5	47
Low Fat Granola: 1/2 cup, 2 oz	190	3	39
w. Raisins, 3/4 cup, 2 oz	220	3	47
Mueslix: Apple & Almond, 3/4 c.	200	5	39
Raisin & Almond, 2/3 cup	200	3	40
Nut & Honey Crunch, 1¹/4 c., 2 oz	220	2.5	46
Nutri-Grain: Almond, 1¹/4 c., 2 oz	180	3	38
Golden Wheat, 3/4 cup, 1 oz	100	1	24

Breakfast Cereals (Cont)

Kellogg's (Cont)	C	F	Cb
Pop Tarts: Crunch, 1 cup	130	1	29
Toaster Pastries, average, 1 oz	210	6	37
Mini Pastries, aver., 1 pouch	170	7	31
Pastry Swirls, 2.2 oz	260	11	37
Product 19, 1 cup, 1 oz	100	0	25
Raisin Bran, 1 cup	200	1.5	47
Raisin Bran Crunch, 1¹/4 c., 2.1 oz	210	1	50
Raisin Squares, 3/4 cup, 2 oz	180	1.5	41
Rice Krispies, 1¹/4 cup	120	0	29
Treats, 3/4 cup	120	1.5	26
Razzle Dazzles, 3/4 cup, 1 oz	110	0	25
Smacks, 3/4 cup	100	0.5	24
Smart Start Multigrain, 1 c., 1.8 oz	180	0.5	43
Special K, 1 cup	110	0	22
Strawberry Squares, 3/4 cup, 2 oz	170	2	40
Temptations: Fr. Van. Alm., 3/4 c.	100	1.5	21
Honey Rst. Pecan, 2/3 c., 1 oz	120	0.5	24
La Loma: Ruskets, 2 biscuit, 1 oz	110	0	22
Mueslix: Crispy Blend, 2/3 c., 1.9oz	200	2	44
Nabisco: 100% Bran, 1/3 cup, 1 oz	70	1	21
Cream of Wheat:			
Banana Nut Bread, 1 pkg, 1.4 oz	150	1.5	32
Muffin; Cobbler, 1 pkg, 1.3 oz	140	1	32
Cocoa Blasts, 1 cup	130	1	29
Fruit Wheats, 1/2 cup, 1 oz	90	0	23
Shredded Wheat: 1 biscuit	80	0.5	19
Spoon size, 2/3 cup, 1 oz	90	1	23
Shredded Wheat'n Bran, 2/3 cup	90	0	23
Shredd. Wheat w. Oatbran, 1 oz	100	1	22
Team Flakes, 3/4 cup, 1 oz	110	0	24
Nature's Path: Corn Flakes, 3/4 c.	115	0.5	26
Heritage: all varieties, 3/4 c., 1 oz	115	0	24
Heritage Muesli, 1/2 cup, 2 oz	215	3	41
Honey'd Raisin Bran, 3/4 cup, 1 oz	110	0	25
Mesa Sunrise: all variet., 3/4 c., 1 oz	130	2	25
Millet Rice, 3/4 cup, 1 oz	120	1	25
Multigrain, 2/3 cup, 1 oz	110	0.5	24
New Morning			
Fruite-O's, 1 cup, 1oz	120	1	25
Bran Flakes; Crispy Rice, 1 c., 1 oz	110	1	23
Cocoa Crispy Rice, 1 cup, 2.1 oz	210	1.5	45
Corn/Honey Frost. Flakes, 1 c.	120	1	25
Ginky O's; Orig. Otios, 1 c., 1 oz	120	1	21
Granola Clusters, 3/4 c., 1.9 oz	200	2	42
Otiola: Blueberry, 1 cup, 1.9 oz	200	1.5	41

New Morning (Cont):	C	F	Cb
Otios: Cocoa, 1 cup, 1.76 oz	170	1.5	21
Apple Cinnamon, 1 cup, 1 oz	90	1.5	21
Honey Almond, 1 cup, 1 oz	100	1	22
Original, 1 cup, 1 oz	120	1	22
Raisin Bran, 1 cup, 30g	90	0.5	22
Ultimate Oat Bran Flakes, 1 c., 28g	110	1	21
Nutlettes: 1/2 cup, 1.8 oz	140	1.5	15
Pillsbury: Toaster Strudel, 54g	180	8	26
Post: Alpha Bits, 1 cup	110	1	24
Cocoa Pebbles, 7/8 cup	115	1	25
Great Grains, 2/3 cup, 1.8 oz	210	5	39
Fruit & Fiber, 1 cup	210	3	46
Grape Nut 'O's, 1 cup, 1.1 oz	120	0	28
Grape Nuts; Raisin, 1/4 cup	105	0	23
Honey Bunches of Oats, 3/4 cup	120	1.5	25
Honey Nut Shredd. Wheat, 1 c.,1.8oz	200	2	43
Natural Bran Flakes, 2/3 cup	90	0	23
Oat Flakes, 2/3 cup	105	1	22
Oreo O's, 3/4 cup	110	2.5	21
Raisin Bran, 2/3 cup, 1.4 oz	120	1	32
Waffle Crisp, 1 cup	130	3	24
Pritikin: 10-Grain, 1¹/2 c., 1 oz	110	1	24
Quaker			
Ready to Eat: Oat Bran, 1¹/4 cup	210	3	41
Cap'n Crunch, aver. all types, 3/4 c.	105	1.5	22
Life, all types, 3/4 cup	120	1.5	26
Oatmeal Squares, 1 cup	225	2.5	45
100% Natural Granola, 1/2 cup	220	9	31
Lowfat, 2/3 cup	210	3	44
w. Raisins, 1/2 cup	230	9	34
Popeye: Puffed Rice; Wheat, 1 cup	50	0	12
Quisp, 1 cup	110	1.5	23
Shredded Wheat, 3 bisc.	220	1.5	50
Toasted Oatmeal, 1 cup	190	2.5	39
Unprocessed Bran, 1/3 cup	30	0	11
Quaker by the Bag:			
Apple Zaps; Fruitany O's, 1 cup	120	1	27
Cocoa Blasts, 1 cup	130	1	29
Frosted Flakers, 3/4 cup	120	0	28
Frosted/Honey Nut Oats, 1 cup	110	1	24
Frosted Oats/ Sweet Crunch, 1 cup	110	1.5	23
Fruitangy Oh's, 1 cup	120	1	27
Honey Crisp Corn Flakes, 3/4 cup	110	0	27
Marshmallow Safari, 3/4 cup	120	1.5	25
Rice Crisps, 1 cup	110	0	26

Quaker (Cont)

Grits: Per Packet

	C	F	Cb
Regular: All types, aver., 1/4 cup	130	0.5	31
Instant: All types, average	100	1	22

Instant Quaker Oatmeal: Per Pkt

	C	F	Cb
Oatmeal: Regular, 1 oz	100	2	19
Cinnamon & Spice, 1 1/2 oz	150	2	33
Cookie Blast, average, 1 1/2 oz	160	2.5	32
Maple/Br.Sug; Rais./Spice	160	2	33
Raisin/Date/Walnut, 1 1/4 oz	140	2	27
Average other varieties	135	2	27
Dinosaur Eggs, 50g pkt	200	4	37
Kid's Choice: 1 pkt, aver., 1 1/2 oz	160	2.5	32
Sea Adventures, 1 pkt, 1 1/2 oz	190	4	37

Quick'n Hearty (Microwave Oatmeal): Per Pkt

	C	F	Cb
Regular, 1 oz	110	2	19
App.Spice; Cinnamon Dble Raisin	170	2	35
Br.Sugar Cinnamon; Honey Bran	150	2	30
Quaker/Hot: Multigrain, 1/2 cup	130	1.5	29
Oat Bran, 1/2 cup	150	3	25
Whole Wheat Hot Nat. 1/2 cup	130	1	30
Oats: Quick/ Old Fash., Steel, 1/2 c.	150	3	27

Other Quaker Brands

	C	F	Cb
Honey Graham Oh's, 3/4 cup	110	2	23
King Vitaman, 1 1/2 cup	120	1	26
Kretschmer: Wheat Bran, 1/4 cup	30	1	18
Wheat Germ, all types, 2 Tbsp	50	1	6
Mother's: Hot Cereals, 1/2 cup	130	1.5	27
Oatbran; Oatmeal, 1/2 cup	150	3	3
Sun Country Granola: Almd, 1/2 c.	270	9	38
w. Raisins & Dates, 1/2 cup	260	8	43

Ralston: Bran Flakes, 3/4 cup, 1 oz	110	1	24
Chex Multi Bran, 1 1/4 cup, 2 oz	220	2	46
Cocoa Crispy Rice, 1 c., 1 3/4 oz	200	1	45
Cookie Crisp, 1 cup, 1 oz	120	2	25
Frosted Flakes, 3/4 cup, 1 oz	120	0	28
Hot Ralston, 1/2 cup, 1.5 oz	150	1	31
Muesli: Blueberry, 1 cup, 2 oz	200	3	41
Cranberry, 3/4 cup, 2 oz	200	3	40
Strawberry, 1 cup, 2 oz	210	3	41
Raisin Bran, 3/4 cup, 2 oz	190	1	41
Sun Flakes, 3/4 cup	110	1	33
Tasteeos, 1 1/4 cup, 1 oz	130	3	22

Stone-Buhr: Bran, 1/4 c., 0.5 oz	65	0	14
7 Grain, 1/3 cup, 1 1/2 oz	140	2	31

Uncle Sam: Wheat/Flaxseed, 1 c.	190	5	38

US Mills: Aver. all varieties, 1 oz	110	1	23

Grains & Flours

Per 1/2 Cup (8 level Tbsp)

	C	F	Cb
Amaranth, 1/2 cup, 3 1/2 oz	350	6	60
Arrowroot, 1/2 cup, 2 1/4 oz	230	0	57
Barley: Regular, 1/2 cup, 3 1/4 oz	325	2	56
Pearled, raw, 1/2 cup, 3 1/4 oz	350	1	78
Flakes, 1/2 cup, 1 1/2 oz	150	0.5	33
Buckwheat: Regular, 1/2 c., 3 oz	290	3	61
Groats, roasted, dry, 3 oz	285	2	60
Roasted, cooked, 3 1/2 oz	90	0.5	19
Flour, whole-groat	200	2	42
Bulgur: Dry, 1/2 cup, 2 1/2 oz	240	1	54
Cooked, 1/2 cup, 3 1/4 oz	75	0.5	17
Carob Flour, 1/2 cup, 1.8 oz	95	0.5	25
Corn kernels (blue/yellow), 3 oz	300	4	66
Corn Bran, 1/2 cup, 1.4 oz	85	0.5	32
Corn Flour/Masa, 2 oz	210	2	44
Corn Grits:			
Dry, 1/2 cup, 2 3/4 oz	290	1	62
Cooked, 1/2 cup, 4 1/4 oz	75	0.5	16
Corn Germ, toasted	245	13	21
Cornmeal: Average All Types			
3 Tbsp, 1 oz	100	0.5	22
1/2 c., 2.2 oz	220	2	46
Mixes: same as above	220	2	46
Cornstarch: 1 Tbsp, 8g	30	0	7
1/2 cup, 2 1/4 oz	230	0	57
Couscous: Dry, 3 1/4 oz	345	0	72
Cooked, 4.1 oz	60	0	12
Farina: Dry, 3 oz	325	1	70
Cooked, 4.1 oz	60	0	13
Flax Seeds, 2 oz	280	20	22
Garbanzo (Chick Pea), 1/2 c., 2 oz	200	3	35
Matzo Meal, 1/2 cup	260	1	55
Millet: raw, 1/2 cup, 3 1/4 oz	375	4	76
Cooked, 1/2 cup, 4 1/4 oz	145	1	29
Oat Bran: Raw, 1/2 cup, 1.7 oz	115	2	31
Cooked, 1/2 cup, 4 oz	115	1	33
Oats, rolled/oatmeal:			
Dry, 1/2 cup, 1.5 oz	155	3	28
Cooked, 1/2 cup, 4.2 oz	75	1	13
Polenta: See Cornmeal			
Made Up, 1/2 cup, 5 oz	220	2	24
Potato flour, 1/2 cup, 3.2 oz	315	0	72
Psyllium Husks, 1 Tbsp (5g)	10	0	7
Quinoa, 1/2 cup, 3 oz	320	5	53
Eden, 1/2 cup, 3 oz	340	5	62
Rice: See Next Page			

Grains & Flours (Cont)

	C	F	Cb
Rice Bran, 1/3 cup, 1 oz	90	6	14
Rice Flour, 1/2 cup, 2 3/4 oz	290	2	63
Rice Polish, 1/2 cup	220	7	39
Rye Grains:			
1/2 cup, 3 oz	280	2	59
Flakes, 1/2 cup, 1 1/2 oz	150	0.5	32
Flour, dark, 2 1/4 oz	210	2	44
Medium light, 1.8 oz	185	1	40
Semolina, 1/2 cup, 3 oz	305	1	61
Sorghum, 1/2 cup, 3.4 oz	325	3	72
Soybean Flakes, 1/2 cup, 1 1/2 oz	190	8	14
Soy Flour, 1/2 cup, 2 oz	250	11	18
Tapioca, pearl, Dry: 1/2 cup, 2. 7oz	260	0	67
3 Tbsp, 1 oz	100	1	26
Teff (Seed) Flour, 2 oz	200	0.5	41
Tortilla Flour Mix, 1/2 cup, 2 oz	225	12	37
Triticale, 1/2 cup, 3.4 oz	325	2	70
flour, whole-grain, 1/2 cup	220	1	47
Wheat: Average, 1/2 cup, 3 1/2 oz	320	2	28
Wheat Bran, unproc., 1/2 c., 1 oz	65	1	20
Wheat Flakes, 1/2 cup, 1 1/2 oz	160	0.5	32
Wheat Germ: Crude, 2 oz	200	8	29
toasted, 1/2 cup, 2 oz	215	12	28
Wheat Flour: Whole grain, 2.1 oz	205	1	44
White, all types, 1/2 c., 2.2 oz	220	0.5	46

Also See *Arrowhead Mills Cereals* ~ Page 88

"I got the idea while down at the bank."

ENGLEMAN

Brown Rice

Average Short or Long Grain

	C	F	Cb
Raw/Dry: 1/2 cup, 3 1/2 oz	350	2.5	72
1 cup, 7 oz	700	5	144
Cooked: Hot, 1/2 cup, 3 1/2 oz	110	0.5	23
1 cup, 7 oz	220	1.5	46
Cold, 1/2 cup, 2 1/2 oz	90	0.5	19

White Rice

	C	F	Cb
Raw: Short/Med. Grain, 1 c., 7 oz	720	1	156
Long Grain, 1 cup, 6 1/2 oz	670	1	144
Glutinous, 1 cup, 6 1/2 oz	680	1	150
Cooked (Boiled/Steamed):			
Short/Medium Grain:			
Hot, 1/2 cup, 3 1/4 oz	120	0	27
1 cup, 6 1/2 oz	240	0.5	54
Cold, 1/2 cup, 2 3/4 oz	90	0	20
Long Grain: Hot, 1/2 c., 2 3/4 oz	100	0	22
1 cup, 5 1/2 oz	200	0.5	44
Cold, 1/2 cup, 2 1/2 oz	80	0	17
Glutinous, 1 cup, 6 oz	170	0.5	36
Parboiled, ckd, hot, 1/2 c., 3 oz	90	0	20
Precook./Instant: Dry, 1/2 c., 3 1/2 oz	370	0	80
Cooked, Hot, 1/2 cup, 3 oz	90	0	20
Wild Rice: Raw, 1 cup, 5 1/2 oz	570	13	120
Cooked, hot, 1 cup, 5 3/4 oz	165	0.5	35

Rice Dishes

	C	F	Cb
Chinese Fried Rice: 1/2 c., 2 1/2 oz	160	5	21
1 cup, 5 oz	320	13	42
2 cups, 10 oz	640	26	84
Mexican Rice: 1 cup	500	12	90
Taco Bell, 1 serving	190	10	20
Taco John's, 1 serving	350	18	40
Taco Time, 1 serving	160	2	28
Rice-A-Roni ~ See Page 66			
Rice Pilaf: Restaurant, 1 cup	270	7.5	43
Boston Market, 2/3 cup	180	5	32
Denny's, 1 serving	110	2	21
Sizzler, side serving	260	5	47
Rice w. Raisins/Pinenuts, 1 cup	400	11	70
Risotto, 1 cup	420	18	65
Saffron Rice, 1 cup	370	12	66
Spanish Rice, 1 cup	390	9	72
El Pollo Loco, 1 serving	130	3	24
Sticky Thai Rice, 1 cup	750	28	121
Sushi Rice, 1 Tbsp	25	0	6

- Macaroni includes all shapes and sizes; (e.g. spaghetti, fettuccini, shells, tubes, ziti, twists, sheets, cannelloni, manicotti, elbows).
- All regular macaroni products have the same cals/fat/carb. on a weight basis.
- 1 oz Dry = approx. 2¹/₂ -3 oz cooked.

Dry Spaghetti/Macaroni

	C	F	Cb
1 oz quantity	105	0.5	21
1lb box/pkg., 16 oz	1680	7	336
Elbows, 1 cup, 3³/₄ oz	395	2	77
Shells, small, 1 cup, 3¹/₄ oz	340	2	66
Spirals, 1 cup, 3 oz	315	2	61

Cooked Spaghetti/Macaroni

Plain, All Types (no added fat):

	C	F	Cb
Firm/Al Dente (8-10 mins.), 1 oz	42	0.5	8.5
Medium (11-13mins.), 1 oz	37	0.5	7.5
Tender (14-20mins.), 1 oz	32	0.5	7
(Longer cooking increases water absorbed)			
Spaghetti, ¹/₂ cup, 2 ¹/₂ oz	90	0.5	18
Medium serving, 1 cup, 5 oz	185	1	37
Large (restaurant), 2 c., 10 oz	370	2	74
Elbows/Spirals, 1 cup, 5 oz	185	1	38
Small Shells, 1 cup, 4 oz	150	0.5	31
Protein-fortified: Dry, 1 oz	107	0.5	21
Cooked, 1 cup, 5 oz	230	0.5	44
Spinach/Vegetable: Dry, 1 oz	105	0.5	21
Cooked, 1 cup, 5 oz	180	0.5	37
Whole-wheat: Dry, 1 oz	100	0.5	21
Cooked, 1 cup, 5 oz	175	0.5	37

Fresh Pasta (Refrigerated)

Plain/Spinach/Tomato, average:

	C	F	Cb
As purchased, 4 oz	325	2.5	64
Cooked, 1 cup, 5 oz	190	1	38
Home-made, without egg:			
Cooked, 1 cup, 5 oz	175	1	35

Other Spaghetti/Pasta Listings:
Frozen Foods, Pp. 55; Canned, Pp. 64
Restaurant Dishes - Italian, Pp. 156
Spaghetti Sauces - Sauces, Pp. 79
Pasta Roni - Canned/Packaged Foods, Pp. 66

Noodles

	C	F	Cb
Plain/Egg:			
Dry, 1 oz	108	1	20
1 cup, 1¹/₃ oz	145	1.5	28
Cooked, 1 oz	38	0.5	7
¹/₂ cup, 2³/₄ oz	105	1	20
1 cup, 5¹/₂ oz	210	2	40
Yolk Free: *Cooked, Per Cup*			
'No Yolks' *(Foulds)*	210	2	40
Passover Gold *(Manischewitz)*	200	0	42
Chinese:			
Cellophane/Rice, dry, 1 oz	100	0	25
Chow Mein/hard, dry, 1 oz	150	5	17
Japanese:			
Soba, dry, 1 oz	95	0.5	21
cooked, 1 cup, 4 oz	110	0.5	24
Somen, dry, 1 oz	100	0.5	22
cooked, 1 cup, 6 oz	225	0.5	49
Japanese Style Pan Fried:			
Maruchan's Yaki-Sobu,			
1 cup, 5.6 oz	260	3	50
Udon *(Chikara)*, aver., 7.5 oz pkt	250	1	52
Stir Fry/Yakisoba, 1 serve, 3.5 oz	220	2	44

Egg Roll Skins/Won Ton

	C	F	Cb
Egg Roll Skins:			
(Golden Dragon) 1 pce, 1 oz	80	0	18
(Wung Hung) 4 skins, 4 oz	300	0	64
Won Ton Wrappers:			
(Dynasty) 10 wrappers, 2.1 oz	170	1	36
Egg Roll/Spring Roll Wrapper:			
(Dynasty) 3 wrappers, 2.1 oz	170	1	36

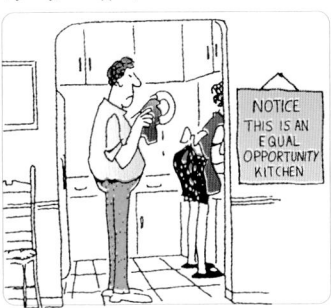

NOTICE
THIS IS AN
EQUAL
OPPORTUNITY
KITCHEN

Breads

Note: All breads have similar calories on a weight basis. However, volume may vary. For example, 1 oz of bread may equal 1 slice regular bread or 2 slices of a lighter bread. It is best to weigh bread used and calculate on 1 oz bread = 70 calories.

Quick Guide   C F Cb

Bread

Average All Varieties:

	C	F	Cb
Thin slice (1/4") 1 oz	70	1	13
Extra thin slice 3/4 oz	55	<1	10
Light thin slice, 0.6 oz	40	<1	7.5
Toasting slice, 1.2 oz	85	1	16
Thick slice (3/8"), 1.5 oz	105	1.5	20
Large thick (1/2"), 2 oz	140	2	26
1-lb Loaf, 16 oz	1120	6	208

Toast has same calories as bread used.

	C	F	Cb
1 thin slice + 1 tsp of fat	105	5	13
1 thick slice (3/8") +2 tsp fat	175	10	20

Breads

	C	F	Cb
Batard (8 oz), 1/4, 2 oz slice	140	0.5	28
Boule, 1/2" thick, 2 oz slice	130	0	29
Bran style, 1 oz slice	70	1	14
Buttermilk, average, 1 oz slice	80	2	13
Caraway Rye, 1 oz slice	70	0	15
Challah, 1 oz slice	85	2	14
Corn Bread, aver., 1 pce., 3 oz	180	7	36
Cracked Wheat Sourdough, 1 1/2 oz	130	0.5	27
Croutons, 2 Tbsp	35	1	6
Dark Bread, 1 oz slice	70	1	14
Date & Nut, 1 oz slice	90	1	14
'Enriched' Breads, aver., 1 oz sl.	75	1	18
5-Grain Honey Whole Wheat, 1 slice, 1 1/2 oz	110	1	23
Foccacia: Plain, 2 oz portion	150	4	23
Cheese & Garlic, 2 oz	170	8	21
Pesto, 2 oz	170	6	21
Tomato & Olive, 2 oz	120	2	20
French Stick, 1 oz slice	70	1	15
French Toast, 1 slice, 2 1/4 oz	160	7	14
Sticks (*Aunt Jemima*), 1 pce, 1 oz	75	3	12
Garlic Bread, 1 pce. w. fat, 1 oz	125	6	14
Garlic Toast, (*Pepp.Farm*), 1.4 oz sl.	160	10	15
Italian Bread, 1 oz slice	75	1	15
Light Bread, aver., 0.8 oz slice	40	<1	7.5
1 oz slice	70	1	13
Melba Toast, 2 pces	25	0	6

Breads   C F Cb

	C	F	Cb
MultiGrain: 1 slice, 1 oz	75	1	14
Fat Free, 1 oz	70	0	15
Nut/Health Nut, 1 oz slice	85	2	15
Oatmeal/Oatbran Bread, 1 oz sl.	70	1	13
Party Breads (*Pepp. Farm*): Rye, 1 sl.	15	<1	8
Dijon; Pumpernickel, 1 sl.	18	<1	3.5
Pita Bread, aver. all types, 2 oz	150	2	30
Mini/Pocket, 1 oz	75	1	15
Poppyseed (Vienna), 0.8 oz sl.	55	1	10
Pumpernickel, 1 oz slice	75	1	15
Cocktail size, 0.4 oz	30	<1	6
Raisin Bread, 1 oz slice	80	1	14
Raisin Walnut, 2 oz slice	160	3.5	29
Roman Meal, 1 oz slice	70	1	14
Country Potato & Oat, 1 1/2 oz	110	1.5	20
Rye, average., 1 thin slice, 1 oz	75	1	13
1 thick slice, 2 oz	150	2	25
Cocktail size, 0.4 oz	25	<1	4
Sandwich Bread, 1 oz slice	70	1	13
Sandwich Pockets: Reg., 2 oz	150	1	30
Sourdough, 1 oz slice	70	1	12
Wheat/Cracked Wheat, 1 oz sl.	75	1	14

Bread Rolls & Buns

	C	F	Cb
Brown 'n Serve, average, 1 oz	80	2	15
Dinner Rolls: 1 small, 1 oz	85	2	15
1 medium (3" diam), 1 1/2 oz	130	3	23
English Muffins, aver., 2 oz	140	2	27
Frankfurter/Hot Dog: 1 1/4 oz	100	2	19
1 1/2 oz size	120	2	23
French: 1 medium, 1.3 oz	110	1	24
1 large, 3 oz	240	2	52
Hamburger: Regular, 1 1/2 oz	120	2	23
Large, 3 oz	240	4	46
Hoagie/Submarine, 4 3/4 oz	400	8	77
Kaiser Roll, 2 oz size	170	3	18
Onion Roll, 2 oz size	170	2	18
Parker House Roll, 0.7 oz size	65	1	12
Party Roll, 1 oz	55	1	10
Sandwich Roll, 1.6 oz size	120	2	23
Soft Pretzel Bun (*J & J*), 3 oz	235	3	50
Sourdough Roll, 1 1/4 oz	100	1	18
Sweet Rolls, 1 oz	100	2	20
w. Icing, average	160	6	20
Wheat Roll: Small, 1 oz	75	0.5	14
Medium, 1 1/2 oz	110	1	20

Quick Guide · C · F · Cb

Bagels

Average All Brands

Plain/Onion:

	C	F	Cb
1 mini/bagelette, 1 oz	80	<1	15
1 small bagel, 2 oz	160	1.5	30
1 medium bagel, 3 oz	240	2	45
1 large bagel, 4 oz	320	3	60
Bagel Chips (New York Style), 4 slices, 3/4 oz	90	2	17
Pizza Bagel, 6 oz each	380	7	60
Bagel Bites (Ore-Ida), 4 pces	190	7	25
Bagel Crisps (Burns Ricker), 1 oz	150	9	28

Bagel Brands

	C	F	Cb
Amy's Kitchen, aver., 3 1/2 oz	235	2	50
Awrey's, 2.7 oz each	190	0.5	41
Cosco Bakery: Plain, 4 oz	300	1	61
Everything, 4 oz	330	3.5	62
Lenders, all flavors, 3.6 oz	280	3	55
Oroweat: Oatmeal, 3.4 oz	270	4	49
Multi-Grain, 3.4 oz	260	1.5	51
Sara Lee: Mini, average, 1 oz	80	0	15
Toaster Size, all types, 2.2 oz	160	0.5	33
(95g) 3.4 oz Size: Egg	260	2	50
Other flavors, 3.4 oz	260	1	55
(113g) 4 oz Size:			
Apple Cinnamon	310	1.5	64
Banana Walnut	350	7	61
Chocolate Chip	320	3.5	61
Cranberry Orange	310	1.5	64
Honey & Oat	310	2	61
New York Style, 4 1/2 oz	330	1	69
Sun Dried Tomato Basil	300	1.5	61
The Works	330	3.5	62
Western: All flavors, aver., 3 oz	230	1	47

Bagels ~ see Einstein Bros Bagels, Pp 191
Bagel Sandwiches ~ See Pp 160

Bagel Spreads

	C	F	Cb
Cream Cheese: Plain, 1 oz	80	8	2
Reduced Fat, 1 oz	60	5	2
Flavors: Lox, 1 oz	75	6	1
Raisin Walnut, 1 oz	90	6	8
Strawberry, 1 oz	60	3	7
Sundried Tomato, 1 oz	80	7	2
Vegetable, 1 oz	60	6	1

Bread Products · C · F · Cb

	C	F	Cb
Bread Crumbs, dry:			
Plain or seasoned, 1 oz	110	1	20
1 rounded Tbsp, 10g	35	<1	6
1 cup, 3 1/2 oz	390	5	73
Corn Flake Crumbs, 1 oz	110	1	20
Graham Cracker Crumbs, 1 oz	115	1	21
Keebler, 1 cup, 4 1/4 oz	520	14	84
Bread Dough: Frozen, 1 slice	75	<1	14
Refrigerated, French, 1" sl.	60	1	13
Wheat/White, 1" sl.	80	2	14
Breadsticks: Boboli, 1.75 oz	130	2	22
Stella D'oro: Sesame, (1)	50	2	7
Plain/Onion/Wheat, 1 pce.	40	1	7
Keebler/Lance, 2 sticks	30	<1	4
Salt Sticks, plain, 1 oz	110	1	20
Croutons: Aver. all brands, 1 oz	100	3	17
2 Tbsp, 10g	35	1	6
Coating Mixes:			
Seasoned, average, 1 oz	110	3	20
Featherweight, 1.4 oz pkg	72	<1	17
Pretzels: See Snacks ~ Page 124			
Stuffing: Average, dry miz, 1 oz	110	1	10
Made-up, 1/2 cup, 4 oz	180	9	11

Croissants: *See Page 104*

Rice Cakes

Average All Types/Brands:

	C	F	Cb
Regular size, 1 cake, 9g	35	0	7.5
Hain, Mini, average, 3g each	12	<1	2
Lundberg, all types, 15g each	60	<1	14
Quaker, large, all flavors, 13g each	50	0	11

Taco Shells

	C	F	Cb
Regular size, all types, each	55	3	6
Super Size, each	100	6	10
Mini Size, 1 taco	25	1.5	2
Salad Shell, flour (*Azteca*), 1.4 oz	180	11	19
Tortilla (Soft Taco), each	85	2	15
Corn Tortilla: 6", 1.2 oz each	45	0.5	9
Flour Tortilla: each, 1.75 oz	160	3	28
Lowfat	110	1.5	22
Burritos, 1 tortilla, 2.3 oz	190	5	32
Lowfat	110	1.5	22
Tostada Shells, each	55	3	6

95

Crispbreads

C F Cb

Per Crispbread/Cracker

	C	F	Cb
Ak-Mak: Sesame, 5 crackers, 1 oz	35	0	7
Finn Crisp: Original, rye,1	35	0	7
Other types,1	19	0	3
Kavli Norwegian: Thin,1	17	0	3
Thick,1	20	0	3
Malsovit, Meal Wafers.1	75	4	7
New York Flatbread Crisps, 1	35	0	7
Ry-Krisp: Natural, 1 crispbread	20	0	5
Seasoned,1	30	0	5
Sesame,1	25	1	3
Ryvita: Dark/Light, 1 piece	26	0	4
WASA: Breakfast; Sesame	50	0	9
Extra Crisp; Light Rye	25	0	5
Hearty Rye	45	0	9
Organic Rye	25	0	7
Sourdough Flatbread, 3	50	0	11
Sourdough Rye	35	0	7

Matzos

Manischewitz

	C	F	Cb
American Matzos, 1 board, 1 oz	115	2	22
Passover Matzos, 1 board, 1.1 oz	130	0	27
Passover Egg Matzos, 1.1 oz	130	2	27
Egg 'n Onion Matzo, 1 oz	112	1	23
Thin Salted Tea Matzos, 0.9 oz	100	0	21
Unsalted; Whole Wheat, 1 oz	110	0	24
Dietetic Matzo Thins, 0.83 oz	90	0	19
Crackers: Miniatures, 1 cracker	9	0	20
Passover Egg Matzo, 1 cracker	11	0	20
Matzo Meal, 1 cup, 4³/4 oz	515	2	110
Matzo Farfel, 1 cup, 2.7 oz	180	0.5	60
Grape Matzo, 1 oz each	110	0	25

Paul "Cookie" James — World's Biggest Cookie!

Quick Guide

Crackers

C F Cb

Average All Brands: Per Cracker

	C	F	Cb
Cheese Crackers:			
Plain, 1" square	5	0	0.5
Small, octagonal	10	0	1
Round (2" diam.)	15	0	1.5
Sandwich (Peanut Butter)	35	1	4
Graham, 2¹/2" square,1 cracker	30	0.5	5
Melba Toast, plain, 1 piece	20	0	4
Oyster & Soup crackers, ¹/4 oz	60	2	10
(40 small oysters/20 lge hexagons)			
Rice Crackers: 1 small	9	0	2
Rice Snax (*Amsnack*), ¹/2 oz	60	1	12
Saltines, 2 crackers	25	1	4.5
Snack-type, 1 round cracker	15	0	3
Soda, 1 cracker, ¹/2 oz	60	2	10
Water (*Carr's*), regular, 1 cracker	32	0	7
Bite-size, 1 cracker	13	0	4
Wheat, thin, 1 cracker	9	0	1
Zwieback Toast, 1 piece	30	0	5

Quick Guide

Cookies

C F Cb

Average All Brands: Per Cookie

	C	F	Cb
Biscotti: Almond, 2.5 oz	55	2	8
Chocolate Chip Cookies:			
Small/Thin 0.5 oz	55	3	7
Regular, 1 oz	110	6	15
Large, 2.5 oz (*Mrs Field's*)	280	14	40
Jumbo, 4 oz	450	22	64
Oatmeal/Oatmeal Raisin:			
Small/Thin 0.5 oz	50	1.5	8
Regular, 1 oz	95	3.5	15
Large, 2.5 oz (*Mrs Field's*)	240	9	39
Jumbo, 4 oz	380	14	62
Peanut Butter:			
Small/Thin 0.5 oz	60	3	7
Regular, 1 oz	125	6.5	14
Large, 2.5 oz (*Mrs Field's*)	310	16	34
Jumbo, 4 oz	500	25	54
Lowfat Cookies			
Choc Chip (Lowfat), 1 oz (1)	100	1	21
Oatmeal Raisin (Fat-free), 1 oz (1)	90	0	20
Peanut Butter (Lowfat), 1 oz (1)	105	2	14

Brands

Per Cookie/Cracker (Unless Indicated)

	C	F	Cb
Archway			
Apple/Date-filled Oatmeal	100	3	16
Apricot/Cherry-filled Oatmeal	100	3.5	16
Aunt Bea's Pound Cake Cookie	90	3.5	14
Coconut Macaroon	100	6	12
Chocolate Chip: Regular	130	6	19
Sugar Free	110	5	16
Fat-Free: Lemon Nuggets (4)	110	0	27
Cinnamon Honey Heart (3)	110	0	25
Devil's Food Cookie (1)	70	0	16
Oatmeal Raisin (1)	110	0	25
Sugar Cookies (1)	100	3	16
Frosty Lemon	110	4.5	17
Fruit & Honey Bar	100	3.5	17
Ginger Snaps: Regular (5)	140	4.5	22
Reduced Fat (5)	140	3.5	24
Iced (5)	170	7	26
Lemon Snaps (5)	150	7	20
Molasses	100	3	18
Oatmeal: Regular; Raisin	110	3.5	17
Iced	120	5	19
Pecan	140	7	16
Ol' Fashioned Peanut Butter	120	6	15
Old Fashioned Windmill	90	3.5	14
Peanut Jumble	110	6	13
Pecan Icebox	120	1.5	15
Ruth's Oatmeal	110	4	17
Holiday Favorites: Nougat (3)	170	12	16
Coconut Macaroon 22g each	100	6	12
Austin: *Per Serving*			
Big Munch Wafer Bar, each	200	2.5	24
Cheese/Toast/Wheat Crackers, w. filling			
all types, average	200	2.5	29
Reduced Fat	170	1.5	25
Sandwich Cookies, all types	240	2	36
Smackers Crackers, all types	130	1	32
Zoo Animal Crackers, all types	125	1	20
Zoo Animal Pretzels	200	0	40
Bakery Wagon			
Iced Molasses, lowfat	90	1.5	18
Iced Oatmeal	120	4.5	18
Lemon Heaven	120	3.5	20
Peanut Butter	130	6	15
Sugarless Molasses	120	3	21
Fat-Free: Cobbler	70	0	16

	C	F	Cb
Barbara's Bakery			
Animal Cookies, each	16	0.6	2
Cheese Bites, all types, 26 crackers	120	1.5	24
Coconut Almond, 1 bar, 1 oz	120	4.5	20
Crisp Cookies, all types (1)	80	4	11
Espresso Bean; Lemon Yog., 1 bar	120	3.5	22
Fat Free: Mini, all types, each	18	0	4
Fig Bars, average	60	1	15
Rite Lite Rounds, 5 crackers	55	0.5	12
Roasted Peanut, 1 bar, 1 oz	130	4.5	20
Snackimals, 1 cookie	15	0.5	2
Wafer Crisps (3)	60	1	12
Wheatines, all types, 1 large square	50	1.5	10
Breadshop: Animal Cookies	8	0	1.5
Bremner			
Wafers: All varieties, 1 wafer	10	0.3	2
Breton: Low Sodium Wheat (3)	70	3	8
Vivant Vegetarian	60	2.5	9
Cape Cod: Choc Chip Cranberry	140	6	20
Carr's: Cheddar (3)	80	4	8
Croissant (3)	70	3	10
Wholewheat Crackers (2)	80	3.5	11
Cheeze-It: Heads & Tails (31), 1 oz	140	6	18
Dare: Breton Wheat (3)	60	3	8
Delicious: Butter Finger (3)	130	6	18
Land O' Lakes (2)	120	6	15
Raisinets Oatmeal (3)	140	4.5	22
Skippy Peanut Butter (3)	150	10	13
Dominick's			
Grahams: Cinnamon (8)	140	5	22
Fudge (3)	140	7	19
Honey (8)	150	6	22
Lowfat (9)	120	1.5	25
Saltine Crackers (5)	60	2	10
Sugar Wafers (5)	140	7	25
Unsalted Tops (5)	70	2	10
Cookies: Choc Chip: Chewy (1)	100	5	14
Chunky (1)	80	4.5	10
Reduced Fat (3)	150	6	23
Old Fashioned: Assort.; Oatmeal	80	3.5	11
Pecan Shortbread	100	6	11
Sandwich Cremes: Chocolate	70	2.5	11
Vanilla	80	3	13
Striped Shortbread (3)	160	4	21
Vanilla Wafers (6)	160	6	23

Per Cookie/Cracker (Unless Indicated)

Entenmann's	C	F	Cb
Chocolate Brownie (2)	150	2	21
No Fat, 2 cookies	100	0	24
Original Choc Chip (3)	150	7	20
Soft Baked: Choc Chip	100	5	13
Gourmet English Toffee	100	5	13
Milk Choc Chip	100	5	13
Oatmeal Raisin, Fat Free (2)	100	0	23
White Choc Macadamia Nut (1)	100	6	12

Estee			
Chocolate Chip; Fudge Cookies	38	2	5
Coconut Cookies, Oatmeal Raisin	35	1.5	5
Fig Bars, each	50	0.5	11
Sandwich Cookies	55	2	6
Shortbread	35	1	5
Vanilla; Lemon	35	1.5	5

Famous Amos			
Butter Shorties	80	4.5	10
Chocolate Chip (1)	32	1.5	5
4 cookies, 1 oz	130	7	19
with Pecans (1)	35	2	4.5
Choc Cake Sandwich (3)	150	7	23
Choc Chip & Pecans (4), 1 oz	140	8	18
Chocolate Chunk	80	4	10
Oatmeal Raisin (4), 1 oz	135	5	20
Pecan Shorties	90	5	10
Vanilla Sandwich (3)	160	6	23
Lowfat: Iced Lemon (7), 1.1 oz	130	1.5	25
Iced Gingersnaps (7), 1.1 oz	120	1.5	25

Frookie			
***Cookies:** Average all types*	45	2	7
Animal Frackers	10	0.3	1.5
Apple Cinnamon Oatbran	45	2	7
Fruitins: Apple; Fig	60	1	12
Large Frooks: All types	120	4	18

Grandma's			
Choc Chip; Nutty Fudge	190	9	25
Fudge Choc; Oatmeal Apple	170	6	27
Old Time Molasses	160	4	29
Peanut Butter varieties, aver.	190	9	23
Cookie Bits: Average, (9)	150	7	22
Honey Buns: *Per Bun*	410	21	48
Sandwich: Fudge Vanilla (3)	150	4	25
Fudge; Vanilla (3)	180	5	32
Wafer, 4 cookies	160	6	26

Hain	C	F	Cb
Cheese Bites (22)	120	1.5	23
Cookie Jar Bits (Rice Cakes):			
Average all flavors, 17 bits	60	0.5	12
Mini Rice Cakes: Plain (8)	60	0	13
Oyster Crackers, Fat-Free (36)	60	0	13
Veg/Rice/Sesame Crackers (11)	140	6	19
98% Fat-Free, all types (11)	110	0	23

Health Valley			
Graham: Amaranth; Oat Bran	15	0	3
Original Amaranth/Oat Bran	20	0.5	4
Healthy Pizza, all flavors (6)	50	0	11
Lowfat, all flavors (6)	60	1.5	10
Original Rice Bran	18	0.5	3
Whole Wheat, all flavors	10	0	2
Cookies (each):			
Apple Spice; Hawaiian Fruit	35	0	8
Apricot Delight; Date Delight	35	0	8
Healthy Biscotti, all flavors	60	1.5	12
Healthy Choc./Chips, all flavors	35	0	8
Jumbo, all flavors	80	0	19
Raisin Oatmeal	35	0	8
Raspberry Fruit Center	70	0	18
***Tarts:** All types, 1 tart*	150	0	35

Hy-Top			
Assorted Cookies (5), 1 oz	120	4	19
Assorted Sandwich Creme, aver.	80	3	12
Chewy-a-riffic	90	3.5	12
Chip-a-riffic (3)	170	9	23
Chocolate Chip (5), 1 oz	110	5	16
Cookie Time Assortment	80	3	12
Honey Cinnamon Grahams (2)	120	4	21
Oatmeal	80	3.5	11
Iced Oatmeal	70	3	11
Pecan-a-riffic	100	5	11
Sugar	80	3	12
Vanilla Wafers (8), 1 oz	130	5	21

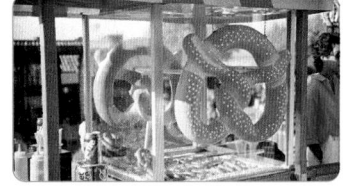

Per Cookie/Cracker (Unless Indicated)

Jewel	C	F	Cb
Animal Crackers (9)	140	3.5	25
Chip-A-Riffic (3)	180	9	24
Choc/Vanilla Sandwich Creme (2)	130	5	20
Chocolate Chip: Regular (3)	170	9	23
Chewy (1)	90	3.5	12
Chunky (1)	80	4.5	10
Choc Chunk, 1 1/2 oz	200	9	26
Chocolate Sandwich Creme (2)	120	5	19
Cinnamon Grahams (8)	140	5	22
Cookie Jar Assortment (3)	150	9	23
Duplex Sandwich Creme (2)	120	5	19
Fudge Creme Wafer (3)	150	8	18
Fudge Marshmallow	110	4	18
Oatmeal	80	3.5	11
Oatmeal Old Fashioned	80	3.5	11
Peanut Butter (2)	140	5	21
Peanut Butter Chip, 1 1/2 oz	210	12	21
P'nut Butter Fudge Wafer (2)	140	8	14
Saltine Crackers; Unsalted Tops (5)	60	1.5	11
Striped Shortbread (3)	170	8	20
Sugar Wafers (5)	140	7	20
Unsalted Top Crackers (5)	70	2	10
White Choc Macadamia, 1 1/2 oz	200	10	26

Keebler	C	F	Cb
Crackers:			
Club Partners, all types (4)	70	3	9
Cracker Paks S'wiches, aver. (1)	190	11	20
Graham Selects: Honey (8)	140	4	23
Cinnamon/French Vanilla (8)	110	1.5	24
Cinn. Crisp; Old Fashioned (8)	130	3	23
Munch'ems: Average (30)	130	4	22
Toasteds: Reduced Fat (5)	60	2	10
Regular varieties (5)	80	3	10
Town House: Regular (5)	80	4.5	10
Reduced Fat (6)	70	2	11
Wheatables: Orig., 7-Grain (12)	140	6	20
Orig. Reduced Fat (13)	130	4	21
Cookies:			
Chips Deluxe: Regular (1)	80	4.5	9
Rainbow (1)	80	4	11
25% Reduced Fat (1)	70	3	11
Chocolate Lovers (1)	90	5	11
Classic Collection: Sandwich	80	3.5	12
Plentiful Peanut Butter	75	4	9
Elfin Delights: Devil's Food (fat free)	70	0	14
Choc./Creme (reduced fat)	55	1	10

Keebler (Cont)	C	F	Cb
Danish Wedding (4)	120	5	20
Fudge Shoppe:			
Fudge Stripes (3)	160	8	21
Reduced Fat (3)	150	5	23
Deluxe Grahams, Reg.(3)	140	7	19
Reduced Fat (3)	120	5	19
Other varieties, average (3)	150	8	21
Fudge Sandwich (2)	120	6	16
PB Fudge Sticks (1)	75	4	9
Pecan Sandies: 25% Red. Fat	70	3	10
Regular varieties, average	80	5	9
Iced Animal, (6)	150	5	24
Krisp Kreem, (5)	140	7	19
Soft Batch, all types, each	80	3.5	10
Wafers: Golden Vanilla Wafers (8)	150	7	20
Reduced Fat Chocolate (8)	130	3.5	25

Lance: Big Town, 1 pkg	C	F	Cb
Lance: Big Town, 1 pkg	250	11	38
Chocolate Chip, each	130	6	18
Oatmeal, each	130	6	18
Creme, each	240	10	35
Apple Bar, each	190	6	32
Peanut Butter, each	140	8	14
Peanut Butter Creme Wafer, 1 pkg	230	12	26
Fig Bar, each	180	3.5	34
Fat Free: Apple/Cranberry, ea.	160	0	38
Dunking Sticks, each	180	10	22
Crackers (Food Service):			
Saltines, 2 pack	25	1	4
Other Crackers, average, 2	30	1	6
Melba Toast, aver., 2 slices	25	0	6
Bread Sticks, 2	25	0	5

Lenell	C	F	Cb
Almonettes (2)	80	4	10
Deluxe Assortment (2)	90	5	11
Icebox Pinwheels (2)	90	5	11
Jelly Stars (3)	100	5	13
Peanut Butter (3)	100	5	13

Lil' Dutch Maid	C	F	Cb
Butter; Chip Delight (2)	80	3	11
Coconut Macaroons (2)	130	5	20
Creme: Chocolate/Duplex (2)	90	3	13
Strawberry/Vanilla, (2)	90	4	13
Oatmeal (2)	70	3	11
Iced Oatmeal (2)	80	3	11
Sugar (2)	80	4	10

Per Cookie/Cracker (Unless Indicated)

Little Debbie	C	F	Cb
Apple Flips	150	5	24
Chse Crackers w. P'nut Butter (4)	140	8	16
German Choc Cookie Rings	140	8	18
Ginger Cookies	90	3	15
Marshmallow Pies, each	160	6	27
Nutty Bar (2), 2 oz	310	18	32
Toasty Crackers w. P'nut Butter (4)	140	7	16
Yo-Yo's	130	6	21
Peanut Clusters, each	190	11	23
Figaroos, each, 1.5 oz	150	3.5	31
Peanut Butter & Jelly Sandwich	130	5	22

Lotte			
Chocolate (13), 1 oz	190	10	13
Koala Vanilla (13)	190	11	15
Koala Yummies (13), 1 oz	200	11	13
Peanut Butter (13)	190	10	11
Strawberry (13)	190	10	14

Lu Marie Lu			
Le Petit Beurre (4)	150	4	25
Le Petit Ecolier (2)	130	6	17
Le Truffe (4)	170	9	20
Pim's, Orange (2)	90	2.5	17

Mrs Fields' Cookies			
Per 1 Cookie, 2.5 oz			
Butter; Butter Toffee	290	12	40
Chewy Fudge	300	14	40
Coconut Macadamia	280	13	39
Debra's Special; Milk Choc	280	12	39
Milk Choc w. Walnuts	320	17	37
Milk Choc Macadamia	320	18	38
Oatmeal Raisin	240	9	39
Peanut Butter	310	16	34
Pumpkin Harvest	270	14	31
Semi-Sweet Chocolate	280	14	40
with Pecans	300	16	37
with Walnuts	310	16	38
Triple Chocolate	300	14	41
White Chunk Macadamia	310	17	37
Nibblers: *Per 2 Cookies, 1 oz*			
Debra's Special	100	4.5	13
Milk Choc w/Walnuts	120	6	14
Milk Chocolate; Peanut Butter	110	6	15
White Chunk Macadamia	120	7	13

Per Cookie/Cracker (Unless Indicated)

Mama's	C	F	Cb
Cremes: All varieties (3)	150	6	23

Manischewitz			
Matzo Boards ~ See Page 96			
Biscotti: Toffee Crunch Macaroons	50	2.5	7
Choc. Chip Cappucino	70	2.5	10
Chocolate Macaroons, each	45	2	8
Matzo Cracker, Miniatures	9	0	2
Whole Wheat Crackers	9	0	2

Marie Lu			
Original Biscuit (3)	170	6	25

Matt's			
Choc Chip	140	6	19
Oatmeal Raisin	120	4	20
Peanut Butter	140	6.5	18

Mother's Brand			
ABC Cinnamon Grahams (1)	12	0.5	1.5
Almond Shortbread	60	4	5
Animal Parade, 1 oz (29g) pkg	140	5	21
Butter Flavor; Vanilla Wafers	24	1	4
Checkerboard Wafers	20	1	3
Chocolate Chip: Cookies	80	4	10
Cookies (bag)	30	2	4
Cookie Parade Assortment, each	35	1.5	5
Chocolate Chip Parade	35	1.5	5
Angel Cookies	60	4	7
Circus Animal Cookies	25	1	3
Cocodas Coconut; Fudge 'n Chip	30	2	4
Dinosaur Grrrahams: Average	75	3	12
Double Fudge	90	4.5	8
Duplex Creme	55	2.5	8
English Tea/Taffy Sandwich	90	3.5	13
Fig Bars: Regular; Wheat	65	2.5	10
Flaky Flix Fudge/Vanilla	70	3.5	8
Gaucho Peanut Butter S'wich	95	5	11
Iced Raisin; Macaroon	80	4	9
Oatmeal Cookies: Regular	55	2.5	9
Iced; Chocolate Chip	65	2	11
Oatmeal Raisin Cookies	30	2	4
Oatmeal Walnut Choc. Chip	65	3	9
Royal Grahams; Walnut Fudge	70	4	8
Striped Shortbread Cookies	55	2.5	7
Sugar Cookies	70	3	10

Per Cookie/Cracker (Unless Indicated)

Murray	**C**	**F**	**Cb**
Butter Cookies (8)	130	4	20
Sugar Free: Lemon Sandwich (3)	120	6	20
Creme Sandwich (3)	120	5	21
Shortbread (8)	120	4.5	20
Oatmeal (6)	120	4	23
Peanut Butter (6)	130	7	17
Wafers: Lemon/Strawb./Vanilla (8)	150	8	21
Ginger Snap Cookies (6)	110	4	21

Nabisco

Crackers: Per Cracker, Unless Indicated

	C	**F**	**Cb**
Air Crisps: Ritz, 1 oz (23)	140	5	22
Potato varieties, 1 oz (22)	120	3.5	21
Pretzel Original, 1 oz (23)	110	4	21
Wheat Thins, 1 oz (23)	130	4.5	21
Bacon Flavored Thins (7), $^1/_2$ oz	80	4	9
Better Cheddars: Reg; Low Salt	7	0.3	1
Cheese Nips (29), 1 oz	140	6	20
Chicken in a Biskit (7), $^1/_2$ oz	80	5	9
Garden Crisps (7), $^1/_2$ oz	60	2	10
Oysterettes (19), $^1/_2$ oz	60	2.5	10
Ritz; Wheatsworth; Stoneground (1)	16	1	2
Ritz Bits S'wiches: Chse (14), 1.1 oz	170	10	17
Cheese, 1$^3/_4$ pkg	270	16	28
Royal Lunch (1)	50	2	8
Snackwell's Red. Fat Fr. Onion (32)	120	2	24
Sociables (7)	80	4	9
Swiss (7), $^1/_2$ oz	70	3.5	10
Tid Bit, cheese (16), $^1/_2$ oz	70	4	8
Triscuit Thin Crisps (14)	130	5	20
Triscuit Wafers: All types	20	1	1
Uneeda, Unsalted Tops	30	1	5
Vegetable Thins (7), $^1/_2$ oz	80	4.5	9
Waverly (5)	70	3.5	10
Wheat/Oat Thins: (8), $^1/_2$ oz	70	2	10
Big Wheat Thins (11)	140	6	20
Zings! 1 pkg, 1.8 oz	240	11	34

Cookies:

	C	**F**	**Cb**
Barnum's Animal Crackers	12	0.5	23
Biscos: Sugar Wafers	17	1	24
Waffle Cremes	35	2	22
Brown Edge Wafers	28	1	4
Bugs Bunny Graham Cookies	12	0.5	5
Cameo Creme Sandwich	65	2.5	10
Choc Cherry Bar, 1 bar	130	2	26
Chocolate Chip Bite Size	10	0.3	2

Nabisco (Cont):

Per Cookie/Wafer

	C	**F**	**Cb**
Chocolate Chip Honey Grahams	5	0.2	1
Chocolate Snaps	17	0.5	3
Chocolate Wafers (Red. Fat)	14	0.2	3
Chips Ahoy: Chewy	60	3	8
Choc. Chip; Sprinkled; Red. Fat	50	2	7
Chunky	80	4	10
Mini	12	0.5	2
Soft Cookies (2-Pack), 1 cookie, 39g	160	7	26
Other types, average	95	5	11
Cookie Break; Van. Crm. S'wich	53	2	8
Famous Chocolate Wafers	28	1	5
Fig Newtons, each	55	1	11
Fat Free, each	35	0	11
Grahams	15	0.5	3
Honey Maid: Grahams, all types (2)	30	0.5	6
Low Fat Cinnamon Grahams (2)	28	0.4	6
Ideal Bars: Chocolate & Peanut	90	5	10
Lorna Doone: Shortbread	35	2	4
Marshmallow Puffs	90	4	14
Marshmallow Twirls	140	6	20
Mystic Mint (1)	90	4.5	9
Newtons: Cobblers, all varieties	50	0	12
Nilla Wafers: Regular; Cinnamon	15	0.5	3
Reduced Fat (1)	15	0.3	3
Nutter Butter: Chocolate	65	4	9
Bites, each	15	0.6	2
Peanut Butter Sandwich	65	3	10
Soft Cookies (2-Pack), 1 cookie, 39g	170	8	22
Oatmeal Crunch	15	0.5	3
Old Fash. Ginger Snaps	30	0.6	5
Oreo: Regular, 3 cookies	160	7	23
Reduced Fat, 3 cookies	130	3.5	25
Double Stuf, 2 cookies	140	7	19
Pecan Passion	90	5	9
Pinwheels: Choc./Marshmallow	130	5	21
Snackwell's Red. Fat Vanilla Creme	65	1.5	10
Teddy Grahams Snacks: All types	5	0.1	1

Pepperidge Farm

	C	**F**	**Cb**
American Collection: Sante Fe	120	4.5	18
Average other flavors	140	7	16
Biscotti: Figaro	110	4	16
Caruso; La Scala; Tosca	90	3	13
Chocolate Chunk Minis (4)	150	8	20
Fruit Cookies: Cherry Cobbler	70	2.5	11
Average other flavors	50	2	7

Per Cookie/Cracker (Unless Indicated)

Pepperidge Farm (Cont)	C	F	Cb
Distinctive: Bordeaux; Pirouette	35	2	5
Brussels	50	2.5	7
Brussels Mint; Milano	65	3	8
Chantilly Hazelnut Raspberry	80	3	12
Chessman; Toy Chest Butter	40	1.5	6
Double Choc. Milano	75	4	8
Endless Choc. Milano	180	10	21
Geneva	55	3	6
Hazelnut Milano	65	3.5	8
Lido	90	4.5	11
Linzer Strawberry Filled	100	4	15
Milk Choc. Bordeaux	60	3	7
Milk Choc. Milano	170	9	21
Mint/Orange Milano	70	4	8
Goldfish: Plain, 55 pces, 30g	140	6	19
Chocolate (19)	140	5	22
Choc. Chunk; Van.; Cinnamon (19)	150	7	21
International: Esprits Noir	90	5	10
Chocolat A L'Orange; Medaillon	75	3	12
Nantucket: Choc Chunk Minis (4)	150	8	20
Old Fashioned: Hazelnut	55	2.5	7
Brownie; Butterscotch Oatmeal	55	3	6
Chocolate Chip; Irish Oatmeal	45	2.5	6
Gingerman; Molasses Crisps	30	1	5
Lemon Nut Crunch	60	3	6
Oatmeal Raisin	55	2	8
Pecan Shortbread	70	4.5	7
Shortbread	70	3.5	8
Sugar	45	2	7
Sausalito: Choc Macadamia (4)	160	9	18
Soft Baked: Caramel; Choc Chunk	130	6	13
Choc. Macadamia/Walnut	130	6	16
Oatmeal Raisin	110	4	17
Vanilla Raspberry Tart	60	1.5	12

President's Choice			
Animal Crackers (14)	150	5	25
Butter Pecan (2)	190	13	17
Choc Chip Pecan (2)	160	9	18
Decadent: Choc Chip, all var., (2)	160	8	19
Family Arrowroot (5)	140	4	25
Grandma's Butter First (2)	180	10	20
Peanut Butter First (3)	160	9	18
Peanut Butter Persuasion (2)	160	8	18
Raisins First (2)	120	6	15
Temptations: Key Lime (2)	150	7	20
Other varieties (2)	140	5	21

Pirouline	C	F	Cb
Pirouline, 8 rolls, 1 oz	130	3.5	23

Sinful			
All Butter Raisin & Oatmeal (2)	130	6	20
Butter w. Soft Creme Raspberry (1)	70	3	11
Choc w. Vanilla Creme (2)	120	5	16
Chocolate Chip (2)	150	7	19

Salerno			
Almond Windmill (2)	120	4.5	17
Bonnie Shortbread (4)	160	7	22
Butter Cookies: Original (6)	160	7	22
Reduced Fat (6)	150	5	22
Coconut Bar (2)	150	8	18
Creme Wafer Sugar-free (5)	190	13	18
Dinosaur Graham	70	2.5	11
Farm Animal Crackers (13)	140	5	22
Grahams: Cinnamon (2)	130	3.5	22
Chocolate (2)	130	3	24
Iced Oatmeal (2)	120	5	18
Mini Butter: Flavored (25)	150	6	20
Angel/Chocolate Creme (9)	140	6	20
Mini Dinosaur (15)	140	5	21
Mint Creme Patties (2)	130	7	16
Oyster Crackers: Regular (42)	60	1.5	11
Fat-Free (42)	60	0	12
Royal Crispy Stix (3)	150	8	18
Royal Stripes (3)	180	8	24
Saltine Crackers: Regular (5)	60	1.5	11
Fat-Free (5)	50	0	11
Unsalted Tops (5)	60	1.5	11
Santa's Favorites, aniseed (6)	150	5	22
Scooter Pie Choc Marshmallow	140	5	23
Sugar Wafers, assorted (5)	180	11	20
Vanilla Wafers (7)	130	5	21

Snackwell's			
Caramel Delights	70	2	13
Chocolate Chip (2)	20	0.5	3
Choc/Creme Sandwich; Oatmeal	55	1.5	10
Streusel Squares	150	3	31

Stella D'Oro			
Almond Toast Cookie	55	1	10
Angel Bars	80	5	7
Anginetti (4)	140	4	23
Anisette Sponge (2)	90	1	19
Anisette Toast (3)	130	1	27
Apple Pastry	80	3	14
Breakfast Treats	100	3	16

Cookies (Cont) • Refrigerated

Stella D'Oro (Cont)

	C	F	Cb
Biscotti (Hazelnut)	100	3.5	15
Castelets, regular/chocolate	70	3	9
Dutch Apple Bars	110	3	19
Egg Biscuits, Low Sodium	40	1	7
Egg Jumbo	50	1	9
Fruit Delight Apple Cinnamon	70	0	17
Golden Bars; Love Cookies	110	4	16
Kichel, low sodium	7	0.4	0.5
Lady Stella Assortment (3)	130	5	19
Margherite, chocolate/vanilla	70	2.5	11
Peach Apricot/Prune Pastry	90	4	14
Swiss Fudge	70	3	9

Sunshine

Crackers:

	C	F	Cb
Animal Crackers	10	0.3	2
Cheez-It Crackers	6	0.3	0.5
Big Cheez-It	12	1	1
Hi-Ho Crackers	17	1	2
Reduced Fat	14	0.5	2
Krispy: Saltines	12	0.3	2
Oyster & Soup, 17 crackers	60	1.5	11

Cookies:

	C	F	Cb
All American: Butter; Lemon	30	1	4
Mini Chip-A-Roos	35	1.5	4
Ginger Snaps	20	0.5	3
Golden Fruit	80	2	14
Hydrox (Reduced Fat) Sandwich	50	2	7
Sugar Wafers: P. Butter; Vanilla	43	2	5
Vanilla Wafers, each	20	1	3
Vienna Fingers (2)	140	6	21
Reduced Fat (2)	130	4.5	22

Voortman

	C	F	Cb
Lemon Lucullan Delights (1)	110	5	16
Mini Chips, 1 oz (5)	135	6	19
Mini Wafers, 1 oz (5)	150	8	19

Waldbaum's

	C	F	Cb
Champagne Biscuits Saviordi (4)	110	0.5	25

Weight Watchers

	C	F	Cb
Apple Raisin Bars, each	70	2	14
Chocolate Chip (2)	140	5	22
Choc. S'wich Cookies (2)	140	3.5	23
Fruit Filled, 1 bar	70	0	16
Oatmeal Raisin (2)	120	2	22
Vanilla Sandwich Cookies	140	3	25

Thaw, Bake & Serve

	C	F	Cb
Big Country: Aver. all types (1)	100	4	15

Cookietree: *Per Cookie*

	C	F	Cb
Buttersugar; Cinn. Apple Oatmeal	120	5	17
Choc. varieties; Pecan/Macadam.	130	7	17
Cookie w. M&M's; Dble Fudge	120	6	17
Fat Free varieties, average	125	0	28
Peanut Butter/Chocolate	130	7	17
Raisin Oatmeal	110	3.5	17

Guiltless Indulgence (1.3 oz Cookie)

	C	F	Cb
Fat Free varieties, aver.	120	0	28
Lowfat Fudge/Choc., aver.	130	2	28

Grands!: *Per Biscuit*

	C	F	Cb
Blueberry; Golden Corn	210	9	28
Butter Tastin'; Buttermilk	200	10	24
Reduced Fat	190	7	27
Cinn. Raisin; Extra Fluffy; Wheat	200	8	28
Extra Rich	220	12	25
Flaky; Homestyle	200	10	25
Southern Style	200	10	24

	C	F	Cb
Hungry Jack: Aver. all types (1)	100	4.5	14

Jewel

	C	F	Cb
Buttermilk Biscuits (2)	100	1.5	20
Old Fashioned Biscuits (2)	100	1.5	20

Pillsbury Cookies: *Per 1 oz*

	C	F	Cb
Buttermilk; Country, each	50	1	3
M & Ms	130	6	17
Choc. Chip/Dbl Choc Chip Chunk	140	7	17
Choc. Chip. Reduced Fat	110	4	18
Chocolate Chip w. Walnuts	130	7	16
Holiday, all types (2), 1 oz	130	7	16
Oatmeal Choc. Chip; Reeses	125	6	16
Peanut Butter	120	6	18
SnackWells, Choc. Chip, Red. Fat	110	3	19
SnackWells, Chocolate Fudge	90	1.5	18
Sugar (2), 1 oz	130	5	20
Tender Layer Buttermilk	160	4.5	9
One Step Pan Cookies	130	6	19

Toll House (*Nestlé*)

	C	F	Cb
Choc Chip	140	6	20
Reduced Fat Choc Chip	130	3.5	23
Choc. Chip White; Chunk	150	6	22
Peanut Butter Choc Chip	150	7	20
Sugar	120	5	18

Cakes, Pastries, Croissants

Ready-to-Eat

	C	F	Cb
Angel Food:			
Plain, no oil, 2 oz	120	0	25
Plain with oil, 2 oz	160	1.5	25
w. Cream Frosting	230	7	37
Apple Fritters, 3 oz	360	22	38
Apple Pie: See Pies/Tarts Page 107			
Baklava, 1$\frac{1}{2}$" square, 1$\frac{1}{2}$ oz	110	6	13
Banana w. Butter Cream, 3 oz	300	13	40
Black Forest, 3 oz	230	10	34
Brownie, 3.5 oz	420	25	52
Bundt, 3 oz	300	17	35
Carrot Cake: Plain, 3 oz	230	8	41
w. Cream Cheese Frosting	380	21	42
Cheesecake: Small serving, 3 oz	260	18	24
Large serving, 5 oz	430	30	40
w. Lowfat Cheese/fruit, 3 oz	150	8	30
Cheesecake Factory: 1 sl., 7 oz	700	48	56
Lite, 1 slice, 7 oz	570	28	60
Denny's Cheesecake, 1 slice	470	27	48
Cherry Cobbler, 5 oz	350	10	62
Chocolate Cake: Plain, 2 oz	220	11	40
w. Chocolate Frosting, 3 oz	320	15	42
& Cream Filling, 3$\frac{1}{2}$ oz	360	21	43
Cinnamon Crumb Cake, 4 oz	450	23	57
Cinnamon Roll, Large, 6 oz	630	27	87
Coffee Cake, 3 oz	230	7	38
Cream Cheese Crumb, 4 oz	410	20	52
Cream Puff (custard fill), 4$\frac{1}{2}$ oz	300	18	26
Creme Horns, each	190	13	19
Croissants: See Next Column			
Cupcake: Plain, 1$\frac{1}{2}$ oz	140	6	25
w. Frosting	170	7	30
Danish Pastry: Small, 2 oz	220	10	25
Large, 4 oz	440	20	51
Date Nut Roll, $\frac{1}{2}$" slice	80	2	12
Devil's Food, w. Frosting, 3 oz	460	25	55
Donut Holes, 1$\frac{1}{4}$" balls, 2 oz (5)	220	10	30
Donuts: See Page 106			
Eclair, Choc. Cust. fill, 3$\frac{1}{2}$ oz	240	14	23
Fig Bars, average, each	150	3	30
Fig Cake, $\frac{1}{2}$ piece	110	4	21
Fruit Cake, Dark/Light, 1$\frac{1}{2}$ oz	165	7	26
Fudge Nut Brownie, each	340	13	56
Gingerbread: From mix, 3" sq.	200	6	37
Honey Bun, each	330	13	47
Key Lime Pie, 4.5 oz	440	22	54
Kolacky, Apricot/Rasp., $\frac{1}{2}$ oz (1)	60	3.5	8

Ready-to-Eat (Cont)

	C	F	Cb
Lemon Cake,	220	9	40
2$\frac{1}{2}$ oz piece			
Lemon Poppy Seed Creme, 3 oz	310	15	40
Mississippi Mud Pie, 4 oz	380	24	37
Mud Cake, 1 piece, 3$\frac{1}{2}$ oz	350	16	48
Muffins: See Next Page			
Orange Creme (Ring), 3 oz	300	15	40
Pineapple Upside Down, 2$\frac{1}{2}$ oz	230	9	37
Peach Melba, 3$\frac{1}{2}$ oz	300	8	52
Strawberry Creme, 3 oz	290	14	40
Strudel Bites, $\frac{3}{4}$ oz	85	4	12
Pecan Twirls, 1 piece	110	5	16
Pecan Pie, 3 oz	330	13	51
Pies & Tarts: See Page 107			
Pound Cake, 3 oz	420	27	42
Sponge: Plain, 2$\frac{1}{2}$ oz	190	3	36
w. Cream & Strawberry	325	8	38
w. Chocolate Icing	300	12	38
Raisin Bun, 1 bun, 2$\frac{1}{4}$ oz	180	2	37
Strudel, fruit, average, 3 oz	280	8	45
Sweet Roll, average, 1$\frac{1}{2}$ oz	155	7	24
Swiss Rolls, each	170	9	23
Tarts: See Page 107			
Tiramisu, 1 piece, 5 oz	400	29	30
Toaster Strudel, 2 oz	190	10	26
Turnovers, fruit, aver., 3 oz	270	12	36

Croissants

Average All Brands

	C	F	Cb
Plain/All Butter:			
Petite, 1 oz	120	7	14
1 Medium, 1$\frac{1}{2}$ oz	180	10	21
1 Large, 2$\frac{1}{2}$ oz	300	18	35
Sweet: Per Croissant, 3$\frac{1}{2}$ oz			
Almond Croissant	420	25	39
Apple Croissant	250	10	30
Chocolate Croissant	400	24	36
Sandwich (Ham/Cheese), 5 oz ~ See Page 160			
Au Bon Pain: See Page 164			
Burger King: Croissan'wich-See Page 173			
Dunkin' Donuts: Plain	290	18	26
Almond	350	22	34
Chocolate	400	25	37
Sara Lee:			
All Butter, 1$\frac{1}{2}$ oz	180	9	19
All Butter Petite, 1 oz	120	6	13

Quick Guide   C   F   Cb
Muffins: Ready-to-Eat

Average All Types:

	C	F	Cb
Small, 1 oz	80	3	12
Medium, 2 oz	160	6	24
Large, 3 oz	240	9	36
Extra Large, 4 oz	320	12	48
Jumbo, 6 oz	480	18	60
English: Average, 1 muffin	150	2	29

Brands ~ Ready-To-Eat

	C	F	Cb
Awreys			
Blueberry, 2.25 oz	210	9	29
Raisin Bran, 2.5 oz muffin	190	7	30
Jewel: English Muffin, 2 oz	130	1	25
Carl's: Blueberry Muffin	340	14	49
Bran Muffin	370	13	61
Dunkin' Donuts: See Page 188			
Hostess: Mini, average, each	55	3	7
Blueberry; Raspberry, each, 4 oz	440	19	62
McDonald's: Apple Bran	300	3	61
Oroweat:			
Cinnamon Rais., 2.4 oz	170	1	35
Extra Crisp; Sourdough, 2 oz	130	0.5	26
Health Nut, 2.3 oz	170	3	30
Otis Spunkmeyer: *Per Whole Muffin (4 oz)*			
Banana Nut, 4 oz	480	24	60
Cheese Streudel	440	20	60
Wild Blueberry	420	22	48
Our Daily Muffin: Each, 3 oz	120	0	31
Pepperidge Farm: Average	150	3	28
Ralphs: Banana, 4.5 oz muffin	470	21	62
Blueberry, 4.5 oz	410	16	60
Bran & Raisin, 5 oz	380	8	78
Sara Lee: Blueberry	220	11	27
Corn	260	14	30
Snackwell's: Blueberry, 1/6 pkt	120	0	28
Weight Watchers: *Per Muffin*			
Chocolate Chocolate Chip	190	2	39
English Muffin Sandwich	210	5	28
Fat Free, average, all flavors	165	0	39
Low Fat, average, all flavors	175	3	37

Muffin Mixes   C   F   Cb

Prepared: Per Muffin

	C	F	Cb
Betty Crocker: Banana Nut	150	5	24
Cinnamon Streusel	170	7	22
Lemon Poppyseed	190	7	30
Twice the Blueberry	140	4	25
Fat Free, all flavors	120	0	26
Duncan Hines: Blueberry, reg.	120	3	21
Bakery Style: Blueberry	190	6	32
Cinnamon Swirl	200	7	32
Cranberry Orange Nut	200	8	29
Pecan Crunch	220	11	27
Cinnamon Topp. Oatbran Honey	140	5	21
Oat Bran Blueberry	110	4	17
Oatmeal & Apples/Walnuts	210	9	30
Pillsbury: Blueberry Lowfat	160	2	34
Cinnamon	160	4	27
Other varieties	180	5	30
Robin Hood: Blueberry; Corn	160	6	24
Other flavors	170	8	23
Sweet Rewards: Fat Free	120	0	28

Sweet Rolls & Buns

	C	F	Cb
Awreys			
Cinn. Swirl, 2.75 oz sweet roll	300	16	36
Entenmann's			
Cinnamon Bun, 2.15 oz	230	10	32
Reduced Fat, 2.15 oz	160	3	32
Pecan Danish Ring, 1/8, 2 oz	250	15	25
Twist: Raspberry, 1/8, 2 oz	220	11	28
Nonfat, 1/8, 2 oz	140	0	32
Cinnamon Danish, 1/6, 2.2 oz	260	14	31
Lemon Danish, 1/8, 2 oz	210	11	26
Walnut Danish Ring, 1/8, 2 oz	240	15	25
Hostess: Honey Bun: Glazed	320	19	34
Iced/Frosted, 3.4 oz	410	24	42
Jewel Bake Shop			
Cinnamon Swirl Bread, 1 oz sl.	160	2.5	30
Gourmet Cinn. Rolls, 6 oz roll	640	29	88
Little Debbie			
Pecan Spinwheels, 1 oz roll	110	4	16
Mickey: Cinnamon Pastry, 4 oz	200	5.5	35
Cinnamon Nut, 2 1/2 oz	230	8	37
Raisin Cinnamon, 2 1/2oz	200	4.5	35
Pillsbury: Cinnamon Roll, 1.5 oz	150	5	23
Reduced Fat, 1.5 oz	140	3.5	24

Donuts

Quick Guide | C | F | Cb
Donuts

Average All Brands

	C	F	Cb
Plain, 1³/4 oz	210	12	25
Sugared, 1³/4 oz	220	11	27
Glazed, 2 oz	250	12	34
Chocolate Iced, 2 oz	260	14	29

Brands

	C	F	Cb
Buttercumb			
Cinnamon, 1 cake, 1.6 oz	170	6	28
Dolly Madison Donuts			
Regular, 1³/4 oz	270	12	40
Gem varieties, 1/2 oz each	65	3	8
Powdered Mini, 1/2 oz each	60	3	8

Dunkin' Donuts: *See Fast-Foods Section ~ Page188*

	C	F	Cb
Dutch Mill: Plain, 1³/4 oz	210	12	25
Sugared, 1³/4 oz	220	11	27
Glazed, 2 oz	250	12	34
Double-Dipped Chocolate, 2 oz	280	17	31
Entenmann's Donuts			
Country Powdered, 1³/4 oz	240	15	24
Frosted Devil's, 2.4 oz	310	19	34
Glazed Buttermilk, 2¹/4 oz	270	13	35
Light, 2 oz	190	7	31
Light Fantastic Fudge, 2 oz	210	9	40
Light Fantastic Fudge, 2 oz	210	9	40
Milk Chocolaty, 2.4 oz	310	19	35
Rich, Frosted, 3 pces, 2 oz	280	18	26
Hostess Donuts			
Cinnamon Sweet Roll, 2 oz	220	7	36
Regular: Plain, 1 oz	140	7	15
Chocolate Frosted, 1¹/2 oz	180	11	19
Pwd Sugar/Cinnamon, 1¹/2 oz	210	10	25
Old Fashioned; Glazed, 1¹/2oz	180	9	23
Blueberry, 1¹/2 oz	210	13	24
Hostess O's, Raspberry, 2 oz	230	10	34
Donettes: Frosted, 1/2 oz	77	4.5	8
Crumb; 1/2 oz	57	2.5	8
Powdered, 1/2 oz	84	4	12
Jewel			
Cinnamon Spiced, 2 oz	230	15	24
Little Debbie Donuts			
Donut Sticks, 1.6 oz pkg	210	13	21
3 oz pkg	390	23	39

Brands (Cont) | C | F | Cb

	C	F	Cb
Mickey			
Egg Fluff, 2, 1.65 oz	210	11	25
French Twirl, 2, 1.65 oz	240	16	21
Jumbo, aver. all types, 1, 1.5 oz	190	11	21
Mini, 2, 1 oz	130	8	15
Sara Lee Donuts			
Choc. Frosted Mini, 3/4 each	100	5.5	13
Powdered Mini, 1/2 oz each	85	4.5	9
Glazed, 1/2 oz each	110	5	14
Reduced Fat, 1/2 oz each	55	2.5	8
Tastykake Donuts			
Plain, 1¹/2 oz	190	10	22
Cinnamon, 1¹/2 oz	180	8	26
Frosted Rich, 2 oz	260	16	28
Honey Wheat, 2 oz	210	8	32
Powdered Sugar, 1¹/2 oz	180	9	24
Van De Kamp's Donuts			
Old Fashioned: Plain	270	11	40
Chocolate, 2.4 oz	340	22	34
Powdered, 2 oz	240	11	35
Assorted, 2¹/4 oz	280	17	32
Mini Donuts: Chocolate, 4, 2 oz	290	17	32
Crumb, 4	220	8	35
Powdered, 4	250	12	33
Lowfat: Maple Buttermilk, 1	200	2	43
Chocolate Buttermilk, 1	200	2	43
Double Chocolate, 1	190	2.5	41
Powdered, 1	150	1.5	32
Zingers			
Devil's/Vanilla Food, 2 cakes	280	8	50

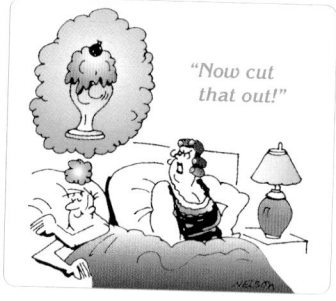

"Now cut that out!"

Quick Guide

Pies

	C	F	Cb
Average All Brands			
1/8 of 9" Pie, 4 oz Serving			
Apple; Blueberry; Cherry	290	13	46
Boston Cream Pie	330	14	55
Chocolate Pie	300	18	35
Custard; Coconut Custard	250	13	27
Lemon Chiffon Pie	360	14	50
Lemon Meringue	270	11	42
Mince Pie	300	13	46
Pecan Pie	470	24	52
Pumpkin Pie	240	13	28
Strawberry Pie	230	9	86

Brands

	C	F	Cb
Per Serving			
Denny's: Apple Pie	430	20	60
Apple Pie w. Equal	370	20	43
Cherry Pie	540	21	83
Chocolate Pecan Pie	790	37	107
Coconut Cream Pie	480	26	58
Dutch Apple Pie	440	20	65
French Silk Pie	650	43	60
German Chocolate Pie	580	33	66
Key Lime/Pecan Pie	600	27	80
Lemon Meringue Pie	460	17	71
Entenmann's: Homestyle Apple,			
1/6 pie, 4.3 oz	340	12	56
Hostess: Fruit; Cherry, 4.5 oz pie	470	22	65
Lemon, 4.5 oz pie	500	24	66
Long John Silver: Per Serving			
Chocolate Cream Pie	280	17	29
Double Lemon Pie	350	18	41
Key Lime Cream Cheesecake	310	19	33
McDonald's: Apple Pie, 2³/4 oz	260	13	34
Mickey			
Apple/Cherry Fruit Pie, aver.	500	30	55
Sweet Rolls: Cinn. Pastry, 4 oz	200	5.5	35
Cinnamon Nut, 2¹/2 oz	230	8	37
Raisin Cinnamon, 2¹/2 oz	200	4.5	35
Mrs Bairds: Apple Pie, 4.2 oz	400	19	56
Cherry Fruit Pie, 4.2 oz	400	19	56
Tastykake: Fruit, average	310	11	50
French Apple	360	12	61
Coconut Creme	390	20	47

Pastry & Pie Crusts

	C	F	Cb
Pie Crust:			
Baked, 9" diameter shell			
1 Pie Shell, 6¹/2 oz	900	60	79
2-crust Pie, 9", 11¹/4 oz	1500	93	137
Betty Crocker, 9", 1/8 shell	110	8	9
Boboli, thin Pizza Crust, 1/5, 2 oz	160	4	24
Jewel, 1/8 of 9" crust	130	8	13
Keebler Graham Cracker, 1/8 of 9"	110	5	14
Mrs Smith's Deep Dish, 9" (1/8)	110	7	11
Nabisco Oreo, 1/6 of 9" crust	140	7	18
Pet-Ritz, all types, 1/8, 3/4 oz	90	5	11
Pillsbury (All Ready), 1/8 pie, 1 oz	120	7	13
Piecrust Sticks, 8 oz	960	64	90
Choux Pastry, raw, 1 oz	60	4	3
Filo Pastry: 4 sheets, 2¹/2 oz	210	2.5	40
Athens: 1/8 pkg, 2 oz	180	1	35
Mini Dough Shells, 2, 8g	45	2	1
Pepp. Farm, 2 sheets, 1¹/2oz	120	1	25
Flaky Pastry, 1 sheet, 6 oz	780	72	18
Puff (*Pepp.Farm*), 1/2 sheet, 4.5 oz	510	33	42
1/6 sheet, 1¹/2 oz	170	11	14
Bake & Fill Shell, 1.7 oz	190	13	16
Pizza Crust, 1/8 whole	90	1	16
Bisquick Baking Mix:			
Original, 1/3 cup, 1¹/2 oz	170	6	25
Reduced Fat, 1/3 cup, 1¹/2 oz	150	2.5	28

Pie Filling

	C	F	Cb
Canned: Average All Brands			
Apple, 4 oz	120	0	28
1 Can, 21 oz	600	0	145
Apricot, 4 oz	150	0	36
Blackberry, Blueberry, 4 oz	120	0	28
Bosenberry, Cherry, 4 oz	120	0	28
Chocolate, Coconut, 4 oz	140	3	33
Lemon, 4 oz	200	2	47
Mincemeat, 4 oz	190	1	45
Peach, 4 oz	120	0	28
Pumpkin, 4 oz	170	0	40
Libby, 1/2 cup	100	0	23
Raisin, 4 oz	130	0	30
Raspberry, Black/Red, 4 oz	190	0	45
Strawberry, 4 oz	120	0	28

Cakes & Pastries - Packaged

Cakes & Pastries	C	F	Cb
Amy's: Apple Pie, 8 oz	280	12	42
Banquet			
Cream Pies: Average, 1/3 pie	350	21	42
Eli's Frozen Cheesecakes: Per 1/8 Pkg, 3 oz			
Cookies N Creme; Choc. Caramel	320	23	11
Keylime	320	22	26
Original, 3 oz	310	22	23
Entenmann's			
All Butter Loaf, 1/6 loaf, 2 oz	210	9	30
Brownie: Ultimate Fudge, 2 oz	220	13	27
Light: Fudge, 1/10 strip, 1.4 oz	110	0	27
Lemon; Coffee, 1/8 strip, 1.9 oz	130	0	28
Cheese Coffee, 1/8 cake, 1.7 oz	160	7	21
Cheese-Filled Crumb Coffee			
1/8 cake, 2 oz	200	9	25
Chocolate Fudge, 1/6 cake, 3 oz	310	14	46
Creme-Filled Choc Cupcakes, 1	160	0	39
Crumb Coffee, 1/10 cake, 2 oz	250	12	33
Golden Loaf, (Light) 1/8, 1.7 oz	130	0	28
Louisiana Crunch, 1/9, 3 oz	330	14	48
Mocha Cake, 1/6 cake, 3 oz	340	17	45
New York Crumb Coffee, 1/10, 2 oz	250	12	33
Ultimate Choc Crumb, 1/9, 2 oz	250	13	34
Ultimate Crumb, 1/10, 2 oz	250	13	33
Grands!: Blueberry Biscuits, 2 oz	210	9	29
Cinnamon Rolls, 3.5 oz roll	300	7	54
Hostess			
Angel Food Cake, 1/8	160	1.5	33
Brownie Bites, each	57	3	7
Carrot Cake, 2 pces, 3.5 oz	300	7	55
Suzy Q's, 2 cakes, 2 oz	230	9	36
Twinkies, 2 pces, 1.5 oz	150	5	25
Per Cake: Chocodiles	240	11	33
Chocolicious	190	7	30
Chocolate/Orange Cupcake, aver.	170	6	28
Crumb Coffee	130	5	19
Dessert Cups, each	100	2	17
Ding Dongs; King Dongs	180	9	24
Ho Ho's, each	125	6	17
Honey Bun: Glazed	320	19	34
Iced/Frosted	410	24	42
Light: Brownie	140	2.5	28
Cupcakes; Twinkies	135	1.5	28
Crumb Cakes	90	0.5	19
Snoballs	180	5	31

Jewel Bake Shop	C	F	Cb
Choc Mini Cupcakes, 1 cake	100	12	30
Cinnamon Swirl Bread, 1 oz slice	160	2.5	30
Creme Horns, 1 horn	190	13	19
Elephant Ears, 2.5 oz	340	22	34
Fancy Jelly Roll, 1/6 roll, 2.7 oz	190	2.5	38
French Torpedo Roll, 2.7 oz	170	1	35
Gourmet Cinn. Rolls, 6 oz roll	640	29	88
Key Lime Meringue Pie,			
1/6 whole, 5 oz	340	12	55
Kroger			
Angel Food Cake, 1/5, 2 oz	150	0	35
Dessert Shells, 2 shells, 1.65 oz	150	1.5	31
Gourmet Rugala, (18g), 0.6 oz	80	5	8
Little Debbie (Fresh)			
Cakes:			
Coffee, 2, 2 oz	230	7	39
Choc Chip Snack 2, 2.4 oz	290	14	42
Chocolate Cup, 1.5 oz	180	9	26
Creme-filled Strawb. Cupcake ,1	200	9	29
Devil Cremes, 1.65 oz cake	190	8	29
Devil Squares, 2 cakes, 2.2 oz	270	13	37
Frosted Fudge , 1.5 oz cake	200	10	25
Swiss Cake Rolls, 2 cakes	260	12	39
Zebra Cakes, 2 cakes, 2.6 oz	330	16	45
Fudge Brownies, 2 oz, 1	270	13	39
Honey Buns, 1.75 oz bun	220	13	24
Muffin Loaves, 2 oz loaf	230	11	30
Oatmeal Creme Pies, 1	170	7	26
Pecan Spinwheels, 1 oz roll	110	4	16
Manischewitz			
Cheesecake, 3 oz	250	19	16
Marie Callender (Frozen)			
Cobbler, all types, 1/4 pie, 4.25 oz	390	19	45
Pepperidge Farm			
Cakes Supreme: Per 3 oz Slice			
Lemon Mousse	290	12	35
Chocolate Mousse	250	10	35
Boston Creme	260	9	32
Cream Cakes Supreme:			
Cream Cheese Carrot, 1/9, 3 oz	320	20	38
Pineap./Strawb. Cr., 2.7 oz slice	240	10	38
Old Fashioned Cakes: Per 3 oz Slice			
Butter Pound	290	13	39
Deluxe Carrot	310	16	39
Turnovers: All types, aver., 3 oz	290	15	48

Pepperidge Farm (Cont)	C	F	Cb
Layer Cakes: *Per 3 oz Slice*			
Chocolate Fudge	300	16	37
Devil's Food; Coconut; Golden	290	14	40
Strawberry Stripe, 1/8	250	11	35
Vanilla	290	13	41
Three Layer Cakes:			
German Choc. 1/8 cake, 2.5 oz	250	13	31
Strawberry Stripe, 1/8	250	11	35
Fruit Squares: *Single, 2.5 oz*			
Apple; Blueberry; Cherry	210	10	27

Rich's	C	F	Cb
Chocolate Eclairs (Frozen), 57g ea.	190	9	24

Sara Lee (Frozen)	C	F	Cb
Cakes: *Per Serving*			
All Butter Pound, 1/6, 2.7 oz	320	16	38
Reduced Fat, 1/4, 2.7 oz	280	11	42
All Butter; Chocolate, 1/4, 2.7 oz	320	16	40
Banana Sundae, 1/10, 3 oz	270	14	32
Butter Streusel Coffee, 1/6, 2 oz	220	12	25
Choc Layer, 1/8, 3 oz slice	340	17	46
Dble Choc Layer, 1/8, 2.8 oz	260	13	33
Free & Light, 1/4, 2.7 oz	200	4	39
Golden Butter, 1/4, 2.7 oz	300	13	41
Pecan Coffee, 1/6, 2 oz	230	12	24
Red, White, Blueb. 1/10, 3 oz	210	8	31
Strawberry, 1/4, 2.7 oz	290	11	44
Dessert Cakes: *Per 1/6 Whole*			
Carrot, 3.2oz	320	17	39
Banana, 2.3 oz	230	8	37
Layer Cakes: *Per 1/8 Whole*			
Strawberry Shortcake, 2.5 oz	180	7	27
Other flavors, average, 3 oz	260	13	32
Cheesecake: *Per Serving*			
Cherry/Strawberry, aver., 4.75 oz	340	12	53
Chocolate Chip, 4.3 oz	410	21	47
Peanut Butter Cup, 3.5 oz	380	22	34
New York Style: Classic, 1/6	500	30	50
Mixed Berry Swirl, 1/6	490	28	52
Choc Chip Cookie Crumble, 1/6	520	27	61
Original: 1/5 whole, 4.3 oz	350	18	39
Classics: Choc. Mousse, 1/5	400	25	37
French, 1/5, 4.7 oz	410	25	41
Strawberry, 1/6 whole	320	14	43
Bars: 1 bar, 2.75 oz	190	14	14
Bites: Choc-Dipped Orig., 5 pces	480	33	40
Tstd Almond, 5 pces	450	29	42

Sara Lee (Cont)	C	F	Cb
Cheesecake Singles: *Per Slice*			
Caramel Choc Pecan, 110g	400	25	37
Strawberry Drizzle, 113g	380	20	46
Cream Pies (9"): *Per Serving*			
Choc. Silk; Coconut Crm, 1/5, 5 oz	500	32	49
Lemon Meringue, 1/6, 5 oz	350	11	59
Homestyle Pies (9"): *Per 4 1/2 oz (1/8 of Pie)*			
Apple; Cherry	340	16	46
Blueberry; Dutch Apple	355	15	53
Mince/Raspberry, averge	390	18	52
Peach	330	13	50
Pecan	520	24	70
Pumpkin	260	11	37
Individual Slices: *Per Slice*			
Apple/Cherry Pie, 4 oz	300	11	47
Carrot; Cookies N Cream, 3.5 oz	335	20	40
Lemon Icebox Pie, 3.5 oz	260	10	41
Southern Pecan Pie, 4 oz	470	23	62
Strawberry Swirl Ch'cake, 3.5 oz	300	17	31
Round Danish: *Per 1/6 Whole*			
Butter Streusel/Pecan	225	12	24
Cheese	180	6	28
Raspberry	200	8	27
Deluxe Cinnamon Roll	320	15	41
Weight Watchers: *Per Serving*			
Brownie à la Mode	190	4	34
Chocolate Mousse	190	5	31
Chocolate Eclair	150	4	25
Choc. Chip Cookie Dough Sundae	180	4	33
Choc. Rapsberry Royale	190	3	39
Double Fudge Brownie Parfait	190	2.5	39
Double Fudge Cake	190	4.5	36
French Style Cheesecake	180	5	28
Mississippi Mud Pie	160	5	24
New York Style Cheesecake	150	5	21
Strawberry Parfait Royale	180	2	35
Triple Chocolate Eclair	160	5	25

Eat it Today. . .
Wear it Tomorrow!

Cakes & Dessert Mixes

Made As Directed **C** **F** **Cb**

Betty Crocker

Cakes (Super Moist): *Per 1/12 Cake (Prep'd)*

	C	F	Cb
Chocolate Chip	270	13	34
Peanut Butter Choc; White	240	10	35
Other flavors, average	250	11	34

Per 1/10 Cake (Prepared):

	C	F	Cb
Carrot	320	13	42
Cherry; Sour Cream	280	12	43
Strawberry Swirl	290	12	43
Light: White	210	3.5	43
Devil's Food; Yellow	230	4.5	43

If using *No Cholesterol Recipe*, deduct 40 calories; and 4 grams fat.

	C	F	Cb
Angel Food Cakes: 1/12 mix	140	0	32

Brownie Mixes: *Per 1/20 Pkg (Prep'd)*

	C	F	Cb
Chocolate Chunk	180	9	24
Dark Chocolate	170	7	25
Fudge	170	7	23
Original Supreme	160	6	27
Peanut Butter; Walnut	180	9	23
Turtle (Caramel & Pecan)	170	8	23

Classic Dessert:

	C	F	Cb
Boston Cream Pie (1/10)	200	4.5	38
Choc. Pudding Cake (1/8)	170	3.5	33
Date Bar, 1/12 mix, dry	160	7	23
Gingerbread Cake (1/8)	230	7	38
Golden Pound (1/8)	290	13	41
Lemon Chiffon (1/16)	140	3	26
Lemon Pudding (1/8)	180	4	33
Pineapple Upside Down (1/6)	400	15	63

Creamy Chilled:

	C	F	Cb
Banana Cream (1/9)	250	11	35
Chocolate French Silk (1/8)	270	11	39
Coconut Cream (1/8)	290	13	38
Cookies & Cream (1/6)	380	16	53
Sunkist Lemon Supreme (1/9)	320	13	52

Stir 'n Bake Mixes: *Per 1/6 Pkg*

	C	F	Cb
Carrot Cake w. Crm Chse Frosting	250	7	46
Chocolate Brownies	220	8	35
Coffee	200	6	36
Devil's Food Cake w. Choc. Frost.	240	8	42

Supreme Dessert Bars: *Per Bar*

	C	F	Cb
Caramel Oatmeal; Choc. Chunk	180	9	24
Strawberry Swirl Cheesecake	180	19	20
Sunkist Lemon	140	4	23
Other varieties, average	170	8	24

Made As Directed **C** **F** **Cb**

Aunt Jemima

	C	F	Cb
Coffee Cake, 1/8 cake	170	5	30

Duncan Hines

	C	F	Cb
Angel Food, 1/12 Whole	140	0	30
Other flavors, average, 1/12	190	5	34
Cookies: All flavors, 1 cookie	65	3	8

Estee

	C	F	Cb
Brownie, 1 pce, 2" x 2"	50	2	12
All cakes, 1/5 cake	200	4	38
Choc. Chip Cookie, 1 cookie	45	2.5	6

Jell-O-No Bake: *Prepared As Directed*

Cheesecakes:

	C	F	Cb
Cherry/Strawberry, 1/8 pkg	340	13	52
Peanut Butter Cup, 1/8 pkg	380	23	44
Real/Homestyle, 1/6 pkg	360	17	48
Cookies & Creme: 1/6 pkg	390	8	29
Double Layer Lemon, 1/8 pkg	260	13	35

Manischewitz

	C	F	Cb
Apple Cake w. real apple, (1/6)	260	10	43

Nancy's

	C	F	Cb
Petite Desserts, 1 tartlets, 0.6 oz	80	4.5	9.5

Pillsbury

Moist Supreme: *Per 1/12 Cake (Prepared)*

	C	F	Cb
Angel Food	140	0	31
Devil's Food	270	14	33
French Vanilla; German Choc.	250	11	34
Funfetti	240	9	38
Other flavors, average 1/12	260	12	35
Streusel Coffee: 1/16 Cake	260	11	37

Bundt:

	C	F	Cb
Hot Fudge, 1/12	350	20	39
Chocolate Caramel Nut, 1/16	290	18	28
Strawberry Cream Cheese, 1/16	300	17	34

Deluxe Brownies: *Per 2" Square*

	C	F	Cb
Fudge, 1/16	150	6	22
Fudge, 1/20	190	9	24
Thick 'n Fudgy: Cheesecake Swirl	170	9	21
Double Choc.	150	6	23
Chocolate Chunk	160	7	22

Deluxe Bar Mixes: *Per Serving*

	C	F	Cb
Apple Streusel	150	6	24
Chips Ahoy	150	5	25
Fudge Swirl Cookie	180	8	25
Lemon Cheesecake	190	10	22
Other flavors, average	175	7	26

Cakes & Dessert Mixes (Cont)

	C	F	Cb
Robin Hood			
Devil's Food, 1/5 cake	310	17	36
Yellow 1/5 cake	280	13	37
Sweet Rewards			
Fat Free, all flavors (1/8)	170	0	40
Reduced Fat, all flavors (1/12)	200	5	37
Brownie Mix: Supreme, 1 pce	150	4	27
Lowfat Fudge, 1/18 pkg	130	2.5	27
Snackwell's			
Brownie: Devil's Food (1/12)	150	2.5	28
Fudge (1/12)	150	2.5	29
Cakes: Devil's Food, 1/6 cake	200	4	38
White; Yellow, 1/6 cake	210	4.5	39
Cookies: Choc. Chip, 1 oz (1/18)	110	3	19
Chocolate Fudge, 1 oz (1/18)	90	1.5	18
Streusel Squares, 1.5 oz piece	150	3	31

Cake Frostings

	C	F	Cb
Betty Crocker			
Rich & Creamy (Ready-to-Spread)			
All flavors, average, 2 Tbsp	150	6	24
Light, 2 Tbsp	120	1	27
Soft Whipped (Ready-to-Spread): 2 T.	100	5	15
Pillsbury: Per 2 Tbsp (approx.1/12 Tub)			
Caramel Pecan	150	8	19
Cream Cheese; Lemon	150	6	24
Chocolate; Choc. Fudge/Mocha	140	6	21
Coconut Pecan	160	10	17
Dark Choc	130	6	20
All other flavors	150	6	25
Decorators, Choc., 1 Tbsp	70	2	11
Sweet Rewards			
Average all flavors, 1 Tbsp	120	2.5	24

Baking Ingredients

	C	F	Cb
Almond Paste:			
(Marzipan), 1 oz	125	7	12
Baking Powder: Regular, 1 tsp	3	0	0.5
Cream of Tartar, 1 tsp	2	0	0.5
Bisquick Baking Mix:			
Original, 1/3 cup, 1 1/2 oz	170	6	25
Reduced Fat, 1/3 cup, 1 1/2 oz	150	2.5	28
Butter/Margarine: 1/2 cup, 4 oz	820	91	0
Carob Flour, 1/2 cup	90	<1	26
Chocolate Baking Bars: *Average All Brands*			
Unsweetened, 1 oz	150	15	8
Grated, 1 cup, 4 1/2 oz	680	68	36
Semi-sweet, 1 oz	160	8	18
Bitter-sweet/White Baking 1 oz	160	9	17
Chocolate Baking Chips: *Average All Brands*			
Milk Choc./Semi Sweet 1 oz	140	8	16
1/4 cup, 1 1/2 oz	210	12	24
1 cup, 6 oz	840	48	96
Cocoa Powder, Baking: *Nestle*, 1 T.	15	1	3
1/3 cup, 1 oz	80	4	12
Hershey's, 1 Tbsp	20	0.5	3
1/3 cup, 1 oz	115	3.5	21
Coconut, dried: Unsweet., 1 oz	190	18	7
Sweetened/flaked, 1 oz	135	9	14
1/2 cup, 1.3 oz	175	12	18
Toasted (*Baker's*), 1 oz	170	13	17
Creamed 1 oz	195	19	19
Coconut Cream (*Coco Lopez*), 2 T.	120	5	5
Cornstarch, 1 Tbsp	30	0	7
Flour: All Purpose, 1 cup, 5 oz	400	0	84
Flavor Extracts, *Average All Brands*			
Imitation, 1 tsp	15	0	3.5
Pure Extract, 1 tsp	20	0	4
Almond, Vanilla, 1 tsp	10	0	3
Fruit Pectin: Swtnd, 1 Tbsp, 1/2 oz	35	0	10
Unsweetened, 1 Tbsp	2	0	0.5
Gelatin, dry, 1/4 oz pkg	30	0	0
Lemon/Orange Peel, 1/4 cup	30	0	4
Nuts & Seeds ~ Page 127-128			
Pie Crusts & Fillings ~ Page 107			
Rennin, 1 pkg (11g)	12	0	3
Vinegar, aver. all types, 1 oz	4	0	2
Whey, sweet, dry, 1 oz	90	<1	20
Yeast: Active, dry, 1/4 oz pkg	15	0	2
Fleischmann's, 0.6 oz pkg	15	0	2
Bakers, compressed, 1 oz	25	0	3
Brewers; Torula, 1 oz	80	<1	11

Puddings, Desserts, Gelatin

Ready-To-Serve | C F Cb

Instant Pudding & Pie Filling
Per 1/2 Cup

	C	F	Cb
Regular: average all flavors	170	4	30
Reduced Calorie: *D-Zerta*	70	<1	12
Estee	70	0	12
Jell-O, sugar-free	80	2	11
Royal, sugar-free	100	2	17
Del Monte Pudding Snacks: Each			
Chocolate; Chocolate Fudge	130	4	24
Butterscotch; Tapioca; Vanilla	120	3	22
Fat Free Vanilla	90	0	20
Dr McDougall's: Rice Pudd., 3 oz	310	1.5	69
Jell-O Pudding Snacks (6 Pack)			
Choc./Caramel, 4 oz (113g) each	160	5	28
Fat Free, 4 oz snack	100	0	23
Chocolate/Vanilla; Van. Swirls	160	5	27
Cheesecake Snacks, aver., 4 oz	150	4.5	25
Jewel: Chef's Kitchen			
Rice Pudding, 1/2 cup, 4.5 oz	230	8	35
Tapioca Pudding, 1/2 cup, 4.5 oz	170	8	35
Kozy Shack: Banana; Van., 4 oz	130	3	22
Lite, 4 oz	110	1	22
Rice Pudding, 4 oz cup	140	3	25
Creme Caramel Flan, 1 cup, 4 oz	150	4	25
Choc./Tapioca Pudding, 4 oz	140	3	25
Manischewitz: Choc., 1/2 cup	110	0.5	26
Passover Gold Noodle, 1/2 cup	140	2	28
President's Choice			
Key Lime Pie (36oz) 1/8 pie, 4.5 oz	440	22	54
Mississippi Mud Pie (36oz) 1/9, 4 oz	380	24	37
Swiss Miss Pudding Snacks			
Swirls, 4 oz	160	6	26
Choc. Pudding Snacks, 3 1/2 oz	150	5	23
Tapioca: 1 pudding, 3 1/2 oz	120	3.5	21
Fat Free varieties, 3 1/2 oz	90	0	20
Weight Watchers (Frozen)			
Chocolate Mousse, 2 3/4 oz	190	5	31
Other Desserts ~ See Page 109			

Pudding Bars (Frozen)

	C	F	Cb
Jell-O Pudding Pops: Regular	80	2	12
Deluxe Chocolate covered	200	10	27

Homemade Puddings | C F Cb

	C	F	Cb
Apple Tapioca, 1/2 cup	150	0	32
Bread Pudding, 1/2 cup	250	8	40
Blancmange, 1/2 cup	140	5	19
Chocolate, 1/2 cup	190	6	30
Corn Pudding, 1/2 cup	135	4	21
Crème Brûlée, 1/2 cup	400	35	16
Plum Pudding, 2 oz	170	3	32
Rennin Dessert, 1/2 cup	115	4	16
Rice with Raisins, 1/2 cup	200	4	38
Sponge Pudding, 3 1/3 oz	340	16	45
Tapioca Cream, 1/2 cup	110	4	15
Trifle, 1/2 cup	180	7	26

Custards

Custard Mix
Jell-O (Americana) Golden Egg:

	C	F	Cb
Dry, 1/6 pkg	80	0	19
Prep. w. 2% milk, 1/2 cup	140	2.5	19
Jello Flan, w. 2% milk, 1/2 cup	140	2.5	20
Royal-Flan: Prep w 2% milk, 1/2 c.	130	2.5	18
Homemade Custard			
Baked, plain, 1/2 cup, 4 1/2 oz	150	7	16
w. skim milk, artif. sweetened	70	3	4
Boiled, 1/2 cup	165	7	18

Meringues

	C	F	Cb
Meringue Swirl, 1/2 oz	50	0	8
Meringue Shell, 1 oz Shell	100	0	16
(Add extra calories/fat/carbohydrate for fillings)			

Gelatin/Jell-O

Gelatin Mix:
Average, (Jell-O, Royal)

	C	F	Cb
Regular, all flavors, 1/2 cup	80	0	18
Sugar Free/Low Cal., 1/2 cup	8	0	0
Creme Gelatin/Parfait: *Per 1/2 Cup*			
Winky: Strawberry (109g)	110	1.5	22
Rainbow (130g)	100	0	24
Reser's: Dessert Parfait (110g)	100	2	19
Mrs Crockett's Kitchen: Str. Parfait	160	4	26
Snack Cups (Del Monte/Jell-O):	70	0	17

Non-Dairy Desserts

Imagine (4 Pack):

	C	F	Cb
Aver. all flavors, 1 cup, 3.75 oz	160	3	34

Pancakes & Waffles

Quick Guide

Pancakes

	C	F	Cb
Plain: *Average All Types*			
Small (3" diam.), 3/4 oz	50	2.5	6
Medium (4" diam.), 1 1/4 oz	80	3	11
Large (5" diam.), 2 1/2 oz	160	6	21
Add Extra for Syrups/Butter			
Pancake Syrup: Regular, 1 Tbsp	50	0	13
1/4 cup	200	0	52
Lite, 1 Tbsp	25	0	6
1/4 cup	100	0	24
Butter/Margarine: Regular, 1 T.	100	11	0
Whipped, 1 Tbsp	70	7.5	0

Restaurant Style Pancakes

	C	F	Cb
Denny's: Hot Cakes, Plain, 3	490	7	95
w. Syrup & Butter	725	17	130
Original Grand Slam Breakfast	795	50	65
w. Syrup & Margarine	1030	60	101
Syrup, 1 serving	145	0	36
Whipped Margarine, 1/2 oz	90	10	0
Hardees: 3 Pancakes (no fat)	280	2	56
w. Sausage Pattie	430	16	56
w. 2 Bacon Strips	350	9	56
IHOP (International House of Pancakes)			
Pancakes (Syrup/Butter extra):			
Buttermilk, 1 (2 oz)	105	3	17
Short Stack, 3	315	9	51
Full Stack, 5	525	15	85
Buckwheat, 1 (2 1/2 oz)	135	5	20
Country Griddle, 1 (2 1/4 oz)	135	4	22
Harvest Grain 'N Nut, 1	160	8	18
Crepes (Egg Pancakes), 1 (2 oz)	100	5	12
Waffles (Plain): Regular, 1 (4 oz)	305	15	37
Belgian: Regular, 1 (6 oz)	410	20	50
Harvest Grain 'N Nut, 1	445	28	40
Jack in the Box			
Pancakes w. Bacon	400	12	60
Pancake Syrup, 1 pkt	120	0	30
McDonalds: Hotcakes, Plain	310	7	53
w. Marg. & Syrup	580	16	100
Perkins: Buttermilk, 3, plain	440	12	70
Harvest Grain: Plain, 3	270	2	56
w. lowcal Syrup	295	2	63
5-Stack w. lowcal Syrup	475	3.5	93

Brands

	C	F	Cb
Aunt Jemima			
Frozen: Lowfat, 3	130	2	33
Original; Blueberry, 3	200	3	40
Pancake & Waffle Mix:			
Original, 1/3 cup, prepared	240	6.5	38
Complete, 1/3 cup	160	2.5	32
Mini Pancakes (13)	240	4	46
Thaw & Pour B'milk Pancake Batter:			
1/2 cup, 4 x 4" pancakes	260	3.5	51
Betty Crocker Pancake Mixes			
Complete Original, 3	200	3	40
Complete Buttermilk, 3	200	2.5	40
Bisquick (Shake 'N Pour)			
Pancake & Waffle Mixes:			
Average, all types, 3	200	3	38
Hungry Jack Pancakes			
Mixes: Per 1/3 Cup (prep.)			
Buttermilk: Complete, 1/3 cup	160	1.5	32
Original, w. 2% Milk, Oil, Egg	290	13	32
w. Skim Milk, Oil, Egg Whites	220	6	32
Extra Lights: Complete	150	2	30
Microwave: Buttermilk, 3	270	4.5	51
Original, 3 pancakes	270	4.5	51
Northern Pines			
Complete Gourmet			
3 x 4" pancakes, 3.5 oz	380	7	71

Waffles

	C	F	Cb
Homemade: 7" waffle, 2 1/2 oz	245	13	26
From Mix: 7" waffle, 2 1/2 oz	205	8	28

Frozen Waffles

	C	F	Cb
Aunt Jemima			
Blueberry, 1 waffle	95	3	15
Buttermilk, 1	100	3	17
Dominick's: 1 waffle	58	1	10
Eggo (*Kellogg's*)			
Chocolate Chip, 1 waffle	90	3	15
Cinnamon Toast, 1	73	3	12
Homestyle, average, 1	110	8	32
Nut & Honey, 1	120	10	31
Nutri-Grain, 1	100	6	17
Special K (fat free), 1	60	0	26
Hungry Jack: Blueberry, 1 waffle	105	4	17
Buttermilk; Homestyle, 1	95	3	15
Mini Funfetti, 1	65	2	11

Sugar, Sweeteners, Jams

Sugar

	C	**F**	**Cb**
White Sugar, granulated:			
1 level teaspoon, 4g	15	0	4
1 heaping teaspoon, 6g	25	0	6.5
1 cube, 1/2"	24	0	6.5
Single portion, 1 packet	25	0	6.5
1 Tablespoon, 12g	46	0	12
1 ounce, 1 oz	110	0	20
1 cup, 7 oz	770	0	203
1 pound	1760	0	464
Brown Sugar:			
1 Tbsp, 13g	50	0	13
1 ounce, 1 oz	109	0	28
1 cup, not packed, 5 oz	540	0	140
1 cup, packed, 7³/4 oz	845	0	218
Powdered/Confectioners:			
Sifted, 1 cup, 3¹/2 oz	385	0	98
Unsifted, 1 cup, 4¹/4 oz	460	0	117
Other Sugars			
Glucose, 1 oz	110	0	27
Tablets (*Dex 4*), 1	15	0	4
Barley/Wheat/Rye Malt,			
1 Tbsp, ³/4 oz	60	0	14
Cinnamon Sugar, 1 tsp	15	0	4
Dextrose, 1 oz	110	0	27
Fructose: 1 tsp	15	0	4
3 Tbsp, 1 oz	110	0	27
Estee, 1 pkg	10	0	2
FruitSource: 1 oz (powder)	110	0	27
Sorbitol, 1 oz	110	0	27
Turbinado Sugar, 2 Tbsp, 1 oz	110	0	27
Unrefined Cane Sugar, 1 oz	110	0	27

Sugar Substitutes

	C	**F**	**Cb**
Diabetic Sweet: 1 pkt	0	0	1
Equal: Tablet/Liquid	0	0	0
Granulated, 1 pkg	4	0	1
NutraSweet Spoonful, 1 tsp	2	0	0.5
Nutra Taste, 1 pkt	0	0	0
Sprinkle Sweet, 1 tsp	2	0	0.5
Stevia, 1 pkt	0	0	0
Sugar Delight, 1 pkt	8	0	2
Sugar Like (Bateman's), 1 tsp	4	0	1
Sugar Twin: 1 pkt	3	0	0
Sugar Substitute, 1 tsp	2	0	0
Sweet 'N Low, 1 pkt	0	0	0
Sweet One, 1 pkt	0	0	0
Weight Watchers Sweetener, 1 tsp	4	0	1

Honey, Jam, Preserves

	C	**F**	**Cb**
Honey			
1 tsp, ¹/4 oz	22	0	5.5
1 Tbsp, ³/4 oz	65	0	17
1 ounce, 1 oz	86	0	23
1 cup, 12 oz	1030	0	269
Single Portion, ¹/2 oz pkg	43	0	11
Jams/Jellies/Preserves			
Regular, 1 tsp, ¹/4 oz	18	0	5
1 Tbsp, ³/4 oz	55	0	16
1 ounce	75	0	22
Single Portion, ¹/2 oz pkg	38	0	11
Smucker's, aver. all types, 1 Tbsp	50	0	13
Apple/Fruit Butters, 1 T., 0.6 oz	20	0	6
Fruit Spreads:			
Regular, 1 tsp	16	0	4
Low Sugar, 1 tsp	8	0	2
Low Cal. *(Featherweight)*, 1 tsp	4	0	1
Jelly: Regular, average, 1 tsp	18	0	4.5
Imitation, Low Calorie, 1 tsp	4	0	1
Marmalade, citrus, 1 tsp	18	0	5

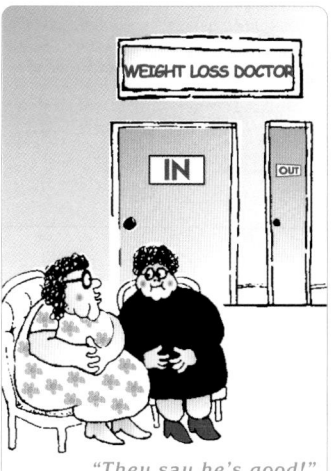

"They say he's good!"

Quick Guide C F Cb

Syrups

Average All Types
(Corn/Rice/Maple/Pancake/Waffle)
Regular/Dark/Light Color:

	C	F	Cb
1 Tbsp	55	0	14
2 Tbsp	110	0	27
1/4 cup	220	0	55
1 cup	880	0	22
Single Portion: 1 oz pkg	115	0	29
1 1/2 oz: pkg	170	0	42
Lite (e.g *Weight Watchers*),			
1 Tbsp	25	0	6
2 Tbsp	50	0	12
1/4 cup	100	0	25

Brands ~ Syrups

Per 2 Tbsp (1 fl.oz Serving)
(For 1/4 cup serving, double the figures.)

	C	F	Cb
Arrowhead Mills: Sorghum Pure	60	0	16
Aunt Jemima:			
Original; Butter Rich	105	0	26
Lite; Butterlite	50	0	13
Bernard Jensen's: Rice Bran	53	0	15
Cary's: Sugar Free	18	0	5
Pure Maple	105	0	26
Cozy Cottage: Sugar Free	10	0	3
Eden: Barley Malt/Wheat	120	0	28
Estee: Maple/Blueberry	40	0	10
Hungry Jack: Regular	100	0	25
Lite	50	0	12
Karo, all types	120	0	30
Knott's Berry Farm: All types	105	0	26
Log Cabin: Regular	100	0	27
Lite	50	0	13
Lundberg: Brown Rice Syrup	85	0	21
Mrs. Butterworth's: Lite	60	0	15
Original; Country Best Recipe	115	0	29
Northern Pines: Maple Leaf	80	0	20
Smucker's:			
Fruit Syrup; Regular	105	0	26
Light	65	0	16
Spring Tree: Maple Syrup	105	0	26
Sucanat: 100% Pure Cane Syrup	60	0.5	14
Tree of Life: Maple	100	0	26
Rice Syrup	120	0	30
Weight Watchers Syrup	50	0	12

Molasses

Average All Brands	C	F	Cb
Dark/Light: 1 Tbsp	55	0	14
1 cup, 11 1/2 oz	880	0	224
Blackstrap: 1 Tbsp, 3/4 oz	47	0	13
1 cup, 11 1/2 oz	750	0	208

Icecream Toppings

Per 2 Tbsp

	C	F	Cb
Hershey: Choc. Fudge	100	4	14
Kraft: Butterscotch	130	2	28
Caramel	120	0	28
Chocolate; Pineapple; Strawb.	110	0	28
Hot Fudge	140	4	24
Marzetti: Caramel Apple	60	7	23
Caramel Apple Reduced Fat	30	3	26
RW Knudsen: All flavors	75	0	19
Smuckers: Butterscotch Caramel	140	1	30
Chocolate Fudge	130	1	28
Dove: Dark Choc.	140	5	22
Milk Choc.	130	4	21
Fat Free, all flavors	130	0	31
Guilt Free, all flavors	100	0	24
Hot Caramel	120	3	28
Hot Fudge	140	4	22
Light Hot Fudge	90	0	23
Marshmallow	120	0	30
Magic Shell Toppings	200	16	25
Microwave: Choc./Fudge	130	2	28
Fat Free	110	0	27
Peanut Butter Caramel	150	4.5	24
Pecans/Walnuts in Syrup	170	10	20
Pineapple; Strawberry	120	0	28
Sundae Syrups, all flavors	110	0	27

Candy, Chocolate

Quick Guide C F Cb

Chocolate

Average All Brands
Milk Chocolate, regular:

	C	F	Cb
Plain/Nuts/Fruit, average, 1 oz	**150**	10	15
1½ oz Bar	**225**	15	23
2 oz Bar	**300**	20	30
4 oz Block	**600**	40	60
8 oz Block	**1200**	80	120
1 Pound, 16 oz	**2400**	160	240
Dark/White Chocolate, 1 oz	**150**	10	16

Chocolate-coated:

	C	F	Cb
Almonds, 5-6, 1 oz	**160**	11	11
Clusters, nut, 2, 1 oz	**160**	11	11
Coffee Beans, 1.4 oz	**180**	10	24
Creme/Cordial Centres, 1 oz	**120**	4	27
Fudge, 1 oz	**125**	5	18
Macadamias, 2-3 pces., 1 oz	**180**	13	11
Mints, 1 med., 11g	**45**	1	9
Nougat & Caramel, 1 oz	**120**	4	21
Peanuts, 12 med., 1 oz	**160**	11	15
Raisins, 30 med., 1 oz	**120**	4	21

Cooking Chocolate:

	C	F	Cb
Sweet/Semi-sweet, 1 oz	**160**	8	18
Chips, ¼ cup, 2½ oz	**210**	12	24
Unsweetened, 1 oz	**150**	15	8
Carob: plain, 1 oz	**160**	11	9

Also See Baking Ingredients: Page 111
Carob Candy: See Page 122

"It's time to curb this inflation"

Brands & Generic

Per Piece/Serving

	C	F	Cb
Abba Zabba, 2 oz bar	250	5	48
Absolutely Almond, 2.5 oz bar	380	23	40
Aero Bar *(Nestle)*, 1.45 oz bar	210	13	26
After Dinner Mints, 1 small	45	1	9
After Eight Mint, each	35	1.2	6
Allen Wertz: Simply Sugar Free			
Coffee Time (decaf), 4	45	15	12
Coffee Toffee, 6	120	3	33
Other types, 4	120	2.5	37
Almond Joy, 1.76 oz bar	240	13	29
King Size, 2	220	12	26
Snack, 2, 1.3 oz	190	10	23
Almond Roca, 1 pce	70	5	6
Almonds, sugar-coated, 7, 1 oz	130	5	20
Altoids *(C & B)*, each	3	0	1
Amazin' Fruit, 1 bag	180	0	41
Andes: Creme de Menthe; Cherry Jubilee			
Choc covered Patty, (3), 1½ oz	180	3	35
Thins, aver. all flav., (8), 1.4 oz	210	13	22
Anthon Berg: Cognac, each	180	8	25
After Dinner Sweet:			
Marzipan w. Madeira, 1.4 oz	175	7.5	26
Marcipan Brod, each	120	7	13
Asteroid *(Nestle)*, 54g	260	10	40
Baby Ruth, King Size, 3.7 oz bar	495	21	67
2.1 oz bar	280	12	36
Fun size, each	100	4.5	17
Snack, 1 bar, ¾ oz	100	5	12
Baci *(Perugino)*, each	85	5	8
Bar None, 1.5 oz bar	240	14	23
Barley Sugar, 1 pce., 0.2 oz	23	0	6
Big Hunt, 2 oz	230	3	47
Bit-O-Honey, 1.7 oz	200	3.5	41
Chews, 6 pces, 1.4 oz	170	3	34
Blow Pops, each	50	0	14
Bonus Bar, 2.1 oz bar	290	16	34
Boston Baked Beans, 30 pces, 1 oz	135	5	22
Brach's: Almond Supremes,11	220	15	18
But'rscotch Disks, 3, 0.6 oz	70	0	16
Choc Bridge Mix, 16, 1.4 oz	190	9	25
Circus Peanuts, each	25	0.6	3
Clusters, 3	220	14	19
Double Dip Choc Peanuts, 15	220	14	19
Golden Butter/Internation. Toffee	25	0.6	5
Lemon Drops, 4, 0.6 oz	50	0	13
Malted Milk Balls, 15	190	9	27

Per Piece/Serving

	C	F	Cb
Brach's (Cont):			
Milk Maid Caramel, 18	170	5	30
Orange Slices Hi-C, each	50	0	13
Breath Savers, all types, each	10	0	2
Brite Crackers, 1 bag, 1.5 oz	140	0	32
Brock: Candy Corn, (10) 0.7 oz	75	0	18
Gummy Bears; Sour Balls, each	26	0	6
Lemon Drops, each	20	0	5
Orange Slices, each	35	0	9
Spice Drops, each	12	0	3
Starlight Mints, each	20	0	5
Toffee, each	25	0.8	5
Bubble Gum ~ *See 'Gum'*			
Buncha Crunch, 1/2 cup, 1.4 oz	200	10	26
Burnt Peanuts, 40 pces, 40g	190	8	32
Butterfinger, King Size, 3.7 oz bar	480	18	75
2.1 oz bar	270	11	41
Fun size, each	100	3.5	14
Mini, each	20	1	7
Snack, 2, 1.3 oz	170	7	27
Butterfinger B.B.'s, 1.7 oz bag	230	10	33
Buttermints, 18 pces, 1 1/2 oz	160	0	40
Butterscotch, 5 pces	115	5	30
Buttons (*Walgreens*), 3, 18g	70	0	16
Chips, 1 oz	150	7	36
Discs (*Sathers*), 3, 0.6 oz	110	0	16
Candy Cane, Medium, 5", 1/2 oz	50	0	12
Candy Corn, 1 oz	110	0	27
4 oz pkt: 24 pces, 1 1/2 oz	150	0	37
Candy Necklaces, 20g each	80	0.5	20
Caramels: each	30	1	6
Chocolate, each	25	0.3	6
Creams, 3 pces, 1 1/4 oz	130	3	23
2.75 oz pkt, 5 pces, 1 1/2 oz	160	3.5	30
Hershey's Classic Caramels:			
Soft & Chewy, 6 pces	160	5	27
Choc Creme Filled, 6 pces	160	6	26
Caramel Nips, each	30	1	6
Caramel Popcorn, 1 cup, 1 oz	120	1.5	26
Caramel Truffles (*Godiva*), 1 pce	110	6.5	11
Caramello (*Hershey's*) 1.6 oz bar	220	10	29
Cellas Choc Cherries, .1 pce	55	2	9
Certs: Breath Mints, 1 pce	6	0	1
Sugar-free, 1 piece	7	0	2
Candy Jar Mix (*Jewel*), 3, 17g	70	0	17
Charleston Chew, 1 bar, 53g	230	7	40
Cherry Sours (*Sathers*), 11, 1 1/2 oz	150	0	38
Chews, all types, 1 oz	110	1	25

Per Piece/Serving

	C	F	Cb
Chocolate Mints, each	55	4	4
Chocolate Parfait Nips, each	30	1	5
Chuckles, each	35	0	10
Chunky Bar (*Nestle*), 1.4 oz	210	11	24
Cinnamon Bears (*Walgreens*), 5	150	0	38
Cinn. Buttons (*Walgreens*), 3 pce	70	0	17
Cinnamon Drops (*Sathers*), 19 pce	150	0	36
Coconut Stacks, 4, 41g	190	6	33
Coffee Go Coffee/Cappuccino, ea.	18	0.4	4
Coffee Rio-Gold, each	15	0.5	3
Collard & Bowser: Eng. Toffee, 2	80	4	12
Corn Nuts, 1/3 cup, 1 oz	130	4	20
Cote d'Or: Bouchee, each	130	8	12
Chokotoff, each	210	9	30
Nougatti	150	8	19
Bar & Nuts,1.3 oz	220	18	12
Cracker Jack, 1.25 oz box	150	2.5	29
Crisped Rice: Almond, 1 bar	130	6	18
Choc Chip, 1 bar	115	4	18
Crows, 7 oz pkg	150	0	37
Crunch: 5 oz bar	725	38	90
King Size, 2.75 oz bar	400	21	51
1.55 oz bar	230	12	29
Fun size, each	50	2.5	7
Snack, 3, 1 1/2 oz	220	11	28
Crunch Berries Treats, 1.6 oz bar	190	4.5	36
Decadence (*NuBar*) Bar, 1.3 oz	140	2.5	30
Dots, 12 dots	150	0	37
Double Dip Stick, 1 stick	16	0.5	3
Dove: Dark/Milk, 1.3 oz bar	200	12	22
Bar, 6 oz	920	56	104
Miniatures, each	30	2	3
Dum Dum Pops (*Spangler*), 1 pop	25	0	6
English Toffee, 1 pce	48	3	5
Eda's Sugar Free, all flav., 5, 1/2 oz	40	0	15
Estee Dietetic Candies:			
Caramels, all flavors, 1 pce.	30	1	5
Chocolate, Dark/ Mint, 1/2 bar	200	14	23
Gummy Bears; Gum Drops, 1 pce.	7	0	1.5
Hard Candies: Butterscotch, 2	25	0	6
Assorted Fruit Lollipops, 5	60	0	15
Peppermint, 3	30	0	7
Mint/Toffee, 5	60	0	15
Lollipop	30	0	8
Milk Chocolate, 1/2 bar, 4 oz	230	17	17
Peanut Butter Cups, 1 cup	40	3	3
Fructose Sweetened, 1 cup	40	2	3
Peanut Brittle, 1/3 box, 1.5 oz	240	9	28

Per Piece/Serving	C	F	Cb
5th Avenue, 2.1 oz bar	290	13	40
King Size bar	460	20	64
Fanny May: Single wrapped pces			
Mint Meltaway Patty, 1.5 oz	250	17	22
Pixie, 1.5 oz	215	12	24
Trinidad, 1.5 oz	205	11	24
Ferrero Rocher, each	75	5	6
3 pces, 1.3 oz	220	15	17
Fifty 50 Snack Bars: P'Nut But, 2	200	14	16
Almond Choc., 7 pce, 1¹/2 oz	210	15	20
Crunch Choc., 7 pce, 1.1 oz	160	11	19
Fruit & Nut Choc., 7 pce, 1¹/2 oz	200	14	21
Milk Choc., 3 pce, ¹/2 bar, 43g	210	14	25
Mini bars, 8 bars, 1 oz	140	9	16
Fondant: Choc-coated, 1.2 oz	130	3	28
Mint, 1 oz	105	0	27
Franklin Crunch 'N Munch:			
All varieties, aver. 1.25 oz	170	7	30
Fran's: Gold Bar, 1.75 oz	260	14	34
Gold Bites (Almonds), 1	130	7	17
Fruit Crystals *(Walgreens)*, 3 pces	70	0	17
Fruit Drops, each	6	0	1
Fruit Gems *(Sunkist)*, 3, 1.1 oz	105	0	26
Fruit Leathers, average, 0.5 oz	45	0	12
Fruit Pastilles, 1 roll, 1.4 oz	100	0	26
Fruit Rolls, 1 roll	80	0	20
Fruit Roll-Ups, ¹/2 oz	50	0	12
Fruit Runts *(Walgreens)*, 1T., ¹/4 pkt	60	0	14
Fruit Waves, 0.5 oz	50	0	12
Fudge: Chocolate/Vanilla, 1 oz	115	3	20
with Nuts, 1 oz	120	4	21
Choco. Marshmallow, 1 oz	120	5	18
w. Nuts, 1 oz	125	5.5	18
Peanut Butter, 1 oz	105	2	21
Ghirardelli: Milk/Dark Chocolate,			
1.25 oz bar	185	12	20
w. almonds, 1.5 oz bar	220	14	25
Choc Nuts & Chews, 1 pce	55	3.5	5
Godiva: Hearts, each	45	2	4
Almond Butter Dome, 1 pce	80	6	6
Bouchee au Chocolate, 1 pce	220	13	23
Cordial Assortment, each	60	2.5	9
Gold Ballotin, 1 pce	70	3.5	4
Milk/Dark/IvoryAssortment, each	75	4	8
Nut & Caramel, each	75	4	6
Truffle Amaretto, 1 pce	110	6.5	12
Golden Almond Bar, 1 bar	520	34	40

Per Piece/Serving	C	F	Cb
Golden 111 Bar, 1 bar	500	30	52
Go Lightly: Box Candies, 4	60	0	15
Bags: Assorted Taffy, 6	140	3	36
Vanilla Caramels, 6	150	6	31
Super Free Choc Crunch, 7, 1¹/2 oz	180	13	23
Goobers Peanuts, 1 pkg, 1.4 oz	210	13	20
Good & Fruity, 1 box, 1.8 oz	140	1	35
Good & Plenty: ¹/5 bar, 1.4 oz	130	0	38
Candy Bar, ¹/5 bar, 1.4 oz	130	0	31
GooGoo Cluster, 1 bar, 1.75 oz	240	11	32
GUM: *Per Piece*			
Bazooka, each	30	0	7
Beechies	6	0	2
Big League Chew	10	0	2
Bubble Gum Balls *(Walgreens)*	5	0	2
Bubble Yum	25	0	6
Sugarless	10	0	3
Candilicious	30	0	2
Carefree (Sugarless/Regular	5	0	2
Chiclets	5	0	1
Clorets, stick	10	0	2
Dentyne	6	0	2
Estee, bubble/regular	5	0	2
Extra *(Wrigley's)*,			
Sugar-Free Bubble Gum, 1	5	0	2
Freshen-Up	13	0	2
Hubba Bubba: Regular	23	0	6
Sugar-free, average	14	0	0.5
Ice Breakers, 1 stick	5	0	2
Sonic Boom Bubble Gum	15	0	3
Sticklets	7	0	2
Trident: Slab	5	0	1
Soft Bubble Gum	9	0	1
Wrigley's, all flavors	10	0	2
Gum Drops, 1 small	15	0	3
1 large, 0.4 oz	40	0	7
6 oz pkt: 4 pces, 1.4 oz	130	0	31
Gummi Bears: 1 bear	17	0	4
8 bears, 1¹/2 oz	140	0	32
Gummi Novelties *(Walgreens)*, 6	150	0	22
Gummi Savers, each	12	0	3
Gummi Sweet Tarts, 1 bug, 1.5 oz	150	0	34
Gummi Watch, 1, 2 oz	105	0	24
Gummi Worms, each	25	0	5
Guylian: No Sugar Added			
Milk Chocolate, 8 squares, 1 oz	126	9	15
Dark Chocolate, 8 squares, 1 oz	117	9	14

Per Piece/Serving	C	F	Cb
Halvah (Joyvah):			
Plain/Marble, 1/2 bar, 2 oz	390	25	18
Choc.coated Sesame, 1/2 bar, 2 oz	380	23	20
Hard Candy, all flavors, 1 oz	110	0	28
1 regular piece	18	0	5
Heath: Original, 1.4 oz bar	210	13	25
Sensations Singles, 1.4 oz	210	14	25
Hershey's:			
Bar, 1.55 oz bar	240	14	25
King Size bar	410	25	38
w. Almonds, 1.45 oz bar	230	14	20
Bites: Almond Joy (20), 40g	220	14	22
Cookies 'n' Creme (20), 40g	210	10	23
Cookies 'N Mint, 1.55 oz bar	230	12	27
Crunchy Cookie Cups, 1.4 oz	210	12	23
Hugs: w. Almonds (9), 1.4 oz	230	13	22
Kisses: Milk Choc./Almond (8)	210	13	23
Milk Chocolate, 1.55 oz bar	200	12	25
2.6 oz bar	400	23	42
7 oz bar, 1/5 bar	200	12	21
Miniatures, 5 pces, 1.5 oz	230	13	25
Nuggets: Milk Choc./Alm. (4)	210	13	23
Cookies 'N Mint, (4)	200	10	24
Cookies & Creme, (4) 1.4 oz	200	11	25
P'nut B. Crispy Rice, 2 bars, 1.1 oz	230	13	25
Special Dark Choc., 1.45 oz bar	230	13	25
Sweet Escapes: 1.4 oz bar, aver.	180	7	27
Choc Toffee Crisp, 1 bar, 18g	80	3.5	12
Triple Choc Wafer, 1 bar, 20g	80	2.5	14
C'mel & P'nut But., 1 bar, 18g	70	2.5	12
Whoppers (18), 40g	190	7	30
Honeycomb: Plain, 1 oz	115	0	27
Choc-coated, 1 oz	125	1	28
Hot Tamales, 1 box, 60g, 2.1 oz	220	0	55
Sathers, 19 pces, 1.4 oz	150	0	36
Ice Blue Mints (Walgreens), 3, 17g	70	0	17
Jawbreakers (Sathers), 3, 17g	70	0	17
Jellies, 3 medium, 1 oz	120	0	30
Jells Raspberry (Joyva), each	70	1	8
Jelly Beans: Small, 22 beans, 1 oz	100	0	24
Regular, 12 beans, 1 oz	100	0	24
1 bean	8	0	2
Jumbo, 1 bean	20	0	5
Jewel, 13 beans, 1.4 oz	140	0	36
Sathers/Walgreens, 17, 40g	150	0	37
Jelly Bellys, each	4	0	1
35 pces, 1.4oz	140	0	37

Per Piece/Serving	C	F	Cb
Jelly Rings, (Jewel), 3, 1.5 oz	160	0	39
Jolly Rancher: Candy (3), 0.6 oz	70	0	17
Jolly Jellies, 7 oz	120	0	30
Sugar Free, 4 pces, 0.5 oz	35	0	14
Junior Mints, 1.6 oz box	180	3	38
16 pces, 1.4 oz	160	2.5	34
Juicefuls: Red Raspb., (3), 0.6 oz	60	0	15
Assorted Fruits, 1 pce	20	0	5
Jujubes, each	3	0	0.5
Juju Mix (Sathers), 11 pce, 1 1/2 oz	150	0	36
Juju Toys: (Jewel), 6, 1.5 oz	150	0	37
(Walgreens), 11 pce, 1.5 oz	150	0	36
Jujufruits, each	10	0	2
Kit Kat: 2.6 oz bar	365	21	50
King Size, 2.8 oz bar	410	22	48
1.5 oz bar	215	12	27
Multipack, each	80	4	10
Snack, 3 (2 pce bars), 1.65 oz	240	12	30
Krackel, 2.6 oz bar	390	21	45
Snack size, 0.35 oz	55	3	5
Kudos: 1 oz bar, average	120	5	20
Lance: Popscotch, 1.2 oz pkg	160	6	24
Chocolaty Peanut Bar, 2 oz bar	320	18	30
Peanut Bar, 1.8 oz pkg	260	14	24
Lemon Drops, 3, 1/2 oz	50	0	12
Sugar Free (Walgreens), 5, 1/2 oz	35	0	14
Lemonhead, 10, 1/2 oz	60	0	14
Licorice: Average all types, 1oz	100	0	25
Bites (Switzer), each	12	0	1
Chews (Panda), each	10	0	2
Tid Bits, each	5	0	1
Twists: Black/Red, aver. 1 pce	30	0	7
American Licorice Company:			
Stick, (1) 0.5 oz	45	0	11
Choco Sticks, (4) 1.4 oz	145	0	35
Red Bites, 1.4 oz	140	0	34
Laces, 1 pce	35	0	8
Super Red Ropes, 1 rope, 2 oz	200	0	46
Vines, 1 pce	70	0	17

You can begin to control what you eat when you write it down everyday.

Per Piece/Serving	C	F	Cb
Lifesavers:			
Regular, all flavors, 1 candy	9	0	2
1 Roll (14 candies), 1.14 oz	130	0	32
Large size, 1 candy	15	0	4
Sugar-free Delites: *Per Candy*			
Orchard Fruits; Summer Blend	5	0	2
Butter Toffee; European Collect.	9	0.5	3
Gummi Savers, 1.5 oz roll	140	0	32
Lollipops Fruit, 1 pce, 0.4 oz	45	0	11
Lik-m-aid (Nestle), 1.7 oz	60	0	15
Lindt: Lindor, Balls, average	73	4	8
Dark Choc Truffles, each	70	6	4
Lollipops, each, 0.2 oz	20	0	7
Lollipops C Pops (Glenny's), each	35	0	8
Mamba, 9 pces, 1$\frac{1}{2}$ oz	160	2	36
M&M's:			
Milk Chocolate, 1 pce	4	0.2	0.5
20 pces, 0.6 oz	80	4	10
34 pces, 1 oz	135	6.5	17
68 pces, 2 oz	270	13	34
Almond Choc., 1.3 oz pkg	200	11	21
1.5 oz pkg	230	13	25
Crispy, 1.5 oz	200	9	30
King Size, $\frac{1}{2}$ pkg, 1.6 oz	240	12	28
1.5 oz pkg	220	11	26
Mini Milk Choc.Candies, 1 tube	180	8	24
1.5 oz pkg	70	3	7
Peanut: 1.7 oz pkg	250	13	30
Fun Size, 0.7 oz pkg	110	5	13
Peanut Butter/Choc., 1.5 oz	220	12	26
1.6 oz pkg	240	13	27
Fun Size, 0.7 oz pkg	110	6	12
Mars Bar:			
All varieties, 1.8 oz	240	13	31
Fun size, 1 bar	95	5	12
Marshmallows: Firm/Soft, 1 oz	90	0	23
Regular size, 6 pce, 33g	110	0	26
Mini-Marshmallow, $\frac{1}{2}$ c., 30g	100	0	24
Choc-coat. Twists (Joyva), ea.	95	2	10
Kraft: Mini, $\frac{1}{2}$ cup	80	0	21
Creme, 2 Tbsp	40	0	10
Jet-Puffed, 5 pces	90	0	23
Funmallows, each	25	0	6
Miniature, $\frac{1}{2}$ cup	100	0	25
Teddy Bear, $\frac{1}{2}$ cup	50	0	12
Marshmallow Egg, 1 egg	110	0	26
Marzipan: 1 oz	140	7	16

Per Piece/Serving	C	F	Cb
Mauna Loa: Choc. 2.5 oz bar	420	29	36
Choc. coated Macadamias, 9	230	17	19
Mega Fruit Gummi, each	10	0	2
Mike & Ike, 1 pkg, 2.1 oz	220	0	55
Milk Choc. (Hershey's): 1.55 oz bar	240	14	25
with Almonds, 1.45 oz bar	230	14	20
Milk Choc. Crisp, 1.45 oz bar	205	11	22
Milk Duds, 13 pces, 1.3 oz	160	6	30
Milk Shake Bar, 1.8 oz bar	220	7	37
Milky Way: 2 oz bar	270	10	41
Fun size, 1.4 oz bar	90	3.5	14
Miniatures, 5, 43g	190	7	30
Snack, 2, 40g	180	7	28
Milky Way Lite, 1.6 oz	170	5	34
Creme Egg, 1.2 oz pkg	190	13	18
Miniatures, 1.4 oz pkg, 5	150	4.5	29
Mints: uncoated, 1 oz	100	0	23
1 small mint ($\frac{3}{4}$" diam)	7	0	2
1 large mint 1$\frac{1}{2}$" diam.)	30	0	7
Mon Cheri (Ferrero), 4 pces, 45g	260	18	20
Mounds, 1.9 oz bar	250	13	31
Mr Goodbar: King Size, 2.6 oz bar	410	25	37
1.75 oz bar	270	17	25
Necco Candy Wafers, 3, 57g	15	0	4
Neuhaus, average all types	80	5	7
Nips (Pearson), all flavors, 2, 14g	60	2	10
Nite Bite, (Glucose Bar))	100	3.5	15
Nougat, 2 pces, 1 oz	115	1	24
Chocolate Covered, 1 oz	120	4	20
Nougat Nut Cream, 3.5 oz	340	31	50
Now & Later (Nabisco), 1 pkg	270	2.5	63
Nutrageous Bar (Reeses) 3.4 oz	520	30	52
King Size, 3.4 oz bar	480	24	54
Oh Henry! 1.8 oz bar	240	10	32
100 Grand, 1.5 oz bar	200	8	30
Orange (Lindt), 6 block, 40g	190	10	24
Orange Slices: (Jewel), 3, 41g	140	0	36
(Walgreens), 3, 43g	150	0	36
Pastel Mints (Walgreens), 33 pce	150	0	38
Patteez (Sweet n' Low), $\frac{1}{2}$ ctn, 5	120	2.5	13
PayDay Bar, 1.85 oz bar	260	13	29
King Size, 3.4 oz	480	24	54
Peanut Bar, 1.6 oz bar	210	14	20
Peanut Butter Bars, 3 pces, 18g	80	1.5	15
Peanut Brittle, 1 oz	130	5	20
Peanut Chews (Goldenberg's), ea.	60	3	21
Peanuts, choc-covered, each	25	1.5	2

Per Piece/Serving	C	F	Cb
Pearson's Mint Patties, 5, 38g	150	2.5	31
Pecan Roll, 1/3 bar, 40g	200	10	26
Peppermints, 7 small, 0.5 oz	50	0	12
Peppermint Twists, 2, 13g	60	0	12
Pez, 1 roll	30	0	6
Planters: Choc. Peanuts, 25, 7 oz	220	13	20
Orig. Peanut Bar, 1.6 oz	230	14	22
Popcorn ~ See Snacks Page 123			
Positively Pecan, 2.5 oz bar	390	24	38
Pralines, small, 0.3 oz	35	2	5
1 large piece, 1.4 oz	180	10	24
Pretzels: choc-covered:			
3 minisize, 1.15 oz	150	5.5	23
1 regular, 1 oz	130	4.5	20
Pretzel Flipz (Nestle), 8, 1 oz	130	5	19
Raisinets, 1 pkg, 1.7 oz	210	8	33
Raspberry Cream, each	80	2.5	5
Reese's:			
Chocolate Bar, 2.8 oz	420	24	43
Candy (Multipack), each	95	5.5	9
Miniatures, each	40	2.5	4
Peanut Butter Bites (18), 39g	210	12	22
Mini, 1 pce	42	2.5	5
Peanut Butter Cups, 1.8 oz cup	280	17	28
Mini, 1 pce	42	2.5	5
Reese's Pieces, 50, 1.4 oz	190	8	24
Snack, 2, 34g	190	11	19
Rice Crunchy Bars: 1 bar, 19g			
Average all flavors	60	0	14
Rice Krispies Treats: 1.3 oz bar	150	3.5	29
Chocolate Chip, 1.3 oz bar	160	5	28
Riesen Choc. Chew, 5, 1.4 oz	180	7	29
Ritter Sport: Plain Choc, 50g	260	16	26
w. Hazelnuts, 1/2 pkg, 50g	290	19	24
Rolo, each	32	1.5	5
Root Beer Barrels, 3, 0.5 oz	60	0	16
Russell Stover Candy: Creams, ea.	60	2	10
Almond Delight, 2 oz	290	17	32
Caramel Bar, 46g	230	11	20
Jelly Cups (P/Nut Butter), 2, 34g	140	9	14
Mint Dream	160	8	19
Pecan Delight (Sugar Free), 2 oz	260	18	27
Pecan Delight, 2 oz bar	310	20	27
Pecan Roll, 50g	260	18	23
Salt Water Taffy (Sathers), 5, 43g	150	2.5	34
Seashells (Guylian) 1 shell	65	4	6
Sesame Crunch, 3 pces	80	4	7

Per Piece/Serving	C	F	Cb
Simply Sugar Free: See Allen Wertz			
Simply Lite:			
Li'l Bits Chocolatey/P'nut Butter, 1/2 ctn, 36 pieces	130	5	18
Sixlets (Hershey), 1 pkg	240	9	37
Skittles, all flavors, 1.5 oz pkg	170	2	39
1.6 oz pkg, each	60	0.5	14
King Size, 2.17 oz, 1 pack	240	2.5	54
Skor Toffee Bar, 1.4 oz	220	14	23
Smarties Candy Rolls, 1 roll	25	0	5
Snackwell's Raisin Dips, 5 oz	160	5	30
Snickers:			
Bar, 2.1 oz bar	280	14	35
King Size, 1/2 bar, 1.2 oz	170	8	21
Munch Bar, 1.4 oz bar	230	15	17
Fun size, each	95	5	12
Miniatures, each	42	2.5	5
Creme Egg, each	170	10	20
Snack, 2, 40g	190	10	24
Sno Caps, 2.3 oz pkg	300	13	48
Soft 'N Chewy Butter Toffee, ea.	32	0.5	7
Sonic Boom Pops (Walgreens), ea.	60	0	14
Sour Brite Crawlers, 13 pces	140	0	31
Sour Punch, all types, 1 pkg	190	9	45
1 straw	20	0	5
Spearmint Leaves: (Jewel), 5, 40g	140	0	35
(Walgreens), 5, 11/2 oz	150	0	38
Spice Drops, 14 pces, 11/2 oz	140	0	36
Spree (Nestle): Snack, 1, 11/2 oz	50	0	13
Starburst:			
Fruit Chews, each	20	0.4	4
2 oz pkg	240	4.5	48
Fruit Twist, each	35	0	8
Fruit Twist, 2 oz pkg	190	1	45
Jellybeans, 1.5 oz	150	0	38
Jellybean Egg, 2 oz	200	0	51
Candy Canes, 0.5 oz cane	70	0	17
Trop. Fruit Chews, 2.7 oz pack	240	5	48
Starlight Mints: 3 pces, 1/2 oz	60	0	16
Suckers (Walgreens), 1 sucker, 11g	45	0	11
Sweet 'N Low: Chews, each	11	0.2	3
Sugar-Free Hard Candy, each	8	0	2
Sweet Escapes: See Hershey's			
Sweet Success Bars, 1 bar	120	4	23
Sweet Tarts (Nestle), 7, 1/2 oz	50	0	13
Symphony: All types, 1/5 bar, 7 oz	220	14	24

Per Piece/Serving	C	F	Cb
3 Musketeers, 2.1 oz bar	260	8	46
Fun size, each	70	2	13
Miniatures, each	25	0.5	5
Snack, 2, 33g	140	4.5	26
Taffy, 1 pce, $^1/_2$ oz	55	0.5	12
Tang-a-Roos: 1 roll	24	0	6
Tarts: *(Walgreens),* 4 pce, 15g	60	0	15
Tails: *(Walgreens),* 8 pce, 15g	60	0	15
Tastetations *(Hershey's):* Pep'mint	20	0	8
Butterscotch; Caramel; Choc	20	0.5	4
Terry's Orange Milk Choc, 1 pce	50	3	5
Tic Tac, all varieties, each	1.5	0	0
Toblerone: 50g (1.76 oz) bar	270	15	32
1 bar, 100g, (3.5 oz)	540	30	63
$^1/_3$ bar, 33g	180	10	21
Toffees: Regular, 1 oz	150	9	15
Tongue Torchers *(Walgreens),* 3	70	0	17
Tootsie Roll Midgies *(Walgreens),* 6	160	3	33
Tootsie Roll Pops, $^1/_2$ oz pop	50	0	12
Truffles: Regular, 1 pce, 0.4 oz	60	4	5
Large *(Godiva),* 0.75 oz	110	6.5	12
Extra Large *(J.Schmidt),* 1$^1/_2$ oz	220	13	24
Turtles *(Nestle),* each	85	4.5	10
Twix: Caramel, 1 oz	140	7	19
King Size: 1 cookie, 3.35 oz	120	6	16
4 cookies	480	24	64
Fun Size, 0.5 oz	80	4	10
2 oz pkg, 2 bars	280	14	37
Peanut Butter, 0.9 oz	130	8	13
Snack, 1 cookie, 16g	80	4	10
Twizzlers Strawberry, 1 oz pce	110	0	30
Velamints: Sugar Free, 1 pce	10	0	2
Werther's Original, 3 pce, 15g	60	1	13
Whatchamacallit Bar, 1.7 oz	220	10	29
Whitman's:			
Assorted, 1 pce	60	3	9
Dark Chocolate, 1 pce	65	3	8
Pecan Roll, 2 oz roll	300	20	26
Sampler, 3 pces, 1.4 oz	200	11	25
Snoopy Treats, 2 pces	190	10	24
Yogurt Candy: Plain, 1 oz	120	6	15
Coated Raisins, 1 oz	120	4	21
York Mints: 1.5 oz patty	145	5	34
Snack size, 0.5 oz	55	1	11
Peppermint Patties, 3	150	2.5	30
Zachary Old Fash. Creme Drops, 3	170	3	36
Zero Bar, 1 pce, 0.7 oz	85	3	14

Carob Candy

Per Piece/Serving	C	F	Cb
Carob: Plain/Natural, 1 oz	160	11	9
Carob coated: Raisins, 1 oz	130	8	15
Almonds/Peanuts, 1 oz	150	10	14
Malt Balls, 1 oz	135	8	15
Caramels, 1 oz	110	4	18
Dates, 1 oz	125	5	20
Soybeans	145	9	16
Trail; Party Mix, 1 oz	140	9	15
Carob Chips, unsweetened, 1 oz	140	7	19
Carob Bars, average all brands:			
Plain/Nut, 1 oz	160	11	13
Fruit & Nut, 1 oz	155	10	14
Mint/Orange, 1 oz	160	11	14
Caroby Natural Touch, 3 oz	450	27	36
Carafection: Cashew Coconut Crunch,			
$^1/_2$ Bar, (42g) 1.5 oz	250	14	5

Cough Drops & Lozenges

Per Piece/Serving	C	F	Cb
Beech Nut, 1 tablet	10	0	2
Hall's, 1 tablet	15	0	4
Hall's Plus, 1	18	0	5
Helps Cough, all flavors, 1	14	0	3
Listerine Loz. (Amer.Chicle)	9	0	2
Ludens Throat Drops, all flavors, 14	10	0	2
Pine Bros, 1 cough drop	10	0	2
Rite Aid, Menthol Cough, 1 drop	12	0	3
*Rolaids/*Sodium Free, 1	4	0	1
Sathers Peppermint Lozenges, 1	13	0	3
Squibb Cough/Throat Loz.'s, 1	16	0	4
Sucrets (Beecham) Lozenges, 1	10	0	2
Wintergreen Loz. (Walgreens), 1	13	0	3
Cough Medications - Page 128			

Cough Medications - Page 128

Real women don't have hot flashes. . . . They have power surges!

Home-Popped Popcorn

	C	F	Cb
Popping Corn Kernels:			
2 Tbsp, 1 oz	100	1	22
(makes approx. 3 1/2 cups)			
Air-popped (no oil), plain, 1 oz	100	0	22
1 cup (6g)	20	0	4
Oil-popped, plain, 1 oz	140	8	10
1 cup (11g)	55	3	4
Popcorn Oil, 1 Tbsp	120	14	0

Microwave Popcorn

Average All Brands (Popped)

	C	F	Cb
Butter: Regular, 1 cup	35	2	4
Light, 1 cup	25	1	4
Act II Popcorn:			
Butter, 1 cup, 0.3 oz	35	2	4.5
4 cups, popped, 1 oz	140	8	18
Light Butter, 1 cup, 0.2 oz	24	1	4.5
5 cups, popped, 1 oz	120	4	22
Butter Lovers, 1 cup, 0.3 oz	45	3	4.5
3.5 cups, 1 oz	160	10	15
Butter Lovers (Reduced Fat), 1 c.	30	1.5	4.5
4.5 cups, 1 oz	130	6	20
American Fare (K-Mart):			
Butter, 1 cup, 0.3 oz	37	2.5	4
3.5 cups, 1 oz	130	9	14
Light Butter, 1 cup, 0.3 oz	28	1	5
3.5 cups, 1 oz	100	4	14
Healthy Choice: Butter, 6 cups	100	2.5	22
Natural, 6 cups, 1 oz	100	2	22
Newman's Own: Butter, 1 oz	170	11	16
Light Butter Flavor, 3 1/2 cups	110	3	20
Orville Redenbacher:			
Movie Theater Butter, 1 cup	30	2	3
4 cups, popped, 1 oz	120	8	12
Light Movie Theater Butter, 1 cup	20	1	2
4 cups, 1 oz	80	4	8
Double Feature Jumbo, 1 cup	30	2	3
Smart Pop!: Lowfat, 1 cup	15	0	3
Butter Light, 1 cup	20	0.5	3

Bagged Popcorn

Average All Brands (Ready-to-Eat)

	C	F	Cb
Regular: Plain, 1/2 oz pkg	80	5	7
1 oz pkg	160	10	14
Box (store/airport), 2 oz	320	20	28
Bag,(9" high x 5" wide), 3 oz	480	30	42

Bagged Popcorn (Brands)

	C	F	Cb
Act II Popcorn:			
Butter Toffee: 3/4 cup, 1 oz	110	1	27
w. Peanuts, 3/4 cup, 1 oz	120	2.5	24
Caramel w. P'nuts, 3/4 cup, 1 oz	120	2.5	24
Supreme w. Pecans, Almonds, 3/4 c.	130	5	22
Cracker Jack:			
Regular, 1 oz pkg	120	2	33
Fat Free, 3/4 cup, 1 oz	110	0	26
Butter Toffee, 1/2 cup	130	4.5	21
Crunch 'N Munch: 1/2 cup, 1 oz	140	5	22
Caramel w. P'nuts, 2/3 c., 1.2 oz	140	3.5	25
Fiddle Faddle: 3/4 cup, 1 oz	140	6	21
Orville Redenbacher Clusters,			
Butter Toffee, 2/3 cup, 1.1 oz	140	4.5	24
Slimmons (Fat Free): 3/4 c., 1 oz	110	0	25
Weight Watchers: Butter, 2/3 oz	90	2.5	14

Movie Theater Popcorn

	C	F	Cb
Small (7 cups): Plain	400	27	30
with Butter	580	47	30
Medium (16 cups): Plain	900	60	70
with Butter	1170	90	70
Large (20 cups): Plain	1150	76	90
with Butter	1500	116	90

Potato Chips/Crisps

Average All Brands

	C	F	Cb
Regular: Plain or flav'd, 1 chip	9	1	1
17 chips, 1 oz bag	150	10	15
4 oz quantity	600	40	60
Pringles, 12 crisps, 1 oz	150	10	15
6.75 oz can	1000	65	100
Ruffles, Buffalo Style, 1 oz	160	10	14
Reduced Fat:			
Pringles (Right Crisps), 1 oz	140	7	20
Crunch Tators, 1 oz	140	7	19
Kettle Fry (Eagle), 1 oz	150	8	16
Lowfat/Baked varieties, 1 oz	110	1.5	23
Fat Free (*Childer's/Louise's*), 1oz	100	0	22
Pringles (Fat Free), 1 oz	70	0	15
Lay's Wow!, 20 chips, 1 oz	75	0	18
Ruffles Wow!, 17 chips, 1 oz	75	0	17
Cheddar Sour Crm,15, 1 oz	75	0	16

Tortilla Chips *See Next Page*

Pretzels

	C	F	Cb
Average All Brands			
Hard Baked Pretzels:			
1 oz	**110**	2	22
Sticks, thin, 2 1/4" (9/oz), 1	**12**	0	3
Twists, thin, 1/4" thick, (5/oz), 1	**25**	0.2	5
Dutch (2 3/4" x 2 5/8") 1/2 oz, 1	**55**	1	11
Fat Free: Snyders (1), 1 oz	**100**	0	22
Utz Wheels/Nuggets, 1 oz	**100**	0	22
Rold Gold: Sticks, 48, 1 oz	**100**	0	23
Sourdough Nuggets, 12, 1 oz	**100**	0	23
Thins, 12, 1 oz	**110**	0	24
Twists, 16, 1 oz	**110**	1	22
Tiny Twists, 18, 1 oz	**100**	0	23
Low Fat: *American Fare* Mini Twists, 1oz	**120**	1	23
Rold Gold: Crispy Thins, 9, 1 oz	**110**	0.5	22
Choc-coated: (*Nestlé*), 1 oz	**130**	4.5	20
Soft Pretzels (Twists) average:			
Plain: Regular, 2.5 oz	**190**	0	41
King Size, 5 oz	**390**	0	83
Big Cheese, 5 oz	**380**	7	61
Peanut Butter filled (*Tr. Joe's*) 1oz	**160**	7	18
Toffee (*Crunch 'n Munch*), 12	**120**	1	25
Auntie Annie's: Original	**340**	1	72
with Butter	**370**	4	72
Dipping Sauces: *Per Single Serving*			
Caramel/Chocolate	**135**	4	27
Cheese	**70**	5	2
Philadelphia Light: Plain	**45**	3.5	1
Average other flavors	**70**	6	3
Snyder's of Hanover: Logs (7) 1oz	**120**	1	21
Homestyle (15), 1 oz	**120**	1	24
Super Pretzel: Jalapeno, 5 oz	**360**	0	78
Bavarian Twist, 3 oz	**210**	3	41
Cinnamon Raisin w. Icing, 5 oz	**420**	4	76
Sweet Dough Twist, 3.7 oz	**300**	3	60

Tortilla Chips

	C	F	Cb
Tortilla Chips: Average, 1 oz	**150**	8	22
(1 oz = approx. 11 chips or 12 strips)			
Utz: Lowfat Baked, 8 chips, 1 oz	**120**	1.5	23
Doritos: 18 chips, 1 oz	**140**	6	20
Light, 13 chips, 1 oz	**130**	5	20
Wow! Nacho Cheesier, 1 oz	**90**	0.5	16
Keebler Suncheros Light, 1 oz	**150**	8	18
Kettle: Average, 1 oz	**140**	6	18
Padrino Reduced Fat, 1 oz	**130**	4	22

Snacks

	C	F	Cb
Bacon Cheese Crackers, 1 oz	**140**	6	14
Banana Chips, 1/3 cup, 1 oz	**140**	7	18
Beef Jerky: Average, 1 oz	**70**	1	0
Beef Sticks (*Frito-Lay's*) 0.3 oz	**50**	4	1
Biscuit Mix: Aver., 1/2 cup, 1.1 oz	**180**	9	20
Bugles: Original, 1 1/3 cup, 1 oz	**160**	9	18
Baked Bugles, 1 1/2 cup, 1.1 oz	**130**	3.5	23
Cajun Jerky, 1 1/2 oz	**150**	6	6
Carrot Chips (*Hain*)	**160**	9	26
Cheddar Lites (*Health Valley*) 1 oz	**120**	3	21
Cheese Balls, 1 1/8 oz pkg	**190**	13	17
Cheez Mania (*Planters*), 35, 1 oz	**160**	3	15
Cheez Balls: 45 balls, 1 oz	**150**	10	15
Reduced Fat, 45 balls, 0.73 oz	**100**	4.5	13
Cheese Crackers, 1 oz	**130**	6	18
Cheese Filled (*Frito-Lay's*)	**210**	11	24
Cheese Curls, 1 1/4 cup, 1 oz	**160**	9	19
Reduced Fat (*Utz*), 1 oz	**140**	6	21
American Fare, 1 1/4 cup, 1 oz	**140**	5	22
Cheese Puffs, average, 1 oz	**150**	10	15
Lowfat, 1 oz	**140**	5	20
Health Valley, 1 1/2 cup	**110**	3	21
No Fries, 1 oz	**110**	0	23
Cheese Straws, 4 pieces	**110**	7	8
Cheese Twists: 23 twists, 1 oz	**150**	8	19
Cheetos: Regular all flavors	**160**	10	15
Light, cheese flavored	**140**	6	19
Chex Mix: *General Mills,* 1.1 oz	**150**	10	15
Bold 'N Zesty (40% less fat), 1/2 c.	**140**	6	20
Chedder (50% less fat), 1/2 c.	**130**	5	20
Traditional (60% less fat), 2/3 c.	**130**	4	21
Chex (*Ralston*) 2/3 cup, 1 oz	**130**	5	20
Cheez Curls/Doodles, 1 oz	**160**	10	16
Churros (*Mex. Pastry*) 10", 1.2 oz	**140**	9	12
Cinna Chips (*T.J. Cinn.*) 3, 1 oz	**110**	4	19
Combos (Oven Baked): *Per 1/3 cup, 1 oz*			
Cheddar Cheese Crackers	**150**	8	16
Cheddar Cheese Pretzels	**130**	5	19
Corn Chips: Aver. all types, 1 oz	**160**	10	15
8 oz bag	**1280**	80	120
Doritos, (12), 1 oz	**150**	7	20
Corn Crunchies/Spirals, 1 oz	**160**	10	15
Corn Crisps (*Pringle*), 1 oz	**140**	7	18
Corn Nuts, 1/3 cup, 1 oz	**130**	4	20
Corn Puffs (*Health Valley*) 2 c. 1 oz	**120**	1.5	25
Dunkaroos, 1 tray, 1 oz	**130**	5	20

Snacks (Cont) | C | F | Cb

	C	F	Cb
French's Potato Sticks, 3/4 c., 1 oz	180	12	16
Funyun's Onion flavor., 1 oz	140	7	18
Goldfish (*Pepperidge Farm*) 1 oz	140	7	18
Gold-N-Chees (*Lance*), 1³/8 oz	180	7	25
Lance Sandwich: Bonnie, pkg	160	7	23
Capt. Wafers; Choc-O-Mint, pkg	190	10	23
Sour Dough w. Cheddar, pkg	240	15	23
Other varieties, average, 1 pkg	200	10	22
Munchos, 16 pieces, 1 oz	160	10	16
Nabisco: Oreo, 1.3 oz	160	7	24
Chips Ahoy, 1.3 oz	150	5	25
Sweet Crispers (18), 1 oz	135	3	25
Nibblers (*Snyder's*): Regular (13)	130	3	23
Sourdough Fat Free (16)	120	0	25
Onion Rings (*Lance*), 1 pkg	120	6	16
Oriental Mix (rice snacks), 1 oz	155	7.5	15
Original Party Mix (*Flavor House*):			
¹/3 cup, 1 oz	160	10	13
Party Mix (*Flavor Tree*) ¹/4 cup	160	11	14
Pork Skins/Rind: *Baken-ets,*1 oz	160	10	0
*Grande, *²/3 cup	80	5	0
Lance, 1 pkg	65	4	1
Potato Puffs (*Health Valley*), 1 oz	110	3	21
Potato Sticks (*French's*), ³/4 c., 1.1oz	180	12	16
Ranch Puffs (*No Fries*), 1 oz	110	0	23
Rice Chips: Bar-B-Q/Onion, ¹/2 oz	70	3	9
Santitas (*Frito Lay*), 1 oz	140	6	20
Sesame Sticks, 1 oz	155	8	15
Snack Crackers (*No Fries*), 1 oz	110	0	24
Soy Nuts, dry roasted, 1 oz	130	6	9
Spicers Wheat Snacks, 1¹/2 oz	150	7.5	18
Sunchips (*Frito Lay*), 1 oz	140	7	18
Toast/Cheese Crackers, 1 pkg	205	10	23
Tostitos, average, 1 oz	140	8	18
Trail Mix (Nuts/Seeds/Dried Fruit):			
Regular, 3 Tbsp, 1 oz	130	8	13
Tropical, 3 Tbsp, 1 oz	120	5	19
w. Chocolate Chips, 1 oz	140	9	13
Turkey Jerky Teriyaki (*Oberto*)	80	0.5	0
Vegetable Snacks/Chips, 1 oz	130	4	24
Weight Watchers: Chse Curls, ¹/2 oz	70	2.5	10
Apple Chips: ³/4 oz pkg.	70	0	18
Yogurt Raisins, 1 oz	120	4	21

Granola & Sports Bars | C | F | Cb

Per Bar	C	F	Cb
Advantage Bar, 60g	240	10	2
Amway: Positrim Food Bar,			
Cocoa Almond, 1 wrap (2 bars)	190	7	28
Peanut Butter, 1 wrap (2 bars)	210	9	28
Arbonne: Nutrition Bar, 50g	190	4.5	24
Balance + Bar, 50g (1.76 oz)	200	6	22
Snack, Honey, Peanut, 21g	100	3	11
Barbara's Bakery: Real Fruit	50	0	13
Cereal Bars, fruit filled	110	0	27
Granola Bars	80	2	15
Bariatrix: Nutra Bars, 47g	170	5	23
Proti Bars (15g Protein), 41g	130	5	15
Right Choice Bars, 40g	140	3	24
BioX Bio Protein: 81g	300	7	37
Boost: Choc./Strawb. Crunch	190	6	30
Burn-IT: 50g bar	180	3	13
Cap'N Crunch, all types, 0.8 oz	90	2	17
Carnation Breakfast Bars, 35g (1.2 oz):			
Granola (Honey/Choc), average	130	2.5	26
Choc Chip/P.nut Butter, chewy	150	5	24
Clif Bar: 2.4 oz, 68g bar	250	6	40
Balance Bar, aver., 1 bar	200	7	22
Crunch: P'nut Butter, 1 bar	250	4	45
Choc. Chip P'nut, 1 bar	250	6	40
Luna: 48g bar	180	5	24
Real Berry; Apple Cherry, 1 bar	250	2	52
Edgebar, 2 oz, 57g bar	220	2	42
Energia Bar, 2.25 oz	230	2	41
Ensure Choc Fudge Bar	130	3	20
Entenmann's: Multi-Grain, 1.3 oz	140	3	25
Extreme Ripped Force, 45g	160	3	33
Fi-Bar Nectar Granola Bars, 1 oz	100	0	22
Chewy & Nutty Bar, 1.2 oz	140	4.5	23
Fi-Pro-Tein (*R-Kane*), 1.2 oz bar	107	1	16
Figurines Diet Bar, aver., 1 bar	110	6	12
Fruitein Energy Bar, 1.3 oz	130	3	18
Gatorbar, 2.25 oz	210	1	26
GeniSoy: Peanut Butter Fudge	230	5	31
Other varieties, average	220	3.5	32
Glucerna: Nutr'l Bar, 38g	140	4	24
Grandma's: FF Cereal Bar	160	0	39
Hain: Mini Munchies Rice	90	1.5	17
Hardbody, 2.5 oz, 71g	280	7	41
Health Valley: Fruit/Granola Bars	140	0	34
Cereal: Strawberry Cobbler	130	2	27
Continued Next Page			

Per Bar	C	F	Cb
Healthy Recipes (Novartis)	150	4	21
HeartBar, Orig., Cranberry, 50g	190	3	27
HMR Benefit Bar, 1.1 oz	160	5	22
IDN (Nu Skin): AppSignal, 2 wafers	25	0	5
Glycobar, 42g (1.48 oz)	170	5	28
ProGRAM-16 Bar, 65g (2.28 oz)	250	5	34
Isopure, 60g	260	7	34
Jewel Granola Bars: Cereal	140	3	27
Choc Chip/P'nut Butter	130	4.5	20
Lowfat varieties	110	2	22
Jolt Bar (Nutra Tech) 40g	140	3	24
Kudos: M&M's	90	2.5	17
Snickers, 23g	100	3.5	16
Choc Chip/Fudge; P. Butter, 28g	125	5	20
Lean Body, 76g	300	6	15
Met-Rx Food Bars, average, 100g	320	3	50
Source One: Per pkg, all types	190	3	30
MightyBite Choc. bar, 25g	100	4	11
Mountain Lift Energy Bar	220	4.5	34
Myoplex Plus Deluxe, 90g	340	7	43
Nature Valley Granola: Oats	180	6	27
Lowfat varieties	110	2	21
NiteBite (Time-release Glucose Bar)			
Choc. Fudge; P'nut Butter, 25g	100	3.5	15
NuBar Decadence, 1.3 oz	140	2.5	30
Nutiva (Hemp, Sunflower), 40g	205	14	15
Nutra Blast, average, 47g	160	4	27
Nutri-Grain: Cereal/Twist bars	140	3	27
Low Fat Granola Bars, 21g	80	1.5	16
Fruit-full Squares, 49g bar	180	4	35
Optizone, 50g	190	6	20
Perfect Rx Nutrition Bar, 100g	340	3	50
Planters: Peanut Bar, 1.6 oz	230	11	22
Pounds Off Bar: All flavors	220	4	35
Power Bar: Harvest, 2.3 oz	240	4	45
Athletic: All varieties, 65g	230	2.5	45
Perform. Energy: O'meal Raisin	230	2.5	44
PR Bar Ironman, 49.6g	200	6	22
Pro-Amino, 78g	296	7	40
Promax: Dble Fudge Brownie, 75g	270	5	34
Other flavors	280	5	36
Protein Plus, 78g	290	4	38
Prozone Nutrition Bar, 50g	195	6	18
Pure Protein Sports Bar, 78g (2.75 oz):			
Chewy Choc Chip, 1 bar	285	5	16
Peanut Butter, 1 bar	280	7	9
Other varieties, average	270	4	15
Quaker: Chewy Granola Bars			
Choc Chip; P'nut Butter	120	3	20
Fruit & Oatmeal	140	3	26
Other varieties, average	110	2	22
Restart: Peanut Butter, 1.25 oz	140	4	10
Strawb. Banana; Chocolate	130	2.5	21
Rice Krispies Bar (Kellogg's), 28g	120	4	20
Coco Pops Bar, 22g	100	3.5	16
Treats Squares, 22g	90	2	18
Slim-Fast Bars, 1.2 oz	140	5	20
Meal on the Go, 56g	220	5	35
Snac Bar, 42.5g	180	5	24
Snackwell's: Cereal Bars	120	0	29
Hearty Fruit & Grain	130	3	26
Chewy Granola, Fudge-Dip., 1 oz	130	3	24
Source One (Met-Rx), 1 pkg, 62g	190	3	30
Spirutein Energy Bar, 1.4 oz	150	4	19
Energy: Cocoa, 65g (2.3 oz)	210	3	41
Steel Bar, 3 oz, 85g	330	6	52
Steel Pro, 85g	330	6	15
Stoker: Real Apple Oat, 65g	210	3	41
Sweet Rewards: Choc. Chip	110	2	23
Brownie; Fat Free	120	2	30
Sweet Success (Nestlé): Choc Bars	100	3.5	23
Snack Bars, 33g (1.2 oz)	120	4	23
Thermo Speed Bar, 85g	280	5	24
Think! Interactive Bar, 2 oz, 56g	220	3	43
Thunder Bar, all flavors	220	2	44
Tiger's Milk: 35g Bar	130	2.5	24
Peanut Butter	140	5	19
Peanut Butter & Honey/Crunch	150	6	19
Protein Rich	145	5	18
Tiger Sport, 65g	230	2	43
Twinlab: Ultra Fuel, 2½ oz	230	0	42
Ironman Triathlon, 56.8g	230	7	25
Ultimate Protein Bar:			
Choc./Dream; P'nut Butter, 78g	280	6	20
Berries 'N Yogurt, 40g (1.4 oz)	140	3	14
Chocolate Choc Dream, 40g	140	2.5	10
Ultra Slim-Fast:			
Rich Chewy Caramel, 1 oz	110	3.5	22
Peanut Butter Crunch, 1 oz	120	4	20
Universal Muscle, 56.7g	280	5	35
Verve (Wholefoods Mkt), 2.4 oz	240	5	41
White Lightning, 85g	320	5	27
Zone Force, 50g	190	6	21
Zone Perfect, 50g	200	7	22

Per 1 oz Unless Indicated	C	F	Cb
Acorns, raw 1 oz	105	7	12
Almonds, Dried/Dry roasted:			
Whole, 24-28 med., 1 oz	170	15	7
1/2 cup, 2 1/2 oz	420	37	17
Chopped, 1/2 cup, 2 1/4 oz	380	34	16
Sliced, 1/2 cup, 1 2/3 oz	280	25	12
Choc. coated (5-6), 1 oz	160	11	14
Oil rstd. (Blue Diamond), 1 oz	175	17	3.5
Almond Meal (partially defatted)			
1 cup (not packed), 2 1/4 oz	260	11	11
Honey roasted, 1 oz	170	13	8
Brazil Nuts, 8 medium, 1 oz	185	19	3.5
Cashews, Dry or Oil roasted:			
14 large/18 med./26 small, 1 oz	165	14	10
1/2 cup, 2.4 oz	400	33	23
Honey roasted, 1 oz	170	12	10
Chestnuts, aver. all: Dried, 1 oz	105	1	22
Raw/Fresh, 5-6 nuts, 1 oz	60	0	13
Canned, water chestnuts			
sliced/whole/drained, 1 oz	23	0	5
Coconut:			
Flesh (no shell), 1 oz	100	10	4
Raw: 1 pce. (2"x2"x1/2"), 1.6 oz	160	15	7
1/2 medium (4 1/2" diam.)	650	62	30
Dried (Desiccated):			
Unsweetened, 1 oz	187	18	17
Sweetened, shredded, 1 oz	140	9	13
Grated, 1/2 cup, 1.3 oz	185	12	18
Cream (can.), 1/2 c., 5.2 oz	285	26	12
Milk (canned), 1/2 c., 4 oz	225	24	3
Water (center liq.), 1/2 cup,4 1/4 oz	23	0	4.5
Filberts or Hazelnuts:			
Shelled, 18-20 nuts	180	18	4.5
Chopped, 1/4 cup	180	18	4.5
Ground, 1/4 cup	120	12	3
Ginko Nuts, can., 14 med., 1 oz	32	0	6
Hickory, 30 small nuts	190	18	5
Macadamia Nuts, shelled:			
Raw, 7 med./14 small, 1 oz	200	21	4
1/2 cup, 2.3 oz	460	48	10
Oil roasted, 1 oz	205	22	3.5
1/2 cup, 2.4 oz	490	52	8
Choc. coated, 2-3 pces, 1 oz	180	13	15
Mixed Nuts: 18-22 nuts, 1 oz	175	13	7
Planters: Dry roasted	170	15	7
Honey roasted (dry rst'd)	170	13	7
Oil roasted, all types	180	16	7
Kettle: Choc Lover's Mix, 1 oz	130	17	16

Per 1 oz Unless Indicated	C	F	Cb
Nut Toppings:			
Chopped, 1 Tbsp, 1/4 cup	40	4	1.5
Peanuts:			
Raw/Dried: In shell, 1 oz	117	10	3
Shelled, 1 oz	160	14	4.5
Boiled: 1/2 cup, 1.1 oz	102	7	7
Roasted, 30 lge./60 sml., 1 oz	165	14	6
1 cup, 5.1 oz	840	71	31
Chopped, 3 Tbsp, 1 oz	165	14	6
Planters: Oil Roasted, 1 oz	170	15	5
Beer Nuts, 1 oz pkg	180	14	7
Choc-coated, 1/2 cup, 2 1/2 oz	380	25	36
Cocktail, oil roasted, 1 oz	170	14	5
Dry Roasted, 1 oz	160	14	6
Honey roasted, 1 oz	170	13	8
Honey/Dry roasted, 1 oz	160	13	7
Spanish Oil Roasted, 1 oz	170	14	5
Sweet 'n Crunchy, 1 oz	140	8	16
Pecans:			
Kernel halves, 1 oz	190	19	5
(20 Jumbo or 31 large halves)			
1 cup halves, 3.8 oz	720	73	20
Chopped, 1/2 cup, 2 oz	380	30	10
Oil roasted, 1 oz	195	20	4.5
Honey roasted, 1 oz	200	18	5
Pilunits, dried, 1/4 cup, 1 oz	205	23	1
Pinenuts, dried, 1 Tbsp, 10g	50	5	1.5
Pistachios:			
Unshelled, 1/2 cup, 2 oz	165	14	7
Shelled, 1/4 cup, 45 nuts, 1 oz	165	14	7
Lance, 1 1/8 oz package	180	14	8
Planters: **Dry Roasted**, 1 oz	170	15	6
Fruit 'n Nut Mix, 1 oz	150	9	13
Nut Topping, 1 oz	180	16	6
Tavern Nuts, 1 oz	170	15	6
Sesame Nut Mix:			
(Planters), 1 oz	160	12	8
Soybean Nuts:			
Dry roasted, 1 oz	130	6	9
1/2 cup, 3 oz	390	18	28
Oil roasted, 1 oz	140	7	9
Walnuts:			
Black, 15-20 halves, 1 oz	175	16	3.5
Chopped, 1/4 cup	190	18	4
Ground, 1/4 cup	120	12	2.5
English/Persian:			
14 halves, 1 oz	185	18	5
Chopped, 1/4 cup	195	19	5

Seeds, Peanut Butter, Supplements

Seeds

	C	F	Cb
Alfalfa Seeds, sprout., 1/2 c., 1/2 oz	5	0	1
Caraway, Fennel, 1 tsp	10	0.5	1
Cottonseed Kernels, rst., 1 Tbsp	50	4	2
Flax Seeds, 3 Tbsp, 1 oz	140	10	11
Lotus Seeds, dried, 1/2 c., 1/2 oz	50	0.5	10
Poppy Seeds, 1 tsp	15	1	1
Pumpkin & Squash Seeds: whole:			
Roasted/Tamari, 1 oz	125	5.5	3
1/2 cup (32g)	140	6	3.5
Dried, 1 oz	155	13	5
Safflower Kernels, dried, 1 oz	150	11	10
Sesame Seeds: Dried, 1 Tbsp, 9g	50	4.5	2
Roasted/Toasted, 1 oz	160	14	7
Sunflower Kernels/Seed:			
Dry roasted, 1 Tbsp, 8g	45	4	1.5
1/4 cup, 1 oz	160	14	6
Oil roasted, 1/4 cup, 1 oz	180	17	6
Watermelon, dried, 1/4 cup, 1 oz	160	14	4.5

Quick Guide
Peanut Butter

Average All Brands:

	C	F	Cb
1 tsp, 6g	35	3	1.5
1 Tbsp, 0.6 oz, (17g)	105	8.5	3.5
2 Tbsp, 1.2 oz, (34g)	210	17	7
1 oz Quantity (28g)	170	14	6
1/2 cup, 5 oz	850	70	30
Jif "Sensations" Berry Blend, 1 T.	100	8.5	5
Chocolate Silk, 1 Tbsp, 0.6 oz	95	7.5	7
Peanut Wonder, 1 Tbsp	50	2	5.5
Smucker's Honey Swtnd., 1 Tbsp	100	8	4
Goober Grape/Strawb., 1 Tbsp	90	5	4
Skippy, honeynut, 1 Tbsp, 16g	95	8	4

Other Nut & Seed Butter

	C	F	Cb
Almond Butter, 1 Tbsp, 1/2 oz	105	9	2.5
Almond Butter Honey Roasted	90	7	5.5
Beanut Butter, 1 Tbsp, 1/2 oz	88	5.5	7
Cashew Butter, 1 Tbsp	92	7	4.5
Cashew Peanut Date Butter	95	7	4
Hazelnut Butter, 1 Tbsp	100	10	2.5
Pecan Butter, 1 Tbsp	110	11	3.5
Pistachio Butter, 1 Tbsp	100	8.5	5
Sesame Butter/Tahini, 1 tsp	30	3	1
1 Tbsp, 1/2 oz	90	8.5	2
Sunflower Seed Butter, 1 Tbsp	95	8	4

Supplements

	C	F	Cb
Aloe Vera Juice, undil., 2 fl.oz	5	0	1
Cod Liver Oil, 1 Tbsp	120	13	0
Evening Primrose Oil, capsules, 1	5	0.5	0
Fiber Supplements: Tabs, 1	1	0	0
Bios Life 2, 1 packet	10	0	2
Metamucil, 1 packet	5	0	1
Regular, 1 rounded Tbsp	34	0	8
Sugar-Free, 1 Tbsp	6	0	1
Fish Oil Capsules, aver., each	10	1	0
Flax Oil Capsules, 2	10	1	0
Garlic Tablets/Capsules, each	3	0	1
Lecithin Granules, 1 Tbsp, 10g	50	5	1
Protein; Powders, aver., 1 oz	100	0.5	0
Tablets, 20 tabs., 1/2 oz	70	0	0
Seaweed: Dried, 1 oz	85	0.5	22
Soaked, drained, 1 oz	15	0.5	3
Spirulina, 1 tablet	2	0	0.5
Vitamins/Minerals: Tabs/Caps, 1	2	0	0
Vitamin E Capsules, each	5	0.5	0
Yeast: Tablets, 2 tabs.	4	0	0.5
Flakes, 1 heaping Tbsp, 1/3 oz	30	0.5	4
Powder, 1 heaping Tbsp, 1/2 oz	50	0.5	6

Cough & Pharmaceutical

	C	F	Cb
Cough/Cold Syrups: 1 tsp	36	0	9
Regular, average, 1 Tbsp	120	0	30
Sugar-free, 1 Tbsp	0	0	0
Cough Drops/Lozenges ~ See Page 122			
Antacids: Average, 1 tablet	4	0	1
Liquid, 1 Tbsp	6	0	1
Sudafed Syrup, 1 tsp	14	0	3
Tylenol Liquid: Child, 1 tsp	17	0	4
Extra Strength, 1 tsp	11	0	3

𝒩ut eaters are healthier and live longer say medical researchers.

Nuts are a nutritious source of protein, vitamins, minerals and fiber.

Their fat and fiber content can help to lower blood cholesterol, but watch the quantity if overweight.

Weights As Purchased	C	F	Cb
Acerola, 1 cup, 20 pcs, 3¹/2 oz	30	0	7.5
Apples: whole, average all varieties:			
1 small (4 per lb), 4 oz	70	0	17
1 medium (3 per lb), 5¹/2 oz	90	0	23
1 large (2 per lb), 8 oz	135	0	34
I extra large, 11 oz	185	0	46
without skin, ¹/2 medium	35	0	9
Caramel Apple, 1 medium	170	0	42
Nut Coated, 1 medium	230	5	46
Apricots: 1 small (12 per lb)	17	0	4
1 medium (8 per lb), 2 oz	25	0	6
1 large (5-6 per lb), 3 oz	35	0	8
Atemoya, ¹/3 cup	95	0	22
Avocado (w/out seed/skin):			
Average, ¹/2 medium, 3¹/2 oz	160	15	6
1 salad slice, ¹/2 oz	25	2	1
Mashed/Puree, 2 Tbsp, 1 oz	50	4.5	2
¹/4 cup, 2 oz	90	9	5
Californian, ¹/2 medium, 3 oz	150	15	6
Mashed/Puree, ¹/2 c., 4 oz	200	20	8
Florida, ¹/2 medium, 5¹/2 oz	170	13	14
Mashed/Puree, ¹/2 c., 4 oz	125	10	10
¹/2 cup cubed, 3 oz	95	8	8

Note: Avocados are nutritious and contain no cholesterol. Fat is mainly monounsaturated and benefits blood cholesterol. Excellent substitute for butter or margarine on bread.

	C	F	Cb
Banana: 1 small (4 lb), 4 oz	55	0	12
1 medium (3 per lb), 5 oz	80	0	18
1 large (2¹/2 per lb), 7 oz	105	0	24
W/out skin, 1 medium., 3¹/4 oz	80	0	18
¹/2 cup, mashed, 4 oz	105	0	24
Berries: Average all types,			
(Black/Boysenberries/Blueberries)			
¹/2 cup, 2.5 oz	40	0	10
1 pint, 14 oz	220	1	56
Breadfruit, ¹/2 cup, 4 oz	115	0	28
Cantaloupe, ¹/2 med. (5" diam.)	100	0	25
1 slice, 2.5 oz (w/out skin)	20	0	6
1 cup pieces/balls, 5.5 oz	55	0	13
Carambola (Star Fruit), 1 med	50	0	4
Cassava, ¹/3 cup	120	0	27
Cherimoya (Custard Apple), 5 oz	130	0	33
Cherries: Sweet, 8 fruit, 2 oz	40	0	10
¹/2 lb (30 cherries)	145	0	38
Sour, 8 fruit, 2 oz	25	0	6
¹/2 lb (30 cherries)	100	0	23

Weights As Purchased	C	F	Cb
Coconut: Fresh, 1 piece, 1 oz	100	10	4
Shredded, fresh, ¹/2 cup	140	14	6
Sweetened, dried, ¹/2 cup	235	16	22
Crabapples, ¹/2 cup slices, 2 oz	40	0	9
Cranberries, ¹/2 cup, 2 oz	20	0	5
Currants: Per ¹/2 cup			
European Black, raw, 2 oz	35	0	8
Red & White, raw, 2 oz	30	0	7
Custard Apple, raw, 4 oz	115	1	27
Dates ~ See Dried Fruits			
Durian, flesh, 4 oz	140	2	26
Elderberries, ¹/2 cup, 2¹/2 oz	55	0	13
Feijoas, 1 medium, 2¹/2 oz	35	0	7
Figs, green/black: 1 med., 2 oz	40	0	10
1 large, 3 oz	60	0	15
Fruit Salad, fresh, average,			
¹/2 cup, 3¹/2 oz	60	0	15
1 cup, 7 oz	120	0	30
Gooseberries, raw, ¹/2 c., 2¹/2 oz	30	0	7
Grapefruit: average all types,			
¹/2 fruit, 8¹/2 oz (4¹/2 oz flesh)	40	0	10
1 cup sections w. juice, 8 oz	75	0	17
Grapes: Average, 1 cup, 5¹/2 oz	100	0	24
1 small bunch, 4 oz	70	0	15
1 medium bunch, 7oz	125	0	31
1 large bunch, 16 oz	285	0	71
Granadilla, flesh, 4 oz	95	0	23
Groundcherries, ¹/2 cup, 2¹/2 oz	35	0	8
Guava: 1 fruit, 4 oz	80	0	15
¹/2 cup, 3 oz	40	0	9

Continued Next Page

Fresh Fruit (Cont)

Weights As Purchased	C	F	Cb
Honeydew, 1 wedge (7"x2" wide),			
8 oz (with skin)	45	0	10
1 cup cubes/balls, 6 oz	60	0	14
Honey Murcots, 1 only, 5 oz	45	0	11
Jaboticaba, flesh, 4 oz	75	2	15
Jackfruit, flesh, 1/8 average, 4 oz	105	0	25
Jambos (Brazil Cherry), flesh, 4 oz	35	0	8
Java-Plum, 4 plums, 1/2 oz	25	0	6
Jujube, 3 oz	65	0	16
Kiwifruit, 1 medium, 3 oz	45	0	11
1 large, 4 oz	60	0	15
Kumquats, 5 medium, 31/2 oz	60	0	15
Kiwano, 1/2 medium, 5 oz	35	0	8
Langsat, Duku, 1 medium, 2 oz	25	0	5
Lemon, 1 medium, 4 oz	20	0	5
1 wedge, 1 oz	5	0	1.5
Peel, 1 Tbsp	4	0	0.5
Limes, 1 only, 2 oz	20	0	7
Loganberries, froz., 1/2 c., 21/2 oz	40	0	9
Logans, 5 fruit, 1/2 oz	10	0	2.5
Loquats, 4 fruit, 21/4 oz	20	0	6
Lychees, 4 fruit, 21/4 oz	25	0	6
Mamey Apple, 1 whole, 3 lb	430	4	100
1/4 fruit (1 cup flesh), 7 oz	100	1	24
Mandarin, 1 small, 3 oz	25	0	6
1 medium, 4 oz	35	0	8
1 large, 6 oz	55	0	13
Mango, flesh, 1/2 cup sl., 3 oz	25	0	6
1 whole, medium, 11 oz	140	0	34
Melons: Average all types			
1 cup, cubes/balls, 6 oz	60	0	14
Monstera Deliciosa (Taxonia),			
Edible part, 4 oz	50	0	11
Mulberries, 20 fruit, 1 oz	15	0	3
Nashi Fruit (Asian Pear),			
1 medium, 41/2 oz	50	0	11
Nectarines, 1 medium, 4 oz	50	0	12
1 large, 51/2 oz	70	0	17
Oheloberries, 1/2 cup, 21/2 oz	20	0	5
Olives (Pickled): Green, 10 lrg, 11/2 oz	45	5	0.5
Ripe, Grk. Style, 10 med., 1 oz	70	7	2
Ripe (Black), Californian:			
1 small/medium	4	0.5	0.3
1 large/extra large	6	0.5	0.5
1 jumbo	7	0.5	0.5
1 colossal	9	1	0.5
1 super colossal	13	1	1

Weights As Purchased	C	F	Cb
Oranges, average all varieties:			
1 small, 5 oz (with skin)	50	0	12
1 medium (3" diam.), 7 oz	70	0	17
1 large, 10 oz	100	0	24
Flesh only, 1 cup, 6 oz	80	0	19
Californian Valencia,			
1 medium (23/4" diam.), 6 oz	60	0	15
Californ. Navels (3" diam.), 7 oz	60	0	15
Sunkist Navel, 14 oz	130	0	32
Florida Orange, 1 medium, 7 oz	70	0	17
Peel, 1 Tbsp	0	0	0
Papaya, 1/2 cup, cubed, 21/2 oz	30	0	7
1 medium, 16 oz	120	0	28
Passionfruit, 1 medium, 11/4 oz	20	0	4.5
PawPaw (see Papaya)			
Peaches: 1 med. (4 per lb), 4 oz	35	0	8
1 large, 6 oz	55	0	13
Pears: Bartlett, 1 small, 4 oz	60	0	15
1 medium, 6 oz	90	0	22
1 large, 8 oz	120	0	30
Bosc, 6 oz	90	0	22
D'Anjou, 1 medium, 8 oz	120	0	30
Red Pear, 5 oz	80	0	20
Seckel (Wash'ton), 21/4 oz	35	0	9
Asian (Nashi), 7 oz	80	0	20
Pepino, 1/2 medium, 4 oz	20	0	4
Persimmons: Native, 1 oz	30	0	7
Japan. (21/2"d. x 21/2"h), 7 oz	120	0	30
Seedless (Maui), 1 md., 5 oz	100	0	25
Pineapple (flesh only), 1 slice			
(3/4" thick, 31/2" diam.), 3 oz	40	0	10
1 cup, diced, 51/2 oz	80	0	20
1 medium, 11/2 lb	525	0	130
Pitanga, 3 fruit, 1 oz	6	0	1
Plaintains, 1/2 cup slices, 21/2 oz	90	0	22
Plums, average all types:			
Mini/Damson, (1" diam.), 1/2 oz	8	0	2
Small (13/4" diam.), 2 oz	30	0	7
Medium (21/4" diam.), 3 oz	45	0	10
Large (21/2" diam.), 4 oz	65	0	15
Pomegranates, 1/2 fruit, 5 oz	55	0	13
Pummelo, flesh, 1/2 cup, 4 oz	35	0	8
Prickly Pears, 1 fruit, 5 oz	50	0	11
Quinces, 1 medium, 31/2 oz	55	0	14
Rambutan (Rambotang),			
Red/Yellow, 1 med., 2 oz	15	0	4
Raspberries, 1/2 cup, 2 oz	30	0	7

Weights As Purchased

	C	F	Cb
Rhubarb, raw, 1/2 cup, 2 oz	15	0	3
Sapodilla (Chico), 1 md., 7 1/2 oz	140	2	34
Sapotes, 1/2 medium, 5.5 oz	150	0.5	38
Soursop, 1 cup pulp, 8 oz	150	0	38
Strawberries:			
1 cup, 5 1/2 oz	45	0	10
6 medium/3 large, 2 oz	15	0	3
1 pint, 12 oz	95	0	22
Chocolate Dipped, 2 medium	45	2.5	6
Sugar Apples, 1/2 cup pulp, 4 oz	120	0	30
Tamarillo, 1 medium, 3 oz	20	0	4
Tamarind: 1 fruit, 1/4 oz	5	0	0
Tangelo: 1 small, 4 oz	30	0	1.5
1 medium, 5 oz	40	0	2
1 large, 7 oz	55	0	2.5
Tangerine: 1 medium, 4 oz	50	0	12
Tangor, 1 medium, 4 oz	35	0	7
Tomato:			
Cherry, 1 med., 3/4 oz	5	0	1
1 small, 3 oz	25	0	6
1 medium, 5 oz	35	0	7
1 large, 7 oz	45	0	9
1 medium slice	5	0	1
Canned Tomatoes/Products ~ Page 78-81			
Tree Tomato (Tamarillo), 3 oz	20	0	5
Ugli Fruit, Tangelo type, 5 oz	40	0	2
Watermelon (flesh only): 1 sl, 8 oz	70	0	15
1 cup cubed, 5 1/2 oz	50	0	12
Wax Jambu (Rose Apple), 2 oz	10	0	2

Dried Fruit

	C	F	Cb
Apples, 5 rings, 1 oz	75	0	18
Apricots, 8 halves, 1 oz	65	0	15
Banana Chips, 1/2 cup, 1 1/2 oz	160	5	18
Banana Flakes, 4 Tbsp, 1 oz	80	0	20
Currants, 1/4 cup, 1 1/4 oz	100	0	24
Dates: 5 medium dates, 1 1/2 oz	120	0	28
Large Calif., 3 dates, 2 oz	160	0	37
1/2 cup, chopped, 3 oz	240	0	57
Figs, 3 medium figs, 2 oz	145	0	34
Longans; Lychees, 1 oz	80	0	19
Mango Slices, 4 strips, 1 oz	70	0	15
Mixed Fruit, 1 oz	70	0	16
Papaya Spears, 1 oz	75	0	17
Peaches, 2 halves, 1 oz	60	0	14
Pears, 3 halves, 2 oz	75	0	17
Pineapple, 1 oz	80	0	18
Prunes: with pits, 1 oz	60	0	14
1 Medium (60/lb)	16	0	4
1 Large (50/lb)	22	0	5
1 Extra Large (40/lb)	27	0	6
Without pits, 4 med., 1 oz	70	0	17
Cooked: w. sugar, 1/2 c, 5 oz	200	0	45
w/out sugar, 1/2 c, 4 1/2 oz	125	0	28
Raisins, 2 Tbsp, 1 oz package	85	0	19
1/2 cup, 2 1/2 oz	215	0	50

Candied Glacé Fruit

	C	F	Cb
Apricot, 1 medium, 1 oz	100	0	25
Cherry, 3 large, 1/2 oz	50	0	12
Citron/Fruit Peel, 1 oz	90	0	21
Fig, 1 piece, 1 oz	90	0	21
Ginger, 1 oz	95	0	23
Pineapple, 1 slice, 1 1/4 oz	120	0	30

Fruit Leather/Rolls

	C	F	Cb
Average All Brands: 1 oz	100	0	24
Fruit By The Foot, 1 leather	80	0	18
Fruit Roll-Ups, 1 roll, 1/2 oz	50	0	12
Stretch Island Leathers, 2 pces, 1 oz	90	0	21
Sunkist Fruit Roll, 1 roll	75	0	18

Other Fruit Confectionery/Snacks/Bars
~ See Snacks/Granola Bars Page 124-126

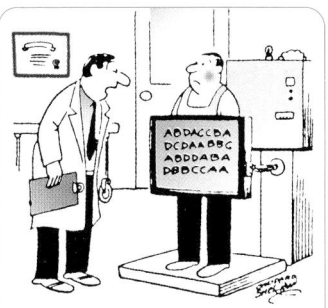

"You have a Vitamin E deficiency."

Canned Fruit & Snacks

Canned Fruit

Solids & Liquids:
Per 1/2 Cup (Approx. 4 1/2 oz)

	C	F	Cb
Apples: sweetened	70	0	17
Apricots: In water/diet	35	0	9
In juice/light	60	0	15
In syrup	105	0	27
Blackberries/Blueberries			
In heavy syrup	115	0	30
Cherries, pitted, in water	55	0	14
In light syrup	85	0	21
In heavy syrup	110	0	28
In extra heavy syrup	130	0	33
Fruit Cocktail: In water/diet	40	0	11
In juice/light	55	0	15
In light syrup	80	0	21
In heavy syrup	95	0	25
Fruit Salad: In water/diet	35	0	9
In juice/Light	60	0	16
In heavy syrup	95	0	25
Gooseberries: Light syrup	90	0	23
Grapefruit: Juice pack	45	0	15
In light syrup	75	0	20
Mixed Fruit: In water/diet	40	0	10
In fruit juices	60	0	15
In light syrup	60	0	15
In heavy syrup	100	0	25
Mandarin Oranges: In water	40	0	11
In light syrup	80	0	21
Peaches (halves or slices):			
In water/diet	30	0	8
In juice/light	50	0	14
In light syrup	70	0	20
drained, 1/2 peach	40	0	11
In heavy syrup	100	0	26
Pears: In water/diet	35	0	10
In juice/light	60	0	16
In heavy syrup	100	0	26
Pineapple:			
(Chunks/Crushed/Spears/Wedges/Slices)			
In own juice	70	0	18
In heavy syrup	90	0	23
Slices, drained, 2 slices			
In own juice	30	0	8
In heavy syrup	45	0	11

Canned Fruit (Cont)

Per 1/2 Cup

	C	F	Cb
Plums: In water	50	0	14
In juice	75	0	20
In light syrup, 3 plums	85	0	21
In heavy syrup, 1/2 cup, 3 plums	160	0	41
3 plums	120	0	31
Prunes: In heavy syrup	120	0	32
4 prunes	70	0	18
Raspberries, in heavy syrup	120	0	30
Strawberries: In water	25	0	7
In heavy syrup	120	0	31
Tropical Fruit Salad:			
In light syrup	80	0	18
In heavy syrup	95	0	21

Fruit Snack Cups

Del Monte Fruit Cups: Per 4 oz

	C	F	Cb
Diced Peaches/Pears/Mixed,			
In heavy syrup	80	0	20
In extra light syrup	50	0	13
In fruit juices	50	0	13

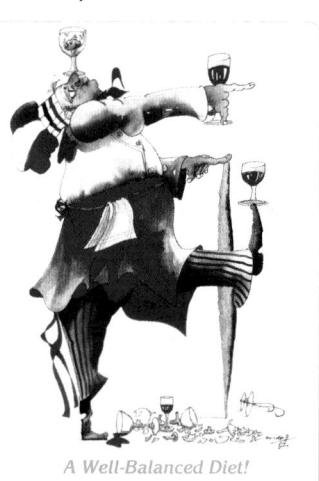

A Well-Balanced Diet!

Vegetables - Fresh or Frozen

Edible Portion (Raw Weight Unless Indicated)	C	F	Cb
Alfalfa Sprouts, 1/2 cup, 1/2 oz	5	0	1
Artichokes, Globe/French:			
1 medium, 4 1/2 oz	65	0	15
Artichoke Heart, 1/2 cup, 3 oz	40	0	10
Asparagus, raw/froz.: 4 med. spears	15	0	3
Cuts & tips, 1/2 cup, 3 oz	25	0	5
Bamboo Shoots, ckd, 1/2 c, 4 oz	15	0	3
Beans: Green/Snap, 1/2 c, 2 oz	20	0	4
Broadbeans, ckd, 1/2 cup, 3 oz	90	0	16
Butterbeans, 1/2 cup, 3 oz	90	0	20
Lima, baby, 1/2 cup, 3 oz	90	0	17
Dry Beans, average all types:			
(Kidney, Brown, Haricot, Lima, Mung, Navy, Pinto, Red, White)			
Raw, 2 Tbsp, 1 oz	95	0.5	18
1 cup, 7 oz	665	3	126
Cooked, 1 oz	35	0	7
1/2 cup, 3 oz	105	0	21
Soybeans: Mature, dry, 1 oz	110	5	7
Dry, 1/2 cup, 3 1/2 oz	385	18	22
Cooked, 1/2 cup, 3 oz	105	6	6
Bean Sprouts, aver., 1/2 c., 3 oz	25	0	3
Beets, cooked, 1/2 c, slices, 3 oz	25	0	6
1 beet, 2" diam., 2 oz	17	0	4
Beet Greens, ckd, 1/2 c., 2 1/2 oz	20	0	4
Bell Pepper: See Peppers			
Black Eyed Peas, ckd, 1/2 c., 2 oz	160	0	32
Bok Choy (Chinese Chard), 3 oz	12	0	2
Broccoli: Raw, 1/2 cup, 1 1/2 oz	12	0	3
1 spear (5 oz edible)	40	0	8
Cooked, 1/2 cup, 3 oz	25	0	5
Brussel Sprouts, ckd, 1/2 c, 3 oz	35	0	7
Cabbage, average all varieties:			
Raw, shred., 1/2 cup, 1 1/4 oz	8	0	1
Cooked, 1/2 cup, 2 1/2 oz	15	0	2
Carrot: Ckd, 1/2 cup sl., 2 1/4 oz	35	0	8
Raw, 1 medium (7 1/2"), 3 oz	33	0	8
Raw, 1 lb, (5-6 med)	175	0	40
4 sticks (4"), 1 1/2 oz	15	0	3
Shredded, 1/2 cup, 2 oz	25	0	6
Cauliflower, cooked:			
3 floret, 1c. 1" pcs, 3 oz	15	0	3
1/2 medium (15 oz raw)	100	0	20
Celeriac, 1/2 cup, raw, 2 3/4 oz	30	0	7
Celery, 1 stalk, 7 1/2", 1 1/2 oz	5	0	1
Diced, 1/2 cup, 2 1/4 oz	10	0	3

Edible Portion (Raw Weight Unless Indicated)	C	F	Cb
Chard (Swiss), 1/2 cup, ckd, 3 oz	20	0	4
Chick Peas (Garbanzo Beans):			
Dry, 1 cup, 6 oz	550	10	92
Cooked, 1 cup, 6 oz	270	4	45
Chicory/Witloof ~ See Endive			
Chicory, Greens, 1/2 cup, 3 oz	20	0	4
Chives, chopped, 1 Tbsp	1	0	0
Collards, 1/2 cup, 3 oz	15	0	4
Corn, yellow/white:			
Raw, kernels, 1/2 c., 2 3/4 oz	65	1	14
Ear (5"x 1 3/4"), 5 1/2 oz	80	1	17
Trimmed to 3 1/2" long	60	1	14
Cooked, kernels, 1/4 c., 1 1/2 oz	35	<1	7
(Also see Frozen & Canned Corn Page 135)			
Cress, Garden, 1/2 cup, 1 oz	10	0	2
Cucumber, 1 whole, 11 oz	40	0	12
1/2 cup slices, 2 oz	5	0	1
Dandelion Greens, 1/2 cup, 1 oz	15	0	3
Eggplant: 1 whole, 4 1/2 oz	40	0	10
1/2 cup, 1" pieces, 1 1/2 oz	10	0	2
1 slice, fried, 1 oz	40	4	10
Endive, Belgian/French:			
1 med. head (6"), 2 1/2 oz	12	0	3
Fennel, 2 oz	10	0	2
Garlic, 1 clove	4	0	1
Ginger, 1/4 cup slices, 1 oz	20	0	4
Crystallized (sugared), 1 oz	95	0	20
Horseradish, 1 pod, 3/4 oz	4	0	1
Jerusalem Artichoke, 1/2 cup	60	0	14
Jicama, raw, 1/2 cup	25	0	5
Kale, 1/2 cup, 2 oz	20	0	4
Kohlrabi, 1/2 cup, cooked, 3 oz	25	0	6
Leek, cooked, 1 whole, 4 oz	40	0	9
Lentils, green/brown: Dry, 1 oz	95	0	17
Dry, 1 cup, 6 1/2 oz	620	0	108
Cooked, 1/2 cup, 3 1/2 oz	115	0	20
Lettuce: 1 c., chop./shred., 2 1/2 oz	10	0	2
Butterhead, 2 leaves, 1/2 oz	2	0	0.5
Cos/Romaine, 1 c., shred., 2 1/2 oz	4	0	1
Iceberg: 1 leaf, 3/4 oz	3	0	1
1 medium head, 15-16 oz	60	0	15
Lotus Root, 10 slices, ckd, 3 oz	60	0	15
Mung Bean Sprouts, 1/2 cup	15	0	3
Mushroom: Raw, 1/2 cup, 1 oz	10	0	2
Cooked, 1/2 cup, 2 1/2 oz	20	0	3
Mustard Greens, 1/2 cup, 1 oz	7	0	1

Vegetables - Fresh or Frozen (Cont)

Edible Portion (Raw Weight Unless Indicated)	C	F	Cb
Okra, ckd., 1/2 cup, slices, 2 3/4 oz	25	0	6
Onions: Raw, 1 medium, 4 oz	40	0	9
1/2 cup, chopped, 3 oz	30	0	7
Dehydrated flakes, 1/4 c, 1/2 oz	45	0	11
Rings, breaded/fried, 2 rings	80	5	9
Ore-Ida, 4 pces	220	11	27
Scallions, 1/2 cup, 2 oz	15	0	4
Spring, 1/4 cup, chopped, 1 oz	6	0	1
Parsley, chopped, 1/2 cup, 1 oz	10	0	2
Parsnips, 1 medium, 4 oz	80	0	20
Cooked, 1/2 cup slices, 2 3/4 oz	65	0	16
Peas: Green, 1/4 cup, 1 1/2 oz	35	0	6
raw, with pods, 1/2 lb	70	0	13
Snow Peas (8-9 pods), 1 oz	10	0	2
Split, dry, hulled, 1 oz	50	0	10
cooked, 1 cup, 7 oz	230	1	41
Peppers: Bell, 1 medium, 5 oz	25	0	6
1/2 cup, chopped, raw, 1 3/4 oz	12	0	3
1 ring (3" diam. x 1/4" thick)	2	0	0
Sweet, 1 medium, 5 oz	35	0	10
Chili: Green/Red, 1 1/2 oz	18	0	4
Habanero, 1 only, 8g	11	0	2
Pigeon Peas, cooked, 1/2 cup	85	1	16
Pimientos, drained, 3 1/2 oz	25	0	5
Poi, 1/2 cup, 4 1/4 oz	135	0	33
Potatoes: Raw (with skin)			
1 Baby, Gourmet, 2 oz	45	0	11
1 small, 3 oz	65	0	15
1 medium, 5 oz	110	0	26
1 peeled, 4 oz	90	0	21
1 large, 8 oz	180	0	41
1 Extra large. (Russet), 12 oz	270	0	62
Mashed w. milk and fat, 1/2 c.	110	4	14
Baked (no fat); large, 10oz raw:			
Plain, with skin, 7 oz	220	0	51
without skin, 5 1/2 oz	145	0	34
With Toppings:			
+ 2 tsp fat	290	8	51
+ Sour Cr./Chives, 2 Tbsp	270	6	53
+ Plain Yoghurt, 2 Tbsp	240	1	55
+ Grated Cheese, 1 oz	330	9	56
+ Cottage Cheese, 2 oz	280	2	56
Roasted (w. fat), 1 small	155	8	36
Garlic Potatoes, 4 oz	120	2	22
Hash Browns: w. Butt. Sce, 2 1/2 oz	125	6	10
Homemade, 1/2 cup, 2 1/2 oz	165	10	10

Edible Portion (Raw Weight Unless Indicated)	C	F	Cb
Potatoes (Cont):			
French Fries: small serve, 2 1/2 oz	220	12	14
medium serve, 4 oz	350	20	22
Froz., uncooked, 18 fries, 4 oz	185	7	22
Oven-heated, 18 fries, 4 oz	185	7	22
Take-Out: 1 cup, 5 oz	440	25	28
McDonald's: Small, 2 1/2 oz	210	10	26
Large, 5.2 oz	450	22	57
Supersize, 6.2 oz	540	26	68
Fried: 18 fries, 3 oz	275	15	16
Au Gratin, 1/2 cup, 4.3 oz	160	9	22
Pancakes, 1 only, 5 oz	90	5	9
Kugel, 5 oz	300	20	26
Puffs, fried, 4 puffs, 1 oz	65	3	37
Scalloped, 1/2 cup, 4 1/4 oz	105	4	13
Stuffed Baked Potatoes:			
See 1-Potato-2 ~ Fast-Food Section			
Ore-Ida Frozen Potatoes (As Purchased):			
Steak Fries, 8 fries, 3 oz	110	3.5	17
Frozen Crispers, 3 oz	220	13	24
Country Fries, 15 fries, 3 oz	120	3.5	19
Crispy Crunchies, 13 fries, 3 oz	160	8	20
Fast Fries, 22 fries, 3 oz	150	6	20
Pixie Crinkles, 22 pces, 3 oz	130	1.5	21
Golden Curls, 17 pces, 3 oz	160	7	22
Golden Fries, 16 pces, 3 oz	120	4	20
Golden Patties, 1, 2.5 oz	140	7	16
Hash Browns: Average, 3 oz	80	0	17
Oven Chips, 7, 3 oz	180	8	25
Potatoes O'Brien, 3/4 c., 2 oz	60	0	14
Season'd Crinkle Cuts, 15, 3 oz	120	3	23
Shoestrings, 3 oz	150	5	22
Sweet Potatoes: 1 patty, 60g	70	0	17
Center Cut: Prime, 2 pce	70	0	16
Petite, 5 pce, 117g	80	0	18
Mashed/Casserole, 1/2 cup	80	0	18
Tater Tots, 9 pces, 3 oz	150	8	20
Taters, 4 pces, 3 oz	150	7	20
Twice Baked, all types, 1, 5 oz	190	7	26
Waffle Fries, 9, 3 oz	150	7	21
Zesties, 12 pces, 3 oz	160	9	21
Potato Salad, 1/2 cup, 4 1/4 oz	180	10	14
Pumpkin, mashed, 1/2 c., 4 oz	25	0	6
Purslane, cooked, 1/2 c., 2 oz	10	0	2
Radish: aver., 10 only, 1 1/2 oz	10	0	2
Oriental, 1/2 c. slices, 1 1/2 oz	10	0	2

Edible Portion
(Raw Weight Unless Indicated)

	C	F	Cb
Rutabagas, ckd., 1/2 c. cubes, 3 oz	30	0	7
Salsify, ckd, 1/2 c. slices, 2 1/2 oz	45	0	11
Sauerkraut, 1/2 cup, 4 oz	25	0	5
Seaweed, aver. all: Dried, 1 oz	50	0	13
Soaked, drained, 1 oz	15	0	4
Nori/Laver, dried, 6 sheets, 1/2 oz	35	0	5
Shallots, chopped, 1 Tbsp	7	0	1
Soybeans ~ See Beans Page 68-70, 133			
(Soy Products/Tofu/Tempeh ~See Pages 67)			
Sorrel, raw, 1/2 cup, 4 oz	23	0.7	4
Spinach, cooked, 1/2 cup, 3 oz	20	0	4
Creamed, 1/2 cup, 4 1/2 oz	140	12	10
Squash: Summer, average			
raw, 1/2 cup slices, 2 1/4 oz	13	0	3
cooked, 1/2 cup slices, 3 oz	18	0	4
Winter, cooked:			
Acorn, 1/2 cup cubes, 3 1/2 oz	55	0	15
1/2 medium (10oz raw wt.)	85	0	22
Butternut, 1/2 c. cubes, 3 1/2 oz	40	0	11
1/4 medium (9oz raw wt.)	95	0	26
Hubbard, 1/2 c. cubes, 3 1/2 oz	50	0	11
Spaghetti, 1/2 cup, 2 3/4 oz	23	0	5
Succotash, ckd, 1/2 cup, 3 1/3 oz	110	1	23
Sweetcorn ~ See Corn.			
Sweet Potatoes: Cooked with Skin			
No fat, 1 only, 4 oz	120	0	28
No skin, mash, 1/2 c., 5 1/2 oz	170	0	40
Swedes, 1/2 cup, 3 oz	45	0	10
Taro, cooked, 1/2 cup, 2 oz	95	0	23
Tomatoes: See Fruit ~ Page 131			
1 small, 3 oz	20	0	5
1 medium, 5 oz	35	0	8
1 large, 7 oz	45	0	10
Cooked, 1/2 cup, 4 1/4 oz	30	0	7
Fried, 1 small, 3 oz	60	4	5
Tomatillo, 1 oz	7	0	1
Turnips: White, ckd, 1/2 cup, 3 oz	15	0	4
Greens, ckd, 1/2 cup, 2 1/2 oz	15	0	3
Water Chestnuts, 4 nuts	40	0	10
1/2 cup slices, 2 1/4 oz	65	0	15
Watercress, 10 sprigs, 1 oz	4	0	1
Yam, raw, 1/2 cup, 2 1/2 oz	80	0	20
Baked Yam, medium, 8 oz	260	0	62
Yardlong Bean, 1 pod, 1/2 oz	7	0	1
Zucchini, 1 medium, 10 oz	45	0	10
1/2 cup slices, cooked, 3 oz	13	0	3

Frozen Vegetables (Mixed)

Birdseye

	C	F	Cb
Brocc./Carrots/W. Chestnuts, 1 cup	35	0	6
Broccoli/Corn/Red Peppers, 3/4 cup	50	0.5	11
Broccoli/Cauli./Carrots, 1 cup	30	0	4
Brussels Sprouts/Cauli./Carrots	35	0	5
Carrots/Corn/Green Beans, 2/3 cup	60	0.5	11
Cauliflower/Carrots/Pea Pods, 1 cup	30	0	5
Chopped Spinach, 1/3 cup	20	0	2
Baby: Corn Blend, 2/3 cup	60	0.5	11
Bean & Carrot Blend, 1 cup	30	0	5
Broccoli Blend, 1 cup	70	1.5	8
Broccoli Florets, 1 cup	25	0	4
Gold & White Corn, 2/3 cup	80	1	15
Pea Blend, 3/4 cup	40	0	7
Sweet Pea, 2/3 cup	70	0.5	12
Pasta Secrets: Primavera, 1 cup	230	10	26
Zesty Garlic, 1 cup, cooked	240	10	31
Stir Fry: Prepared (Includes Pasta)			
Asparagus, 2 cup	90	0.5	16
Green Bean, 1 3/4 cup	100	0.5	19
Voila: Per 1 Cup, Cooked			
Garlic Chicken	260	11	27
Pesto Chicken	250	9	25

Green Giant

	C	F	Cb
Vegetables: Asparagus Cuts, 2/3 c.	25	0	4
Corn: Nibblers, 1 ear	70	0.5	14
Extra Sweet Niblets, 2/3 cup	70	1	13
Sthwestern & Rst Peppers, 3/4 c.	90	1	19
Green Bean Casserole, 2/3 cup	100	5	11
Honey Glazed Carrots, 1 cup	90	3.5	13
Le Sueur Baby Sw. Peas, 2/3 cup	60	0.5	11
Spinach, 1/2 cup	25	0	3
Veges In Lowfat Sauce: Prepared			
Alfredo Vegetables, 3/4 cup	80	3	9
Broccoli & Cheese, 2/3 cup	70	2.5	9
Creamed Spinach, 1/2 cup	80	3	10
Early June Peas, 3/4 cup	100	2	16
Niblets Corn, 2/3 cup	130	3	23
Teriyaki Vegetables, 1 1/4 cup	100	7	7
Create A Meal: Prepared			
Beefy Noodle, 1 1/4 cup	350	14	31
Cheesy Pasta & Veg, 1 1/4 cup	440	23	27
Homestyle Stew, 1 1/4 cup	340	16	34
Lo Mein Stir Fry, 1 1/4 cup	320	7	35
Oven Roasted: Garlic Herb, 1 3/4 c.	360	9	37
Savory Cream, 1 3/4 cup	340	13	27

Vegetables - Canned/Bottled

Frozen Vegetables (Cont)

	C	**F**	**Cb**
Green Giant (Cont)			
Create A Meal:			
Parmesan Herb, $1^3/4$ cup	330	11	37
Skillet Lasagna, $1^1/4$ cup	350	13	33
Sweet & Sour Stir Fry, $1^1/4$ cup	290	7	29
Szechuan Stir Fry, $1^1/4$ cup	310	14	20
Teriyaki Stir Fry, $1^1/4$ cup	230	6	18
Pasta Accents: *Per 1 Cup, Cooked*			
Alfredo Broccoli	210	8	25
Cr. Cheddar w. Broc./Carrots	250	8	30
Garlic Seas. w. Broc/Corn/Carrots	260	10	36
La Choy			
Mixed Fancy Vegetables, $1/2$ cup	12	0	3
Veg-All			
Succotash, $1/2$ cup	80	1	17
Westpac			
Just Add: *As Prepared, Per 10 oz*			
Beef: Oriental Garlic & Ging. $1^1/4$ c.	280	7	25
Chicken, $1^1/4$ cup	290	2	34
Hamburger: Vegetable Stroganoff	320	12	32

Canned/Bottled

	C	**F**	**Cb**
Solids & Liquid			
Artichoke Hearts, plain, 1 oz (1)	30	0	8
Marinated, 1 oz	60	5	2
Asparagus (Tips/Cuts/Spears),			
$1/2$ cup, $4^1/2$ oz	20	0	3
Bamboo Shoots, 1 cup, $4^1/2$ oz	25	0	4
Bean Salad, $1/2$ cup, 3 oz	90	0	23
Bean Sprouts, $2/3$ cup	10	0	2
Beans:			
Green, $1/2$ cup, $4^1/4$ oz	20	0	4
Baked Beans, $1/2$ cup, $4^1/2$ oz	120	<1	18
Butter Beans, $1/2$ cup, $4^1/2$ oz	90	0	20
Italian, cut, $1/2$ cup, $4^1/2$ oz	30	0	7
Kidney Beans, $1/2$ cup, $4^1/2$ oz	105	<1	20
Lima Beans, $1/2$ cup, $4^1/2$ oz	80	0	15
Pinto Beans, $1/2$ cup, $4^1/2$ oz	100	<1	20
Wax Beans, cut, $1/2$ cup, $4^1/2$ oz	20	0	4
(Also see Canned Products ~ Pages 68-70)			
Beets:			
Sliced/Whole, $1/2$ c., $4^1/2$ oz	35	0	7
Crinkle/Pickled (*Del Monte*) $1/2$ c.	80	0	20
Carrots, sliced, $1/2$ cup	35	0	8

Canned/Bottled (Cont)

	C	**F**	**Cb**
Corn: Whole kernel, sweet:			
$1/2$ cup, $4^1/2$ oz	80	0.5	20
Drained Solids, $1/2$ cup, 3oz	65	0.5	15
Creamed style, $1/2$ cup, $4^1/2$ oz	100	0.5	24
Dill Pickles ~ See Page 78			
Eggplant, 2 Tbsp, 1 oz	25	2	5
Garbanzo/Chick Peas, 3 oz	100	2	20
Green Chilies: diced, 2 Tbsp, 1 oz	5	0	1
Hearts of Palm, (1), 1.2 oz	9	0	1
Mushrooms: $1/2$ cup, $2^1/2$ oz	20	0	4
in Butter Sauce, 2 oz	30	1	3
Olive Salad (*Progresso*), drain, 2 T.	25	2.5	1
Onions: Pickled, 1 med., $3/4$ oz	10	0	2
Cocktail, 1 onion	2	0	0.5
Peas, $1/2$ cup, 3 oz	60	0	11
Peppers: Hot Chilli, 1 only, 1 oz	8	0	2
Sweet, undrained, $2^1/2$ oz	15	0	3
Jalapeno, w. liq., $1/2$ c. chopped	17	0	3
Cherry (*Progresso*), dr., 2 T., 1 oz	25	2	2
Fried, drain, 2 Tbsp, 1 oz	60	5	3
Pepper Salad (*Progresso*), dr., 2 T.	15	1	1
Potatoes, $1/2$ cup, 3 oz	55	0	12
Salsa: Average all types, 2 Tbsp	15	0	3.5
Sauerkraut, undrained, $1/2$ c., 4 oz	25	0	6
Spinach, $1/2$ cup, $3^1/2$ oz	25	0	3.5
Straw Mushrooms, $1/2$ cup, 4.3 oz	20	0	3
Succotash: *Per $1/2$ Cup, $4^1/2$ oz*			
w. Cream Style Corn	100	1	23
w. whole kernels, undrained	80	1	17
Sweetcorn: See Corn.			
Sweet Potato, $1/2$ cup, $3^1/2$ oz	105	0	24
Tomatoes, Sundr.: Natural, 5-6 pce	22	0	5
In Oil, drained, 6 pces, $1/2$ oz	60	4	6
Tomato Products ~ See Page 78-81			
Vegetables, mixed, $1/2$ cup, 4 oz	45	0	8
Yams in Light Syrup, $1/2$ cup, 4 oz	105	0	25
Zucchini in Tom. Sce., $1/2$ c., 4 oz	30	0	8

Take-Out Vegetable Dishes

	C	**F**	**Cb**
Appetizers: Caponata, $1/4$ cup	30	1	5
Curried Vegetables, 8 oz serving	400	33	22
Pakoras, 1, 2 oz	110	5	12
Ratatouille, 1 cup, 9 oz serving	200	16	10
Samosa, 2, 4 oz	500	45	25
Succotash, $1/2$ cup	110	1	23
Spring Roll, 2, 3 oz	200	9	28

Salads - Fresh, Deli, Restaurant)

Average All Outlets
Per Serving

	C	F	Cb
Antipasto Salad, 1 cup	140	10	2
Bean Salad, 1/2 cup	110	4	17
Bulgur Salad, 1/2 cup	70	2	12
Caesar Salad, Classic, 1 cup	200	14	15
Side Salad, no dressing	25	0	6
Carrot Raisin: No dress., 1/2 cup	20	0	5
with dressing, 1/2 cup	65	5	5
Chef Salad: Regular, no dressing	620	37	8
w. 2oz 1000 Island	860	61	8
Chicken Salad Platter, 6 oz	200	8	12
Coleslaw: Traditional, 1/2 cup	150	8	18
w. low cal dressing	60	1	12
Corn, Mexican, 1/2 cup	240	12	33
Cucumber, non-oil dress., 1/2 cup	60	0	14
w. Oil dressing, 1/2 cup	140	12	4
Eggplant Salad, 1/2 cup	75	5	7
Fettucini w. veges, 1/2 cup	110	5	15
Garden Salad, no dressing	35	0	8
Greek Salad, 1 cup	120	10	7
Greek Vegetables, 1/2 cup	140	12	7
Lettuce, hearts, 1/4 head	20	0	4
Lobster Salad Platter, 6 oz	200	8	12
Macaroni Salad, 1/2 cup	140	8	16
Nicoise, 1 cup	450	32	18
Pasta Salad, 1/2 cup	160	8	16
Pineapple Coconut Slaw, 1/2 cup	150	10	14
Potato Salad: Dijon	140	7	17
w. Mayonnaise, 1/2 cup	170	10	17
Lowfat, 1/2 cup	110	1.5	21
Rice Salad, 1/2 cup	150	10	13
Saffron Rice, 1/2 cup	130	3	24
Spinach Salad	180	13	13
Tomato & Mozzarella, 1/2 cup	180	14	10
Tabouli, 1/2 cup	150	6	22
Three Bean Salad, 1/2 cup	80	5	9
Tortelini w. Basil Pesto, 1/2 cup	170	10	19
Waldorf w. mayo, 1/2 cup	160	12	12

Signature Salads: *Per 6 oz Serving*
(Supplied to Deli's and Institutions)

	C	F	Cb
Antipasto Salad, 6 oz	510	50	4
Artichoke Salad, marinated	400	41	8
California Medley	120	7	15
Cheese Agnolotti	250	8	23
Chicken Salad	420	33	11
Crabmeat Flavored	450	38	20
Egg Salad	300	23	14

Signature Salads (Cont):

	C	F	Cb
Fresh Button Mushroom	190	16	6
Garden Olive, 6 oz	630	67	3
Ham Salad	400	32	14
Prima Pasta Salad	360	30	18
Seafood Pasta Del Mar	170	10	21
Seafood with Crab & Shrimp	420	34	20
Shrimp Salad	360	32	8
Tuna Salad	450	36	14

Fast-Food Restaurant Chains ~ *See Page 161*

Fresh Salad Packs

Pre-Packaged (Supermarkets)

	C	F	Cb
Dole: Complete: Caesar, 3 1/2 oz	170	13	8
Oriental, 3 1/2 oz	120	6	13
Romano, 3 1/2 oz	150	12	9
Spinach Bacon, 3 1/2 oz	170	10	18
Sunflower Ranch, 3 1/2 oz	160	16	5
Lunch For One: Ranch, 1 kit	350	29	20
Special Blends (no added dressing):			
Aver. all varieties, 2 cups, 3 oz	15	0	3
Regular Salad Packs (no added dressing):			
Classic Coleslaw, 3 oz	25	0	5
Classic Iceberg, 3 oz	15	0	4
Zesty Italian, 7 oz	110	0	4
Fresh Express: *Per 1 1/2 cups*			
Salad Kits: Caesar Salad	170	14	9
Fat Free Caesar Salad	70	0	1
Taco Fiesta	110	8	7
Garden Salad; Italian Salad Mix	20	0	3
European/Riviera Salad Mix	15	0	3
Hearts of Romaine Salad Mix	20	0.5	3
Garnden w. Romaine Salad	20	0	3
Ready Pac: Aver. all types	15	0	2
Weight Watchers			
Caesar/Garden/European, 3.5 oz	60	0	12
Caesar Salad w. cookies, 4 oz	160	3	30
Garden Salad w. cookies, 4 oz	120	1.5	24
European Salad w. cookies, 4 oz	160	3	11

Salad Toppings

	C	F	Cb
Bacon Bits, aver., 1 Tbsp	30	1.5	2
Chow Mein Noodles, dry, 1/2 c.	120	5	13
Croutons, 2 Tbsp, 10g	35	1	6
Olives, 5 medium	25	2	0
Potato Chips, 1 oz	150	10	15
Sunflower Seeds, 1 Tbsp, 8 g	45	4	1.5
Tortilla Chips, 1 oz	150	8	16

Fruit & Vegetable Drinks & Juices

Quick Guide C F Cb

Orange Juice
Per 8 fl.oz Unless Indicated

Average ~ Fresh or Sweetened:

	C	F	Cb
1/2 Cup, 4 fl.oz	55	0	13
Small Glass, 6 fl.oz	82	0	20
Regular Glass, 8 fl.oz	110	0	26
8 3/4 fl.oz Box	120	0	28
10 fl.oz Bottle	140	0	32
11 1/2 fl.oz Can	160	0	36
16 fl.oz Bottle	220	0	52
64 fl.oz Bottle	880	0	208

Other Juices

Average All Brands
Per 8 fl.oz Unless Indicated

	C	F	Cb
Aloe Vera Juice, unsweet., 2 oz	5	0	1
Apple Juice: 8 fl.oz	115	0	30
10 fl.oz Bottle	145	0	36
64 fl.oz	920	0	232
Blueberry Juice, 8 fl.oz	90	0	25
Carrot Juice: Fresh, 6 fl.oz	60	0	14
Sweetened, 6 fl.oz	75	0	17
Cranberry Juice, Cocktail/Blend			
8 fl.oz	120	0	34
Grape Juice, 8 fl.oz	160	0	40
Grapefruit Juice, 8 fl.oz	100	0	23
Lemon Juice: 1 Tbsp	4	0	1.5
1 cup, 8 fl.oz	60	0	21
Concentrate, 1 tsp	0	0	0
Lime Juice, 1 Tbsp	4	0	1.5
Orange Juice, 8 fl.oz	110	0	26
Passion Fruit Juice (Fresh):			
Purple, 1 cup, 8 fl.oz	125	0	34
Yellow, 1 cup, 8 fl.oz	150	0	36
Papaya/Peach Nectar, 8 fl.oz	140	0	35
Pear Nectar, 8 fl.oz	150	0	40
Pineapple Juice, 8 fl.oz	110	0	27
Prune Juice, 8 fl.oz	180	0	43
Strawb./Raspberry Juice, 8 fl.oz	100	0	23
Tangerine Juice, 8 fl.oz	100	0	25
Tomato Juice, 8 fl.oz	50	0	12
Vegetable Juice, 8 fl.oz	50	0	12
Fruit Blends, average, 8 fl.oz	120	0	31
Fruit Nectars, average, 8 fl.oz	140	0	35

Juice Brands C F Cb
Per 8 fl.oz Unless Indicated

Apple & Eve
	C	F	Cb
Naturally Cranberry	120	0	30
Cranberry/Raspberry Apple	120	0	30

Arizona
	C	F	Cb
Crazy Carrot; Lemonade/Pink	110	0	27
Grape/Kiwi/Strawberry	120	0	29
Mucho Mango	100	0	25

Bright & Early
	C	F	Cb
Orange Juice (Chilled/Frozen)	120	0	30
Grape Juice (Frozen)	140	0	33

Campbell's
	C	F	Cb
Tomato Juice, 8 fl.oz	50	0	10
10.5 fl.oz	60	0	12
V-8 Healthy Request, 8 fl.oz	50	0	12
V-8 Splash Tropical Blend, 8 fl.oz	120	0	30

Capri Sun
	C	F	Cb
Average all flavors, 6.75 oz	100	0	28

Chiquita
Frozen Concentrates, prepared:
	C	F	Cb
Average all varieties, 8 fl.oz	130	0	32

Del Monte
	C	F	Cb
Pineapple Juice: Fresh, 8 fl.oz	110	0	27
From Concentrate, 8 fl.oz	130	0	32
Prune Juice, 8 fl.oz	170	0	42
Tomato Juice:			
Fresh, 8 fl.oz	40	0	10
From Concentrate, 8 fl.oz	50	0	12
Snap-E-Tom Cocktail, 6 fl.oz	40	0	10
Fruit Smoothie Blenders: *Per 6.5 fl.oz*			
Mango-Pineapple-Banana;			
Strawberry-Peach-Banana	180	0	45
Peach-R'berry/P'apple-Or.-Ban.	210	0	53

Dole
100% Fruit Juice Blends:
	C	F	Cb
Average all varieties, 8 fl.oz	120	0	29
Fruit Drink Blends:			
Average, 8 fl.oz	130	0	31
Spicy Vegetable Blend, 12 fl.oz	80	0	16

Dominick's
	C	F	Cb
Orange Juice (100% Pure), 8 fl.oz	110	0	27
Tropical Fruit Blend	130	0	32

Fruit & Vegetable Drinks & Juices

Per 8 fl.oz Unless Indicated	C	F	Cb
Eden: Organic Apple, 8 fl.oz	80	0	23
Five Alive: Citrus beverage, 8 fl.oz	120	0	30
Fresh Samantha			
Banana Strawberry	150	1	12
Carrot/Orange; Fresh Tangerine	110	1	8
Colossal C	115	0	10
Grapefruit; Beta Yet; The Big Bang	100	0	8
Mango; Str. Orange; Rasp. Dream	120	1	11
Protein Blast	155	1	10
Spirulina; Desperately Seeking C	130	1	10
Fruitopia			
Average all flavors, 8 fl.oz	120	0	30
Iced Teas ~ See Page 148			
Goya Nectar			
Apricot Nectar, 1 can	130	0	31
Pear Nectar, 1 can	240	0	59
Hawaiian Punch			
Fruit Juicy, Red, 6 fl.oz	90	0	22
Box, 8.45 fl.oz	120	0	30
Hi-C: Orange Juice			
Chilled/Premium Choice, 8 fl.oz	110	0	30
10 fl.oz bottle	140	0	36
Calcium Rich, 8 fl.oz	120	0	33
Other Juices Drinks: Aver., 8 fl.oz	130	0	32
8.45 fl.oz box, average	135	0	33
11.5 fl.oz can	180	0	45
Hood: Grapefruit Juice (Select)	100	0	23
Natural Blenders, average	130	0	32
Orange Juice: Select	120	0	30
Calcium Rich	120	0	30
Jui2ce			
All flavors, 8 fl.oz bottle	95	0	23
Juicy Juice			
Apple Grape, 8.45 fl.oz box	120	0	10
Berry, 8.45 fl.oz box	130	0	30
Punch, 8.45 fl.oz box	140	0	32
Tropical, 8.45 fl.oz box	150	0	26
Kern's Nectars			
Pineapple Coconut Nectar, 6 fl.oz	140	0	26
11.5 fl.oz box	210	0	48
Other nectars, average, 6 fl.oz	110	0	27

Per 8 fl.oz Unless Indicated	C	F	Cb
Kool Aid			
Koolers, average, 8.45 fl.oz	140	0	37
Fruit Drinks, average, 8 fl.oz	100	0	25
Sugar Free, 8 fl.oz	5	0	0
Knott's: Sparkling Ciders, 325 ml	110	0	25
Knudsen			
Fruit Juices: Apple	110	0	28
Apple Blends, all varieties	120	0	30
Black Cherry; Prune	180	0	43
Grape; Pomegranate	150	0	37
Grapefruit	100	0	23
Just Cranberry; Tomato	60	0	14
Orange	100	0	23
Pear	120	0	30
Nectars: Coconut	140	5	26
Other Nectars, average	130	0	36
Blends: Average all flavors	120	0	30
Citrus Juices:			
Rio Red Grapefruit	140	0	35
Lemonade (Natural)	120	0	30
Simply Nutritious: Per 8 fl.oz			
Ginseng Boost	110	0	27
Lemon Ginger Echinacea	120	0	30
Mega C	130	0	31
Mega Green; Gingko Alert	120	0	30
Morning Blend; VitaJuice	120	0	30
Floats: Orange	140	0	33
Spritzers:			
Average all flavors, 12 oz	170	0	43
Lights, all flavors, 12 oz	110	0	28
TeaZers: All flavors, 12 oz	110	0	28
Very Veggie: 8 fl.oz	50	0	10
Krasdale			
Cranberry Apple	170	0	42
Cranberry Juice Cocktail	130	0	32
Cranberry Raspberry	150	0	37
Libby's			
Orange Juice, 8 fl.oz	105	0	25
Juicy Juice, average, 8 fl.oz	140	0	34
Nectars, 1 can, 11.5 fl.oz	220	0	52
Mauna La'i Hawaiian			
All flavors, 8 fl.oz	130	0	32
Mistic (Mega 24 fl.oz)			
Average All flavors, 8 fl.oz	120	0	30
24 fl.oz	360	0	90

Per 8 fl.oz Unless Indicated Ⓒ Ⓕ Ⓒb *Per 8 fl.oz Unless Indicated* Ⓒ Ⓕ Ⓒb

Minute Maid

	C	F	Cb
100% Juices: *Per 8 fl.oz*			
Apple/ Orange Juice	115	0	27
Fruit Drinks/Punch: *Per 8 fl.oz*			
Average all flavors	120	0	30
Chilled Singles: *Per 16 fl.oz Bottle*			
Berry/Tropical Punch	240	0	60
Lemonade/ Orange Juice	220	0	55
Juices to Go: *Per 10 fl.oz Bottle*			
Average all flavors	160	0	40
Boxed Juices: *Per 8.45 fl.oz*			
Cherry Grape; Tropical Punch	130	0	32
Orange Juice; Apple Juice	120	0	31
Berry; Fruit	120	0	31
Calcium Juices: *Per 8 fl.oz*	120	0	27

Mott's

	C	F	Cb
Apple Raspb., Fruit Punch, 10 fl.oz	145	0	36
Apple Cranberry, Grape Apple 10 fl.oz	180	0	42
Clamato Tomato Cocktail, 8 fl.oz	60	0	11
Fruitsations: all flavors, 4 oz	85	0	22
Grapefruit (from conc.), prep.	120	0	28
Juice Paks: All flavors, 8.45 fl.oz	120	0	30
Mini Motts, 4.23 oz	60	0	14
Orange Juice (from conc.)	130	0.5	30

Naked Juice

	C	F	Cb
Apple Juice, 8 fl.oz	120	0	29
Banana Blueberry; Boysenberry	140	2	34
Banana Date	240	4	46
Berry Blast; Wise Guy	130	0	30
Carrot Beet/Celery/Spinach	100	0	21
Chocolate Dream	190	2	38
Grapefruit Juice	110	0	23
Green Machine	140	0.5	35
Mighty Mango; Orange Jce Nirvana	110	0	24
Papaya Strawberry	100	0	24
Protein Drink (6g protein)	170	1.5	33
Protein Zone (17g protein)	220	4	32
Strawberry Banana/Lemonade	140	0	33
Turbo C	110	0	27
Vanilla Creme	150	1	28
Watermelon	80	1	18
Zippitea	80	0	32

Newman's Own

	C	F	Cb
Lemonade, 10 fl.oz	140	0	34

Ocean Spray

	C	F	Cb
Apple Juice (from conc.)	110	0	28
Bl. Cherry; Crazy Kiwi; Mega Melon	130	0	33
Cranberrry:			
Cranberry Grape	170	0	41
Cranberry Juice Cocktail	140	0	34
Light Style (Low Calorie)	40	0	10
Other Cranberry flavors, aver.	150	0	35
Caribbean Colada; Cran-Mango	130	0	32
Cranicot; Cranapple; Cranblueberry	160	0	41
Crantastic Fruit Punch	150	0	37
Fruit/Holiday Punch; Tangerine	130	0	32
Grapefruit:			
100% Juice	100	0	24
Other flavors, average	125	0	31
Lemonade flavors, average	130	0	32
Orange Juice (from concentrate)	120	0	31
Kiwi Strawb.; Summer Cooler	120	0	31

Odwalla

	C	F	Cb
Boyzenberry Mango	140	0	34
C Monster, 16 fl. oz	300	0	72
Fruitshake Blackberry	160	0	40
Grapefruit Juice	90	0	34
Guanaba Dabba Doo!	130	0	30
Lotta Colada	160	0	33
Mango Tango	150	0	37
Mo Beta, 16 fl. oz	280	0	70
Orange Juice	120	0	34
Raspberry Smoothie	140	0	35
Strawberry Banana	100	0	25
Strawberry Go Man Go	100	0	25
Super Protein, 16 fl. oz	400	0	40
Vegetable Cocktail	70	0	18

Orange Julius

Per 16 fl.oz

	C	F	Cb
Orange	265	0	65
Pina Colada	300	0	75
Strawberry	340	0	85
Raspberry Cream Supreme	510	20	82
Tropical Cream Supreme	510	25	71

Realemon - Realime (*Borden*)

Lemon/Lime Juice (from concentrate)

	C	F	Cb
1 teaspoon	0	0	0
2 Tbsp, 1 fl.oz	6	0	2
1/2 cup, 4 fl.oz	24	0	8

Fruit & Vegetable Drinks & Juices (Cont)

Per 8 fl.oz Unless Indicated	C	F	Cb
Santa Cruz			
Natural 100%: Aver. all varieties	120	0	30
Sparkling varieties, 8 fl.oz	150	0	33
S&W: Apple Juice, 8 fl.oz	120	0	30
Orange Juice, 6 fl.oz can	90	0	22
Grapefruit Juice, unswt'd, 8 fl.oz	105	0	25
Tomato Juice, 8 fl.oz	30	0	7
Snapple			
Cranberry Royal, 10 fl.oz	150	0	38
Fruit Drink Blends, 8 fl.oz	120	0	30
Grapeade; Orangeade 8 fl.oz	120	0	30
Orange Juice, 10 fl.oz	130	0	30
Whipped Snapple (Fruit Smoother):			
Aver. all flavors, 297ml bottle	160	0	40
Squeezit			
Average all flavors, 6.75 fl.oz	90	0	23
Sunny D			
Enriched Citrus Beverage (5% Jce)	130	0	31
Sunny Delight			
Florida Citrus, 6 fl.oz	90	0	22
Calcium Rich, 6 fl.oz	150	0	37
Florida Citrus Punch, 6 fl.oz	90	0	22
Sunny Delight Lite, 6 fl.oz	20	0	5
Tropical Fruit Punch, 6 fl.oz	90	0	22
Sunsweet			
Prune Juice/w. Pulp, 8 fl.oz	180	0	43
Tang			
Fruit Box (8.45 fl.oz):			
Average all flavors	140	0	34
Mix: Made up, 6 fl.oz			
Regular (2 Tbsp dry)	90	0	22
Sugar Free	7	0	0
Tree of Life: Black Cherry	180	0	43
Concord Grape	160	0	40
Cranberry Nectar	150	0	38
Other varieties, average	130	0	33
Tree Top: Per 6 fl.oz			
Apple Juice; Apple Citrus/Pear	120	0	30
Apple Cranberry/Grape	130	0	32
Fruit Juice Punch, 10 fl.oz	150	0	37
Grape/Grape Fruit Juice; Sparkling	120	0	30
Orange Juice	120	0	28

Per 8 fl.oz Unless Indicated	C	F	Cb
Tropicana			
Blends: Berry; P'apple, 8 fl.oz	130	0	32
Pure Premium:			
Orange Juice + Fiber	120	0	30
Ruby Red	120	0	28
Season's Best: Orange Juice	110	0	27
7 fl.oz bottle	90	0	23
10 fl.oz bottle	130	0	33
11.5 fl.oz can	140	0	36
Grapefruit Juice, 8 fl.oz	160	0	40
Tropics:			
Average all flavors, 8 fl.oz	110	0	26
Twister: Average, 8 fl.oz	120	0	32
10 fl.oz bottle	150	0	40
11.5 fl.oz can	160	0	40
Light, average, 8 fl.oz	35	0	10
10 fl.oz bottle	50	0	11
V-8 Vegetable Juice			
V-8 Vegetable Juice, average all varieties			
1 cup, 8 fl.oz	50	0	10
11.5 oz Can	70	0	14
Veryfine			
Apple Cranberry	130	0	33
Fruit Punch	140	0	36
Grape Juice (100%)	150	0	37
Grape Drink	110	0	28
Grapefruit Juice (100%)	90	0	20
Pink	120	0	30
Guava Straw.; Lemon Lime	120	0	30
Orange Juice (100%)	120	0	24
Orange Drink	140	0	35
Papaya Punch	120	0	30
Pineapple Orange	130	0	32
Welch's			
Regular Juices:			
Average all blends, 8 fl.oz	160	0	40
Tomato, 8 fl.oz	50	0	10
8.45 fl.oz Box, average	150	0	37
Mini Drinks, 5.5 fl.oz	100	0	25
Frozen Juice Concentrates: Per 8 fl.oz			
(Reconstituted)			
Grape	160	0	41
White Grape Juice Blends	150	0	36
Cranberry/Raspberry	150	0	37
Lite Cranberry/Grape/Raspberry	50	0	13
Other flavors, average	130	0	33

Nutritional Shakes & Drinks

Nutritional Shakes/Drinks

	C	F	Cb
Amway Positrim Drink Mix			
Regular Mix, 1 pkt, 43g	160	4	27
Fat Free Mix, 1 pkt, 65g	230	0	50
Arbonne Int'l Meal Shake	190	4.5	24
Balanced: Diet, 11 fl.oz can	180	1	34
High Protein, 11 fl.oz can	230	3	36
Kids Chocolate, 8 fl.oz can	160	3	30
Bariatrix Shakes, 1 serving	100	2	6
Proti-Max Meal, 67g	250	3	20
Fruit Drinks (High Protein), 20g	70	1	2
Boost: Ready-To-Drink, 8 fl.oz	240	4	41
Boost High Protein, 8 fl.oz	240	6	33
Boost Plus, 8 fl.oz can	360	14	45
Carnation Instant Breakfast			
Powder: 1 reg. envelope, 37g	130	1	28
No Sugar Added, 1 envel., 21g	70	1	12
Ready-To-Drink, aver., 10 oz	220	3	37
Choice dm (Mead Johnson), 8 fl.oz	250	12	25
CEnsure: Regular, 8 oz can	225	6	31
Ensure Bal'd Bkfst, choc pouch	140	0.5	30
Ensure Fiber, 8 fl.oz can	250	6	42
Ensure Light, 8 fl.oz can	200	3	33
Ensure Plus, 8 fl.oz can	360	13	47
Glucerna, 8 fl.oz can	220	11	22
Powder, made up, 1/2 cup	250	9	34
Genisoy: Shake, 1 scoop, 35g	120	0	17
Protein Powder, 1 scoop, 29g	100	0	0
Health Source Soy, 2 scoops, 1 oz	100	1	4
Herbalife, (Thermogetics F.1), 1 oz	100	1	14
HMR 500 Shakes, 1 pkt	100	0	16
HMR 120, 1 serving	120	1.5	16
IDN (Nu Skin): Aloe F'ntain, 2 fl.oz	20	0	5
Amino Build, 3 scoops, 1 1/2 oz	160	1	12
Appeal: French Delight, 2 oz pkt	210	2	33
Swiss Truffle, 2 oz pkt	220	2.5	33
Appeal Lite HT	120	1.5	26
Sports Drinks: See Next Page			
JumpStart: Choc./Van., 42g pkt	150	1.5	27
Prep. with Fat Free milk, 8 fl.oz	240	2	40
Met-Rx: Nutrition Drink Mix, 72g	260	2	22
Metaform: Lean Mass, 2 scoops	140	0	11
Protein Powder, 76g (2.7 oz)	270	2	21
Proton, 45g pkt (1.6 oz)	170	1	15
90% Plus Protein: 3 Tbsp, 1 oz	110	0.5	2
Nutrament (Mead Johnson): 12 fl.oz	360	10	52
Optifast 800: Powder, 1 serving	160	3	20
Ready-To-Drink, Chocolate	160	3	20

	C	F	Cb
Optitrim: Choc./Vanilla			
ProBalance, 8.45 fl.oz	300	10	39
Pro-Cal 100 (R-Kane), 1 pkt	103	2	7
Resource (Novartis):			
Standard 8 fl.oz pak	250	6	40
Plus, 8 fl.oz pak	360	11	52
Diabetic, 8 fl.oz pak	250	11	23
Fruit Beverage, 8 fl.oz pak	180	0	36
Yogurt Flav'd Beverage, 8 fl.oz	250	4	45
Restart: French Vanilla; Choc			
2 level scoops, 1 oz	110	3	8
Rite Aid Nutritional Suppl. 8 oz	250	6	40
Sav-on Nut'l: 8 fl.oz can	360	13	47
Light, 8 fl.oz can	200	3	33
Slim-Fast: All flavors, 1 scoop	100	1	20
Prep. w. Fat Free milk, 8 fl.oz	190	1	32
Sustacal: Liquid, 8 fl.oz can	240	6	33
Basic, 8 fl.oz can	250	9	34
Sustacal Plus, 8 fl.oz can	360	14	45
Powder, 2 oz + water	200	1	36
Sweet Success (Nestle):			
Healthy Shake, 10 fl.oz can	200	3	37
Fruit Flavors, 10 fl.oz	200	0.5	39
Powder, 2 scoops, 32g (1.1 oz)	100	1	25
Total Balance, 9.5 oz can	230	7	25
Twin Lab RxFuel, 1 pkt	250	0	62
Ultra Slim-Fast: Powder, 1 scoop	120	0.5	24
Ready-To-Drink, 11 oz can	220	3	38
Ultimate Whey Designer Prot. 22g	90	1	2.5
Walgreens Nutritional Supplements:			
Advanced Formula, 8 oz can	250	6	40
Plus, 8 oz can	355	13	47
Light, 8 oz can	200	3	33
Weider (Powders):			
Creatine ATP, 2 scoops, 2 oz	230	0	37
Complete Rx, 70g pkt (2.5 oz)	240	2.5	27
Lean Pro, 2 scoops, 50g (1.76oz)	180	1.5	22
Ultra Whey Pro, 1 scp, 30g (1oz)	110	1	2
Women's Natural Replace., 33g	120	1	13
Dynamic: Body Shaper, 35g	140	0.5	22
Muscle Builder, 2 scoops, 45g	190	0	27
Weight Gainer, 4 scoops, 85g	330	0.5	62
Victory Pure Protein: 2 scoops,			
Egg/Beef/Vege. average	140	0	14
Victory Mass 1000, 7 oz	740	2.5	148
Mega Mass 4000, 3 scoops	1640	4	319
Super Mega Mass 2000, 2 sc.	520	1.5	102

Sports Drinks • Smoothies

Sports Energy Drinks

(Fluid Replacement, Carbohydrate Rich) **C** **F** **Cb**
Per 8 fl.oz Unless Indicated

	C	F	Cb
AllSport, all flavors, 8 fl.oz	70	0	18
Amino Force, 22 oz	390	0	75
Blue Thunder, 22 oz	400	0	68
Body Fuel (w. NutraSweet), 8 fl.oz	4	0	1
Body Works (Shasta), 12 fl.oz	90	0	22
Carboplex (Nutra Life), 31g	120	0	30
Cytomax, 8 fl.oz	65	0	13
Exceed (Weider): Powder, 2 Tbsp	70	0	17
Liquid, 12 fl.oz box	105	0	26
Gatorade: ThirstQuencher, 8 fl.oz	50	0	14
ReLode, 1 pkt	80	0	20
GatorLode, 11.6 fl.oz can	280	0	70
GatorPro, 11 fl.oz can	360	6	59
Hydra Fuel (Tury Labs)	65	0	16
IDN (Nu Skin):			
Creatine Blast, 1 scoop, 1$^{1}/_{2}$ oz	130	0	32
Splash C with Aloe, 1 scoop	80	0	20
Sportalyte, $^{1}/_{2}$ pkt (makes 8 fl.oz)	70	0	17
Knudsen, Isotonic Sports	60	0	15
Max, made-up, 8 fl.oz	96	0	24
Met-Rx ORS Endura (Meta genics)	60	0	15
Pedialyte (Abbott)	25	0	6
Powerade, all flavors, 8 fl.oz	70	0	18
Pro-formance, all flavors	100	0	25
Recharge (Knudsen), all flavors	70	0	18
Red Bull Energy Drink, 8.3 fl.oz	113	0	28
Relode Gel, 0.75 oz pkt	80	0	20
Ripped Force, 16 oz	90	0	22
Snapple Sport, all flavors	80	0	20
Sobe (20 fl.oz): Energy; Proline	120	0	32
Elixir 3C: Orange	90	0	24
Cranberry Grapefruit	110	0	28
The Juice, 11 fl.oz	260	0	65
10-K (Suntory)	60	0	15
Thermo Force, 16 oz	260	0	65
Tiger's Milk (mix):			
Energy Booster, 3 heap Tbsp.	120	0	30
Twin Lab Ultra Fuel, 16 oz	400	0	100
Upper Deck: All flavors	80	0	19

Quick Guide

Fruit Smoothies **C** **F** **Cb**

Average All Brands

	C	F	Cb
Fruit Only: 8 fl.oz cup	305	0	25
12 fl.oz	160	0	38
16 fl.oz	210	0	50
24 fl.oz	320	0.5	76
Fruit + Nonfat Milk/Soy:			
12 fl.oz	190	0.5	40
16 fl.oz	250	0.5	53
24 fl.oz	380	1	80
Fruit + Nonfat Frozen Yogurt/Sherbert:			
12 fl.oz	210	0.5	47
16 fl.oz	280	0.5	62
24 fl.oz	420	1	94

Brands - Fruit Smoothies

Jamba Juice (California): Per 24 fl.oz
(Full Listings - See Page 202)

	C	F	Cb
Coffee Colossus	420	0	99
Femme Phenom	500	1.5	11
Lo-Cal Motion	280	1	66
Orange Oasis	430	1	96
Peach Pleasure	480	2	114
Soymilk Splash	380	1	81
The Jamba Powerboost	440	1.5	96
Jera's Juice (Boston): Per 24 fl.oz			
Mango Passion	300	0.5	71
Raspberry Madness	425	1	100
Spring Fever	400	1.5	91
Soy Smoothie	360	4.5	79
Whippy Snapple: Per 10 fl.oz			
Citrus	150	0	39
Pineapple Orange	100	0	41
Fruit Whips: Per 8 oz bottle			
Berry/lemon/Orange/Tropical			
All flavors, 236ml (8 oz)	125	0	29

*D*ehydration limits sporting performance.

*Drink adequate water before, during
and after strenuous exercise.
Lightly sweetened drinks may benefit
endurance athletes.*

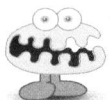

Soft Drinks • Soda

Quick Guide

Cola & Soda Drinks

	C	F	Cb

Average All Brands
Coca-Cola and Pepsi

	C	F	Cb
8 fl.oz Cup	100	0	25
12 fl.oz Can	150	0	37
16 fl.oz Bottle	200	0	50
20 fl.oz Bottle	250	0	63
24 fl.oz (Pepsi)	300	0	75
1 Liter Bottle	400	0	100
2 Liter Bottle	800	0	200

Other Soda Drinks

	C	F	Cb
Club Soda, 12 fl.oz	0	0	0
Club Soda Cream, 12 fl.oz	170	0	42
Diet Soft Drinks: Aver., 12 fl.oz	0	0	0
Ginger Ale, 12 fl.oz	120	0	30
Lemon Lime, 12 fl.oz	220	0	55
Orange, 12 fl.oz	180	0	45
Root Beer, 12 fl.oz	165	0	41
Tonic Water, 12 fl.oz	135	0	34
Mineral Water: Plain, 12 fl.oz	0	0	0
Sweetened/flavored, 12 fl.oz	150	0	37
w. Fruit Juice, 12 fl.oz	120	0	30
Seltzers: Plain/Diet, 12 fl.oz	0	0	0
Sweetened/flavored, 12 fl.oz	150	0	37
w. Fruit Juice, 12 fl.oz	120	0	30

Movie Theater & Take-Out

Average All Flavors
(Figures allow for 25% Ice)

	C	F	Cb
Small, 12 fl.oz	110	0	27
Regular, 16 fl.oz	150	0	37
Medium, 22 fl.oz	210	0	5
Large, 32 fl.oz	300	0	75

Soda Brands

Per 12 fl.oz Unless Indicated

	C	F	Cb
A&W: Cream Soda	165	0	41
Diet Cream Soda/Root Beer	1	0	0
Root Beer	180	0	45
Albertson's: Cola	160	0	43
Lemon Lime	140	0	38
Other flavors, average	170	0	47
Arizona: Lite Choc. Fudge, 8 fl.oz	60	0	14
Strawb. Banana Colada, 8 fl.oz	140	0.5	33
Pina Colada, 8 fl.oz	140	1	34
Lemonade, 15 fl.oz Can	220	0	54

Soda Brands (Cont)

Per 12 fl.oz Unless Indicated

	C	F	Cb
Barq's Root Beer	165	0	41
Big Red: 8 fl.oz	100	0	25
Barrelhead: Rootbeer	165	0	41
Bodyworks (Shasta), all flav.	90	0	23
Canada Dry: Birch Beer; Cactus	165	0	41
Club Soda	0	0	0
Collins Mixer	120	0	30
Ginger Ale, all flavors	135	0	37
Diet, all flavors	0	0	0
Half & Half; Hi-Spot; Wild Cherry	165	0	41
Lemon Sour	150	0	37
Seltzer, all flavors	0	0	0
Sour Mixer	135	0	34
Tahitian Treat	225	0	56
Tonic Water/Twist Lime	150	0	37
Diet	0	0	0
Clearly Canadian, 11 fl.oz, aver.	120	0	30
Coca-Cola:			
Classic	140	0	35
Coke II	160	0	40
Diet Coke; Diet Cherry Coke	1	0	0
Cherry Coke	150	0	42
Cragmont: Cola	165	0	41
Cherry	180	0	45
Diet, all flavors	0	0	0
Crush, all flavors	210	0	52
Crystal Light, all flavors	8	0	2
Diet Rite, all flavors	1	0	0
Doc Shasta	160	0	40
Dr A	150	0	41
Dr Diablo, Cola	140	0	35
Dr Nehi	150	0	41
Dr Pepper: Regular	150	0	40
Diet (Reg.; Caffeine Free)	3	0	0.5
Fanta: Orange; Grape	180	0	45
Ginger Ale	130	0	33
Root Beer	165	0	41
Fresca	4	0	1
Hansen's: Average all flavors	130	0	37
Health Valley: Ginger Ale	150	0	41
Sarsaparilla RootBeer	150	0	41
Rootbeer Old Fashioned	120	0	30
Wild Berry	140	0	35
Hires: Cream; Root Beer	180	0	45
Jolt Cola	150	0	41
Kick (Royal Crown)	180	0	45

Per 12 fl.oz Unless Indicated	C	F	Cb
Knudsen:			
pritzers, average	170	0	43
Lights, all flavors	110	0	28
Lucozade, 7 fl.oz	136	0	34
Manischewitz, Seltzer	0	0	0
Mello Yello: Regular	180	0	45
Diet	5	0	0
Minute Maid: Diet Orange	3	0	0.5
Berry; Black Cherry; Orange	165	0	41
Fruit Punch; Grape	180	0	45
Lemonade	160	0	40
Peach; P'apple; R'berry; Grapefr.	165	0	41
Strawberry	185	0	46
Mountain Dew, 24 fl.oz Bottle	170	0	46
Mr Pibb: Regular	150	0	37
Diet	2	0	1
Mug: Root Beer	160	0	43
Diet	0	0	0
Natural Brew: Apple, Cream	170	0	43
Cafe Mocha, Cherry Amaretto	160	0	40
Ginseng Cola, Ginger Ale	170	0	43
Nehi (Royal Crown): Cream	180	0	45
Ginger Ale, Quinine Water	135	0	45
Other flavors, average	195	0	45
Orangina, 10 fl.oz Bottle	120	0	45
Orbitz, 300ml Bottle, average	130	0	30
Pepsi: Regular; Caffeine Free	150	0	41
Diet Pepsi	0	0	0
One	1	0	0
Wild Cherry	160	0	43
Perrier: Regular or flavors	0	0	0
Ramblin' Root Beer	180	0	45
RC Cola: Regular	160	0	40
Diet Cola	1	0	0
Cherry	165	0	41
Royal Mistic: Punch, 16 fl.oz	230	0	57
'N Juice, average	155	0	38
Sparkling, average, 11.1 fl.oz	115	0	28
Schweppes: Bitter Lemon	165	0	41
Ginger Ale, regular; Raspberry	120	0	30
Ginger Beer; Lemon Lime	150	0	37
Grapefruit	165	0	41
Lemon Sour	165	0	41
Seltzer	0	0	0
Tonic: Regular	120	0	30
Diet	0	0	0
7UP: Regular	140	0	38
Cherry, Gold	155	0	38

Per 12 fl.oz Unless Indicated	C	F	Cb
Santa Cruz: Sparkling, all types	150	0	37
Orange	195	0	48
Sensa (Guarana flavored)	135	0	34
Shasta: Black Cherry	170	0	46
Cherry Cola; Doc Shasta	160	0	40
Club Soda; Diet, all flavors	0	0	0
Cola, regular	170	0	46
Caffeine Free	160	0	40
Fruit Punch, Pineapple	200	0	50
Ginger Ale	130	0	33
Shasta Plus: all flavors	170	0	46
Slice: Lemon Lime	150	0	38
Diet Lemon Lime	0	0	0
Dr. Slice	140	0	40
Fruit; Grape; Pineapple; Red	190	0	51
CherryLime; Slice Cola	160	0	43
Snapple: Average all flavors	180	0	45
Spree (Shasta): all flavors	170	0	43
Sprite: Regular	150	0	37
Diet	4	0	1
Squirt: Regular Soda Citrus	150	0	40
Ruby Red Soda	170	0	46
Sunkist: Average all flavors	210	0	52
Diet Citrus	0	0	0
Diet Orange	7	0	1.5
Surge Citrus	170	0	46
TAB	1	0	0
Upper 10 (RC): Regular	150	0	37
Diet	4	0	1
Vernor's: Ginger Ale	150	0	37
Wink	195	0	48
Welch's: Sparkling, average	180	0	45

Fruitopia

(Contain 10% Fruit Juice): Per 2 fl.oz	C	F	Cb
Apple Raspb.; Trop. Consideration	115	0	45
Lemonade Love; Cranberry Lemon	170	0	43
Pink Lemonade; Tangerine Wave.	175	0	44
Other flavors, average	190	0	47

Kool-Aid, Tang

	C	F	Cb
Bright & Early, 6 fl.oz	90	0	23
Kool-Aid, unsweetened, 6 fl.oz	2	0	0.5
Sugar, sweetened, 6 fl.oz	80	0	20
Sugar Free (NutraSweet), 6 fl.oz	4	0	1
Tang, all flavors, 6 fl.oz	90	0	23
Sugar-Free, 6 fl.oz	6	0	1.5

Coffee

Instant Coffee · C F Cb

	C	F	Cb
Coffee Powder/Granules:			
Regular or Decaffeinated,			
1 level tsp	2	0	0.5
1 rounded tsp	4	0	1
Ground, 1 Tbsp	5	0	1
Brewed/Percolated, 1 cup, 8 fl.oz	5	0	1
Coffee With Milk/Cream/Creamers:			
1 Cup Coffee:			
w. Whole Milk: Dash, 1 Tbsp	10	0.5	1
2 Tbsp, 1 fl.oz	20	1	1.5
w. 2% Milk, 2 Tbsp	15	0.5	1.5
w. 1% Milk, 2 Tbsp	12	0.3	1.5
w. Fat Free Milk, 2 Tbsp	10	0	1.5
w. Half & Half: 2 Tbsp	45	4	1
w. Cream (light coffee): 2 Tbsp	65	6	1
w. *Coffee Mate:* Liquid, reg., 1T.	40	2	5
Liquid Fat Free, 1 Tbsp	15	0	2
Powder, 1 heaping tsp	20	1	2
Sugar ~ Add Extra: 1 heaping tsp	25	0	6
Single portion, 1 pkt	25	0	6

Flavored Coffee Mixes

	C	F	Cb
Caffé D'Vita: 1 tsp	20	1	4
Coffee Essence, 1 tsp	16	0	4
General Foods, Cafe Intl: Regular	60	3	10
Sugar-free, average	30	2	3
Maxwell House: Mocha, 1 envelope	100	2.5	17
Mocha, sugar-free, 1 envelope	60	3	7
Van., Irish Cream, 1 envelope	90	1	20
Chicory: Instant Coffee, 1 tsp	6	0	1
Coffee Essence, 1 tsp	16	0	4

Coffee Substitute Mixes

	C	F	Cb
Roasted Cereal Beverages:			
Cafix Instant Beverage, 1 tsp	6	0	1
Kaffree Roma (Natural Touch), 1 tsp	6	0	1
Postum, Instant Hot Beverage, 1 tsp	12	0	3
Teeccino Caffe, 1 tsp	10	0	2

Bottled Ready-To-Drink

	C	F	Cb
Coffee: Per Bottle			
Main St: Fr. Vanilla, 12 fl.oz	190	3	31
Nescafe: Caffe Latte, 9.5 fl.oz	140	3.5	23
Mocha, 9.5 fl.oz	140	3	26
Starbucks: All types,. 9.5 fl.oz	190	3	40

Coffee Shops/Restaurants

Per 8 fl.oz Cup (Unless Indicated) · C F Cb

	C	F	Cb
Coffee (Regular/Percolated/Filtered)	5	0	1
Americano Drip Coffee, 1 cup	5	0	1
Cafe Au Lait: 1 cup, 8 fl.oz	65	2.5	6
Nonfat Milk, 1 cup	45	0	7
Caffe Latté:			
8 fl.oz cup: w. Whole Milk	100	5	8
w. 2% Milk	80	2.5	8
w. Nonfat Milk	60	0	8
12 fl.oz: w. Whole Milk	180	10	14
w. Nonfat Milk	110	0.5	15
Cafe Mocha (Mochaccino): 1 c.	120	3	15
12 fl.oz	180	4.5	15
16 fl.oz	240	6	15
Cappuccino:			
8 fl.oz cup: w. Whole Milk	70	3.5	6
w. 2% Milk	60	2	6
w. Nonfat Milk	40	0	6
12 fl.oz: w. Whole Milk	110	6	9
w. 2% Milk	80	3	9
w. Nonfat Milk	60	0	9
Mocha, with Cream			
8 fl.oz: w. Whole Milk	180	12	16
w. Nonfat Milk	150	8	16
Tall, 12 fl.oz: Whole Milk	290	18	25
w. Nonfat Milk	230	11	26
Iced Mocha (no cream)			
Tall, 12 fl.oz: w. Whole Milk	190	9	24
w. Nonfat Milk	140	2	24
Espresso: Regular	4	0	1
Doppio (Double)	8	0	2
Espresso Con Panna			
(w. dollop whipped cream)	30	3	1
Espresso Macchiato	15	0.5	2
Frappuccino: Tall, 12 fl.oz	200	3	39
Grande, 16 fl.oz	270	4	52
Frappuccino Mocha:			
Large/Tall, 12 fl.oz	230	3	44
Grande, 16 fl.oz	310	4.5	59
Iced Latte: Similar to Caffe Latte			
Intellicino: 12 fl.oz	150	7	15
Lowfat (2% milk)	120	3.5	5

Irish & Liqueur Coffees

	C	F	Cb
Irish Coffee (no sugar)	175	10	0
Liqueur Coffee, aver. all types	200	10	16

Cocoa & Hot Chocolate

	C	F	Cb
Cocoa:			
(w. Whipping Cream - Starbucks):			
8 fl.oz cup: w. Whole Milk	210	14	19
w. Nonfat Milk	80	8	17
Tall (12 fl.oz): w. Whole Milk	300	20	26
w. Nonfat Milk	120	11	26
Hot Chocolate:			
8 fl.oz cup: w. Whole Milk	200	10	25
w. Nonfat Milk	140	2	25
Tall (12 fl.oz): w. Whole Milk	300	15	38
w. Nonfat Milk	210	3	38

Coffee Extras

	C	F	Cb
Chocolate (Cocoa) Topping, 1/2 tsp	10	0	2
Flavored Syrups, 2 Tbsp	80	0	20
Sugar-free, 2 Tbsp	0	0	0
Hershey's Chocolate Syrup, 2 Tbsp	100	0	24
Half & Half Cream, 2 Tbsp	40	3	3
Light Whipped Cream, 2 Tbsp	30	2	2

Starbucks

	C	F	Cb
Americano:			
Short, 8 fl.oz	5	0	1
Tall, 12 fl.oz	10	0	2
Grande, 16 fl.oz	15	0	3
Venti, 20 fl.oz	15	0	3
Drip Coffee:			
Short, 8 fl.oz	5	0	1
Tall, 12 fl.oz	10	0	1
Grande, 16 fl.oz	10	0	2
Espresso:			
Solo	5	0	1
Doppio	10	0	2
Espresso Con Panna (w. Whipped Cream):			
Solo	30	3	1
Doppio	35	3	2
Espresso Macchiato:			
Solo: w. Whole Milk	15	0.5	2
w. Lowfat Milk (2%)	10	0	2
w. Nonfat Milk	10	0	2
w. Soy Milk	10	0	1
Doppio: w. Whole Milk	20	0.5	3
w. Lowfat Milk (2%)	15	0	3
w. Nonfat Milk	15	0	3
w. Soy Milk	15	0	2

Starbucks (Cont)

	C	F	Cb
Coffee Frappuccino:			
Tall, 12 fl.oz	180	2	38
Grande, 16 fl.oz	240	2.5	50
Venti, 20 fl.oz	300	3	63
Mocha Frappuccino:			
Tall, 12 fl.oz	210	2	43
Grande, 16 fl.oz	280	3	58
Venti, 20 fl.oz	350	3.5	72
Rhomba Frappuccino:			
Tall, 12 fl.oz	240	5	43
Grande, 16 fl.oz	320	7	58
Venti, 20 fl.oz	400	8	72
Chai Tea Latté:			
Short: 8 fl.oz w. Whole Milk	160	7	18
w. Lowfat Milk (2%)	130	3.5	18
w. Nonfat Milk	110	0	19
w. Soy Milk	100	4	13
Tall: 12 fl.oz w. Whole Milk	220	9	26
w. Lowfat Milk (2%)	190	5	26
w. Nonfat Milk	150	0	27
w. Soy Milk	140	5	18
Grande: 16 fl.oz w. Whole Milk	320	13	26
w. Lowfat Milk (2%)	260	7	37
w. Nonfat Milk	210	0.5	37
w. Soy Milk	200	8	25
Venti: 20 fl.oz w. Whole Milk	400	17	46
w. Lowfat Milk (2%)	330	9	46
w. Nonfat Milk	270	1	47
w. Soy Milk	260	10	32
Tiazzi Blended Fruit Juice:			
Mango Citrus/Wild Berry, average			
Tall, 12 fl.oz	180	0	43
Grande, 16 fl.oz	250	0	60
Venti, 20 fl.oz	340	0	81

Rev. Dr Robert Schuller

Inch by inch
Life's a cinch

You'll never win
If you don't begin!

Tea & Iced Teas

Teas | C | F | Cb
Regular: Bag, Loose or Instant			
Brewed, 1 cup, 8 fl.oz	1	0	0
(Add extra for sugar/milk)			
Herbal: Average all varieties, 1 cup	1	0	1
Bigelow: Apple Orchard, 1 cup	5	0	1
Other Varieties	2	0	0.5
Celestial Seasonings:			
Bengal Spice; Spearmint	5	0	0.5
Lemon Zinger	4	0	1
Roastaroma	10	0	2
Other varieties	2	0	0.5
Chai Tea Latté (*Starbucks*): See Previous Page			

Quick Guide
Iced Tea | C | F | Cb
Average All Brands			
Pre-Sweetened: 8 fl.oz	100	0	25
12 fl.oz	150	0	38
16 fl.oz	200	0	50
Unsweetened: 8 fl.oz	2	0	0

Iced Tea Mixes
	C	F	Cb
Per Serving			
4C Instant	90	0	22
Bigelow, Nice Over Ice	1	0	0.5
Celestial Seasonings, Iced Delight	4	0	1
Crystal Light, Sugar Free	3	0	0
Kool-Aid Fruit T's	70	0	17
Lipton: Instant	0	0	0
Instant Lemon/Raspberry	3	0	1
Lemon	55	0	14
Peach/Raspb, Sugar Free	5	0	1
Nestea: 100% Instant	2	0	0
Decaffeinated	6	0	1
Ice Teasers, all flavors	6	0	1
Peach, Raspberry	90	0	22

A woman is like a teabag. You never know her strength until she's in hot water.

~ Nancy Reagan

Bottled & Canned Teas
	C	F	Cb
Per 8 fl.oz Unless Indicated			
Arizona: Green Tea w. Ginseng & Honey	70	0	18
20 fl.oz Bottle: 1 cup, 8 fl.oz	70	0	18
Diet Green w. Ginseng	0	0	0
15.5 fl.oz Can: Average all flavors			
1/2 can, 7.75 fl.oz	95	0	28
w. Ginseng Extract	60	0	15
Herb Tea w. Honey, 8 fl.oz	70	0	17
Honey Lemon, 8 fl.oz	90	0	22
Brisk: 1 liter Bottle: Aver., 1 cup	90	0	24
12 fl.oz Can: Lemon, 1 Can	120	0	33
Raspberry, 1 Can	130	0	35
24 fl.oz Bottle: Lemon, 1 cup	80	0	22
Fruitopia: Average all flavors	110	0	28
Knudsen: Coolers, all flavors	90	0	23
Lipton (16 fl.oz Bottle): *Per 8 fl.oz*			
No Lemon	70	0	18
Lemon	90	0	21
Peach; Raspberry	110	0	26
Mistic: Tropical Cooler, 8 fl.oz	45	0	12
Nestea Iced Tea: Diet Lemon	3	0	0.5
Cool from Nestea, 1 cup, 8 fl.oz	80	0	20
12 fl.oz	120	0	33
Diet Cool from Nestea	2	0	0.5
Lemon/Peach/Raspberry	80	0	20
Sweetened Ice Tea	65	0	17
Oregon Chai: Herbal Bliss, 1/2 cup	70	0	18
Nirvana/Kashmir Green, 1/2 cup	80	0	20
Royal Mistic: Regular, 12 fl.oz	145	0	36
Diet, 12 fl.oz	8	0	2
Schweppes, 8 fl.oz	90	0	22
Shasta, 8 fl.oz	80	0	20
Snapple: Regular, sweetened	70	0	17
Diet/Unsweetened	0	0	0
Lemon; Peach, Raspberry	100	0	25
Sobe: Green Tea, 1 cup	90	0	23
Ssips (*Johanna Farms*), 8.45 fl.oz	100	0	25
Tropicana: Lemonfruit	100	0	25
Diet Lemon Fruit	15	0	4
Peach/Rasp./Tangerine, 8 fl.oz	120	0	28
10 fl.oz Bottle	140	0	35
11.5 fl.oz Can	160	0	40
Twister: Apple Berry, 8 fl.oz	100	0	28
Lemon Citrus	110	0	28
Turkey Hill: Regular	90	0	22
Raspberry Cooler	110	0	28
Diet Decaffeinated	0	0	0

♦ **Health Hazards: Excess alcohol** contributes to obesity, high blood pressure, stroke, heart and liver disease, some cancers, and even impotence.
Concentration and short-term memory are reduced as well as sporting performance.
Other alcohol hazards include stomach upsets, menstrual problems, anxiety, headaches, insomnia, work absenteeism and family arguments.

♦ **Alcohol contributes to obesity** through its high calories and by lessening the body's ability to burn fat. Fat storage is promoted, particularly in the belly - a danger zone. Alcohol can also stimulate appetite.

♦ **Alcohol is potentially more harmful while dieting.** Blood sugar levels may drop with resultant tiredness and further impairment of concentration, reflexes and driving skills - and maybe the dieter's resolve!

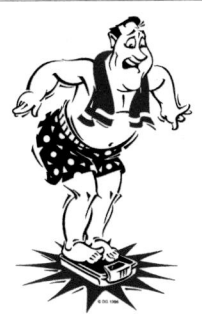

Excess alcohol contributes to obesity and high blood pressure

SAFE ALCOHOL LIMITS

Women: No more than **1 drink** per day.
Men: No more than **2 drinks** per day.
(At least 2 days a week should be alcohol-free.)

1 Drink = 12 fl.oz regular beer, or 5 fl.oz wine,
or 1½ fl.oz spirits (80 proof).
Each drink contains approximately 14g alcohol.

For some people, **safe drinking** will mean no alcohol drinks at all. (Even one drink may impair driving skills, particularly if tired; and 3-4 drinks daily has been linked to brain shrinkage in some social drinkers).

♦ **It is advisable not to drink at all if you are:**
  - pregnant or trying to conceive
  - taking drug medication (unless approved by your doctor or pharmacist)
  - have a condition such as liver or heart disease
  - planning to drive or use machinery
  - studying or needing to concentrate
  - a child or adolescent

♦ **Women and adolescents are more prone** to alcohol's ill-effects due to their lower body weight, smaller livers and lesser capacity to metabolise alcohol.
Note: You cannot save daily drinks for one occasion.
Binge drinking is particularly harmful ~
4 drinks 'in a row' for males or 3 drinks for females.

HOW TO CALCULATE ALCOHOL CONTENT

Percent alcohol on label refers to alcohol volume (ml alcohol/100ml).

100ml = 3½ fl.oz

To convert to grams (weight) of alcohol, multiply the percent volume by 0.8 - since 1 ml of alcohol weighs only 0.8 grams (actually 0.789g).

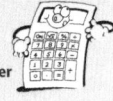

EXAMPLE
12 fl.oz Can Beer
(5% alcohol)

5% alc.volume = 5% of 12 fl.oz
= 0.6 fl.oz
= 18ml alcohol
(1 fl.oz=30ml)

Weight (18ml x 0.8)
= 14.4g alcohol

Beers ◆ Ales ◆ Malt Liquors

Quick Guide **C** **Alc** **Cb**

Beer: **Alc** ~ Alcohol (Grams)

Beer Contains Zero Fat

Malt Liquor/Ale (5.6% Alc. Vol.)

	C	Alc	Cb
12 fl.oz Can/Bottle/Glass	180	16	17
22 fl.oz Can/Bottle/Glass	330	29	32

Regular Beer (5% Alc. Vol.)

	C	Alc	Cb
7 fl.oz Glass	80	8.5	4
12 fl.oz Bottle/Can/Glass	140	14	10
16 fl.oz Bottle/Can	185	19	11
22 fl.oz Bottle	260	26	20
32 fl.oz Bottle	370	37	28
40 fl.oz Bottle	470	47	35

Light Beer (4.2% Alc. Vol.)

	C	Alc	Cb
7 fl.oz Glass	65	7	4
12 fl.oz Bottle/Can/Glass	110	12	5
16 fl.oz Bottle/Can	145	16	8
22 fl.oz Bottle	200	22	11

Low Alcohol Beer (2.3% Alc. Vol)

	C	Alc	Cb
(Example: *Blatz LA*),12 fl.oz	75	7	6

Non-Alcoholic/Near Beer

(Less than 0.5% alcohol by volume)

	C	Alc	Cb
Average All Brands, 12 fl.oz	70	1	16

Beer Brands **C** **Alc** **Cb**

Per 12 fl.oz Serving
Percentage alcohol listed below is by volume - not by weight.

	C	Alc	Cb
Amber Ice (5.3% alcohol)	130	15	6
Anchor Steam (4.6%)	155	13	16
Anheuser Light (3.2% alcohol)	75	9	7
Artic Ice (5.3%)	150	15	8
Artic Ice Light 3.2 (3.9%)	100	11	6
Augsburger Bock (4.9%)	170	14	17
Augsburger Golden/Dark (4.9%)	170	14	17
Augsburger Red (4.9%)	160	14	14
Ballard Bitter (4.7%)	180	14	19
Beck's (5%)	150	14	12
Big Sky (4.8%)	150	14	12
Big Sky Light (4.5%)	105	13	5
Black & Tan (4.5%)	185	13	22
Black Label (5.6%)	155	16	11
Black Label Light (3.7%)	100	11	6
Blackhook Porter (4.9%)	160	14	14
Blatz (4.3%)	135	12	10
Blatz LA (2.3%)	75	7	6

Brands (Cont) **C** **Alc** **Cb**

Beer Contains Zero Fat

	C	Alc	Cb
Blatz Light (3.7%), 12 fl.oz	100	11	3
Blue Moon Ale: Belgian (4.8%)	160	14	13
Honey Blond Ale (5.5%)	200	16	20
Nut Brown Ale (5.1%)	180	15	16
Raspberry Cream Ale (4.9%)	190	14	20
Bud Dry (4.9%)	130	14	8
Bud Light (4.2%)	110	12	7
Bud Ice (5.5%)	150	16	9
Bud Ice Light (4.1%)	95	12	4
Budweiser (4.9%)	150	14	11
Busch (4.9%)	145	14	11
Busch Light (4.2%)	110	12	7
Carling (4.4%)	140	13	10
Carlsberg (5%)	135	13	10
Castlemaine XXXX (4.7%)	140	13	9
Colt 45 MM (5.6%)	155	16	1
Coors (4.9%)	150	14	12
Coors Dry (4.9%)	120	14	6
Coors Light 3.2 (4%)	100	11	4
Corona Extra (4.6%)	130	13	9
Dos Equis Lager (5%)	130	14	9
Elk Mountain Amber Ale (5.5%)	190	16	18
Elk Mountain Red (4.9%)	160	14	13
Extra Gold (4.9%)	150	14	12
Extra Gold 3.2 (4%)	120	11	10
Faust (5%)	170	14	17
First Reserve (4.9%)	170	14	16
Fosters Lager (4.9%)	135	14	9
George Killian's: Irish Brown(5.2%)	185	15	15
Irish Red (5%)	160	14	13
Wilde Honey Ale (5.3%)	170	15	14
Goebel (4.1%)	130	12	12
Goebel Light (3.9%)	110	11	8
Grolsch Premium (5%)	140	14	10
Guinness Draught (4.3%)	155	12	17
Heileman's: Old Style (4.9%)	147	14	12
Old Style Light (4.1%)	110	12	6
Heineken (5.4%)	170	15	15
Heineken Dark (5.2%)	175	15	16
Herman Joseph's			
Special Premium (4.9%)	150	14	12
Highland Ale: Black (5.6%)	180	16	16
Amber (5.2%)	160	15	14
Hurricane (5.5%)	150	16	10
Icehouse, Miller (5.0%)	135	14	9
Icehouse, Miller (5.5%)	150	16	10

Brands (Cont)

Beer Contains Zero Fat
Per 12 fl.oz Serving

	C	Alc	Cb
Keystone Regular/Dry (4.9% alc.)	125	14	6
Ice (5.3%)	145	15	8
Light, 3.2 (4%)	100	10	4
Amber Light (3.8%)	110	11	8
King Cobra (5.9%)	180	17	15
Kirin Lager (Japan) (4.8%)	135	13	9
Labatt's Blue (5%)	145	14	9
Lowenbrau Dark/Special (4.9%)	160	14	15
Magnum Malt Liquor (5.9%)	155	17	23
Meister Brau (4.5%)	130	13	11
Meister Brau Light (4.5%)	105	13	5
Memphis Brown (4.6%)	120	13	6
Michelob: Regular (5%)	160	14	12
Light (4.3%)	135	12	12
Dry (4.9%)	130	14	8
Amber Bock (5%)	160	14	15
Centennial (5.5%)	175	16	15
Classic Dark (5%)	160	14	15
Golden Draft (4.8%)	150	14	13
Golden Draft Light (4.2%)	110	12	7
Hefeweizen (5%)	165	14	14
Malt (5.8%)	160	17	9
Miller, Regular (5%)	150	14	12
Miller Genuine Draft (5%)	145	14	11
Light (4.5%)	100	13	4
Miller High Life (5%)	145	14	9
Miller High Life Ice (5.5%)	142	16	7
Miller High Life Light (4.5%)	100	13	4
Miller Lite (4.5%)	95	13	4
Miller Lite Ice (5.5%)	125	16	4
Miller Lite Ice (5%)	115	14	3
Milwaukee's Best (4.5%)	130	13	11
Milwaukee's Best Ice (5.5%)	135	16	5
Milwaukee's Best Light (4.5%)	100	13	8
Minnesota's Best (4.9%)	140	14	10
Moosehead (5%)	125	14	14
Natural Ice, Budweiser (5.9%)	160	16	10
Natural Light, Budweiser (4.2%)	110	12	7
Natural Pilsner, Budweiser (4.9%)	150	14	12
Newcastle Brown Ale (4.5%)	140	12	13
Northstone Amber Ale (4.9%)	150	14	8
Old Milwaukee (4.5%)	145	13	15
Light (4.3%)	122	12	10
Ice (5.5%)	155	16	10
Red (4.5%)	135	13	11

	C	Alc	Cb
Pabst (5%), 12 fl. oz	155	14	14
Pete's Wicked Ale (5%)	180	14	20
Piels (4.7%)	135	13	10
Piels Light (4.5%)	127	13	9
Primo (4.3%), 12 fl.oz	140	12	13
Ranier (4.6%)	142	13	12
Red Bull Malt (7%)	192	20	17
Red Dog (5%)	150	14	12
Red Hook ESB (5.4%)	175	16	16
Red Hook Rye (5%)	155	14	14
Red Light (4.1%)	105	12	5
Red River Valley (4.9%)	165	14	15
Red Wolf (5.5%)	155	16	12
Samuel Adams (4.6%)	170	13	17
Samuel Adams Lager (4.7%)	180	13	19
Sapporo Draft (Japan) (4.5%)	140	12	12
Schaefer (4.3%)	140	12	12
Schaefer Light (3.9%)	110	11	8
Schlitz Ice (4.6%)	145	13	13
Schlitz Ice Light (4.3%)	120	12	8
Schlitz Malt (5.9%)	180	17	14
Schmidt (4.6%)	142	13	12
Sheaf Stout, 5.7%	180	16	17
Sierra Nevada: Pale Ale (5.6%)	175	16	16
Big Foot Ale (10.1%)	210	29	2
Pale Bock (6.6%)	190	19	20
Porter (6%)	185	17	18
Silver Thunder (5.9%)	165	17	11
Stella Artois, 5%, 330ml	135	14	9
Southpaw Light (5%)	125	14	6
Stroh's (4.4%)	145	13	13
Stroh's Light (4.3%)	115	13	7
Stroh's Signature (4.9%)	160	14	15
Wheat Hook (4.8%)	150	14	12
Winterfest (5.7%)	185	16	18
Zeigenbock (5%)	155	14	13
Zima Clear Malt (4.6%)	150	14	13

Homebrewed Beer: Similar to regular beers, according to alcohol content.

Non-Alcoholic Brews

	C	Alc	Cb
Less Than 0.5% Alcohol			
Average All Brands			
(*Busch, Kaliber, O'Douls, Old Milwaukee NA, Stroh's NA, Sharp's, Haakebeck, Texas Select*)			
12 fl.oz Can/Bottle	70	1	15

Cider • Wine • Liquor

Alcoholic Lemon Brews | C | Alc | Cb

Average All Brands
(4.8% Alcohol)
(Includes Hooper's Hooch, Lusty, Saxer)

	C	Alc	Cb
12 fl.oz Bottle/Can	**150**	13	12

Cider · Alc ~ Alcohol (Grams)

	C	Alc	Cb
Alcoholic Cider: Average,			
5.5% alcohol, Dry, 12 fl.oz	**130**	16	12
Sweet, 12 fl.oz	**160**	16	12
Hardcore Crisp Hard Cider (6% alc)			
12 fl.oz	**190**	17	19
Hornsby's Draft Cider (6% alc)			
12 fl.oz bottle	**170**	17	15
Woodchuck Draft Cider (5% alc)			
Amber, 8 fl.oz	**135**	14	14
Dark & Dry, 8 fl.oz	**120**	14	11
Granny Smith, 8 fl.oz	**110**	14	7

Quick Guide · C · Alc · Cb
Table Wine

Average All Varieties (11.5% Alcohol)

	C	Alc	Cb
4 fl.oz (¹/₂ large wine glass)	**85**	11	2
6 fl.oz (³/₄ large wine glass)	**125**	16	3
¹/₂ Carafe/Bottle, 375ml	**265**	34	6
1 Bottle, 750ml	**530**	68	13

Table Wines

	C	Alc	Cb
Red: Claret/Burgundy/Chianti, 4 fl.oz	**80**	11	0
Sparkling Reds, 4 fl.oz	**90**	11	3
Rose: Medium, 4 fl.oz	**80**	11	0
White: Dry (Chablis/Hock/Riesling), 4 fl.oz	**75**	11	0
Zinfandel Sweet (Moselle/Sauterne), 4 fl.oz	**85**	11	2
Sparkling, 4 fl.oz	**95**	11	4
Champagne: *Per 4 fl.oz Serving*			
Average 1 glass, 4 fl.oz	**85**	11	4
w. Orange Jce (3:1 orange)	**75**	8	4
w. Orange Jce (1:1 orange)	**65**	5	7
Cold Duck, 4 fl. oz	**108**	11	8
Sake: Rice Wine (16% alc.), 4 oz	**125**	15	5
Mulled Wine: (Gluhwein), 4 oz	**180**	14	20
Non-Alcoholic Wine, aver., 4 oz	**50**	0	12
Reduced Alcohol Wine (6%):			
Average all types, 4 fl.oz	**50**	0	12

Dessert Wines | C | Alc | Cb

	C	Alc	Cb
Madeira (18% alc), 2 oz	**85**	9	5
Marsala (18%), 2 oz	**110**	9	11
Port, Muscatel, (18%), 2 oz	**85**	9	5
Sherry (18%), 2 oz			
Dry, 1 Sherry glass	**65**	9	0.5
Sweet/Cream, average	**85**	9	5
Vermouth: Dry (18%), 2 oz	**65**	9	0.5
Sweet (15%), 2 oz	**85**	7	8

Cooking Wine

Average All Brands

	C	Alc	Cb
Red/White, 2 Tbsp, 1 oz	**20**	3	1
Marsala. 2 Tbsp, 1 oz	**35**	4	2
Sherry, 2 Tbsp, 1 oz	**40**	4	2

Cooking with Wine
For alcohol to evaporate, sufficient heat and cooking time (at least 30 minutes) is required.
Red and white table wines would then contain negligible residual calories.
Sweetened wines (marsala/sherry) would contain 10 calories per 1 fl.oz used.
Flambé Desserts: Only surface alcohol is burnt off.

Spirits/Liquors

All Contain Zero Fat
Includes Bourbon, Brandy, Gin, Rum, Scotch, Tequila, Vodka, Whiskey.
Note: All spirits with same proof (alcohol) have similar calories and zero fat.

Average All Brands · C · Alc · Cb

	C	Alc	Cb
80 Proof (40% Alcohol by Volume):			
1 fl.oz	**65**	9.5	0
1¹/₂ fl.oz Jigger	**100**	14.5	0
¹/₂ Bottle, 375 ml	**810**	120	0
1 Bottle, 750 ml	**1620**	240	0
86 Proof (43% Alcohol):			
1 fl.oz	**70**	10	0
1¹/₂ fl.oz Jigger	**105**	15	0
¹/₂ Bottle, 375 ml	**870**	125	0
1 Bottle, 750 ml	**1750**	250	0
100 Proof (50% Alcohol):			
1 fl.oz	**82**	12	0
1¹/₂ fl.oz Jigger	**125**	18	0
¹/₂ Bottle, 375 ml	**1025**	150	0
1 Bottle	**2050**	300	0

Coolers & Premix Cocktails

Zero Fat Unless Indicated
Calorie & Carbohydate estimates given where no data available.

	C	**Alc**	**Cb**
Bacardi Fruit Mixers (Frozen Conc.)			
Made up (2 oz mix + 1 oz Rum + Ice)			
Margarita	160	10	22
Pina Colada	230	10	40
Other varieties, average	200	10	32
(If 2 oz Rum used, add extra 70 cals/10g alcohol)			
Bartles & Jaymes:			
Wine Cooler/Cocktails (5%): *Per 12 fl.oz*			
Berry; Kiwi Strawberry	230	14	35
Fuzzy Navel	250	14	42
Margarita	270	14	47
Oriental Dragon Fruit	250	14	32
Original	200	14	30
Strawberry Daiquiri; Tropical	230	14	39
Malt Based Coolers (3.9% alc.): *Per 12 fl.oz*			
Berry; Black Cherry; Peach	210	11	33
Margarita; Pina Colada	270	11	48
Fuzzy Navel; Tropical	230	11	38
Strawberry Daiquiri	220	11	36
Boone's Farm Wine Coolers:			
Snow Crk Berry; Sun Peach (5%)	150	10	20
Sangria; Strawberry Hill (7.5%)	190	14	23
Breezer By Bacardi (3.2% alc): *Per 12 fl.oz*			
Passionfr.; Calypso Berry	220	9	39
Pina Colada (contains 6g fat)	250	9	33
Strawberry Daiquiri	250	9	47
Tahitian Tangerine	200	9	34
Heublein Premium Classics:			
Long Is. Ice Tea (15% alc), 2 oz	130	7	20
Manhattan (22.5%), 2 oz + ice	160	11	20
Mai Tai (22%), 2 oz + ice	160	11	20
Pina Colada, 4 oz (10g fat) + ice	280	4	40
Jack Daniels Country Cocktails (5.9%)			
Average all flavors, 200ml	170	9.5	25
Jose Cuervo Cocktails (5.9%):			
Margarita/ Lime, 200ml	180	9.5	27
Strawberry, 200ml bottle	170	9.5	25
TGI Friday's Frozen Cocktails (12.5%):			
Per Serving (3 fl.oz Premix & Ice)			
Margarita; Strawberry Daiquiri	145	9	20
Note: All drinks below contain 6g fat/serving.			
B52; Strawberry Shortcake	230	9	29
Mint Choc. Chip; P.Colada	250	9	32
Mudslide; Orange Dream	240	9	31

Premix Cocktails (Cont)

	C	**Alc**	**Cb**
The Club			
(Premix Cocktails): *Per 4oz*			
Long Island Ice Tea; Manhattan	220	16	30
Margar.;Scr'driver; Vod. Martini	210	7	40
Mudslide (9g fat)	270	12	41
P. Colada; Or. Craze; Whisk. Sour	260	10	40

Shooters

Alc ~ Alcohol (Grams)

Kamakazi	150	20	2
Mud Slide	160	13	17
Fuzzy Navel	120	13	7
Pineapple Bomber	130	11	13
Turbo	110	14	3
Shots: Average all types, 1¹/₂ fl.oz	110	14	3

Flavorings/Syrups

Non-Alcoholic, Fat Free

Angostura Bitters, ¹/₄ tsp	3	0	0
Grenadine/Cassis, 2 Tbsp, 1 oz	70	0	17
Lime Juice, 2 Tbsp, 1 oz	10	0	2
Sugar Syrup, 2 Tbsp, 1 oz	70	0	17
Sour Mix, 2 Tbsp, 1 oz	10	0	2
Tonic Water, 8 fl.oz	90	0	22

Cocktail Mix 'N Drinks

No Alcohol Added

Bloody Mary Mix (Mr & Mrs T), 8 fl.oz	40	0	9
Pina Colada Mix: *Daily's,* 3 fl.oz	160	0	37
Mr & Mrs T, 4.5 fl.oz	180	0	43
Margarita Mix (J.Cuervo), 4 fl.oz	100	0	24

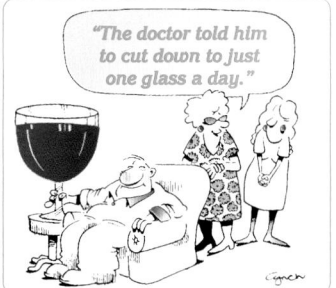

"The doctor told him to cut down to just one glass a day."

Cocktails ◆ Liqueurs

Cocktails ~ Alcohol (Grams)

Zero Fat Unless Indicated
(Made to Standard Recipes)

	C	Alc	Cb
Bloody Mary	120	14	5
Bourbon & Soda	110	15	1
Brandy Alexander (16g fat)	300	16	11
Cerebral Hemorrhage (5g fat)	290	17	32
Collins (w. 2oz gin)	180	20	11
Daiquiri	110	14	3
Gin & Tonic	170	16	14
Harvey Wallbanger (2 oz Vodka)	250	30	11
Highball (1½ oz Whiskey)	110	14	3
Irish Coffee (contains 9g fat)	210	14	8
Leprechaun's Libation	285	31	17
Mai Tai (2 oz Rum)	260	27	17
Manhattan	130	17	3
Martini	160	22	1
Mind Eraser	160	17	10
Mint Julep	165	20	8
Pina Colada (contains 12g fat)	260	14	12
Screwdriver	180	14	20
Spritzer (3 oz Wine)	70	8	3
Tequila Sunrise	190	20	14
Tom Collins	120	16	2
Whiskey Sour	125	15	5

Liqueurs/Cordials

Per 1 fl.oz

Baileys Irish Cream (34 Proof; 5g fat)	95	4	5
Lite (30 Proof; 2g fat)	75	4	4
Cherry Brandy (48 Proof)	80	6	9
Coffee Liqueur (53 Proof)	90	6.5	11
Amaretto (56 Proof)	110	6	17
Benedictine (80 Proof)	90	10	5
Cointreau (80 Proof)	100	10	7
Creme de Cacao (54 Proof)	100	6	15
Creme de Menthe (60 Proof)	120	7	14
Drambuie (80 Proof)	105	10	9
Grand Marnier (80 Proof)	100	10	7
Kahlua (53 Proof)	90	6.5	11
Kirsch (68 Proof)	80	8	6
Midori, aver. all types, (42 Proof)	80	5	11
Ouzo (80 Proof)	90	10	5
Sambuca (84 Proof)	100	10	7
Schnapps (80 Proof)	100	10	7
Southern Comfort (78 Proof)	75	9	3
Tia Maria (64 Proof)	90	8	9
Triple Sec (60 Proof)	80	7	4

Ten Hints to Avoid Harmful Drinking

1. **Add up the alcohol** you typically drink each day and on social occasions. How does this compare with 'low risk' amounts?

2. **Compare the alcohol content** of different drinks and select those with lower content. Request half ounces of alcohol in cocktails and mixed drinks. Dilute them and keep topping off with non-alcoholic drinks.

3. **Try low alcohol** or non-alcohol alternatives such as fruit juices and mineral water. Take your own to parties.

4. **Before drinking alcohol,** quench your thirst with water and non-alcoholic drinks - particularly after vigorous exercise or sport.

5. **Slow the rate of drinking.** Chugging or drinking fast is the major cause of illness and death from alcohol poisoning.

6. **Avoid drinking in 'rounds'.**

7. **Have a non-alcoholic 'spacer'** between drinks (e.g. mineral water, orange juice).

8. **Don't drink on an empty stomach.** Food slows the rate of alcohol absorption.

9. **Keep track of the number of drinks** and know when to stop. Stick to a set limit.

10. **Do not drive, swim, or operate machinery** while under the influence.

Note: Alcohol can be very dangerous when taken with prescription or street drugs or when you are very tired.

Coffee Liqueurs

Average All Types
(Includes Benedictine, Cointreau, Kahlua):

1 serving	200	10	10

Ginseng Vials

Most contain up to 33% alcohol.
A 10ml (⅓ ounce) vial can contain up to 2.5 grams alcohol.

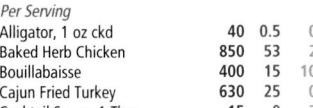

Note: Figures for these dishes are only a guide. Large variations occur with serving size, recipe ingredients and cooking methods.

Chinese & Asian Dishes

Appetizers

	C	F	Cb
Curried Meat Triangles, 1 pce	150	5	12
Dim Sum (Dumplings), 1 ball	65	2	5
Egg Rolls, mini, 3 rolls	100	3	11
Spring Roll, Small, 1 1/2 oz	100	7	10
Medium, 3 oz	200	12	20
Large, 5 oz	350	15	33
Wonton, 1 only	55	3	4
Soup: Clear, 1 bowl	30	1	4
with Noodles	100	3	12
Chicken & Corn	150	8	8
Fortune Cookie: each	25	<1	5

Entrees & Main Dishes
Per Whole Dish (2-3 Serves)

	C	F	Cb
Beef with Broccoli, 16 oz	650	30	31
Beef in Black Bean Sce, 17 oz	530	33	17
Chicken & Almonds, 18 oz	685	50	18
Chop Suey: Chicken, 20 oz	560	37	7
Pork, 20 oz	680	50	12
Chow Mein: Beef/Chick., 24 oz	940	60	50
Crispy Fried Chicken, 8 oz	485	33	12
Lemon Chicken, 10 oz	580	32	25
Omelet: Chick/Shrimp, 16 oz	990	82	10
Sweet & Sour: Fish, 20 oz	1160	58	106
Pork, 18 oz	950	50	92
Duck, 18 oz	1120	71	85
Vegetable Combination, 6 oz	250	17	13
Extra Listings: See Frozen Entrees/Meals.			
Rice: Plain, 1 cup, 5 oz	170	0	36
Fried: 1 cup, 5 oz	320	13	42
Large dish, 16 oz	1010	40	134
Noodles: Chinese Egg, boiled,1 cup	200	3	42

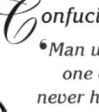

***C**onfucious say:*

'Man who eat with one chopstick never have problem with obesity!'

Cajun & Creole   C F Cb

Per Serving

	C	F	Cb
Alligator, 1 oz ckd	40	0.5	0
Baked Herb Chicken	850	53	2
Bouillabaisse	400	15	10
Cajun Fried Turkey	630	25	0
Cocktail Sauce, 1 Tbsp	15	0	3
Couche-couche, 1/2 cup	80	0	17
Crawfish Bisque	500	10	10
Crawfish, cooked, 2 oz	45	0.5	0
Creole Jambalaya	550	30	15
Dove, cooked, 1 oz	60	3.5	0
Frog's Legs, steamed (2)	45	0	0
Guinea Fowl, flesh, 1 oz, ckd	40	1	0
Hogshead Cheese, 1/4 cup	80	5.5	0
Jambalaya, Shrimp & Crabmeat	520	14	12
Red Beans & Rice	400	17	52
Roasted Quail, w. Bacon on Toast	550	25	15
Remoulade Sauce, 1 Tbsp	55	5.5	1
Shrimp Creole	450	20	10
Stuffed Smothered Steak, w. 1 cup rice	890	50	50
Squab, flesh, 1 oz cooked	60	3.5	0
Turtle, cooked, 1 1/2 oz	60	1.5	0

French Foods

	C	F	Cb
Blanquette d'Agneau (Lamb Stew w. Veg)	800	30	17
Brioche, 1 cake	280	14	34
Bouillabaise (Fish Stew)	400	15	10
Coq au Vin (Chicken in Wine)	800	30	16
Coquilles St. Jacques, fried, 6 lge	300	14	2
Creme Caramel (Caram. Custard)	260	10	38
Crepe Suzette, 1x 6" crepe/sauce	220	10	13
Duck a l'Orange	780	35	47
Escargots (Snails), in garlic but., (6)	200	10	4
Frogs Legs, fried, 4 med. pairs	400	20	10
Lamb Noisettes, fried, 2 chops	500	40	1
Mousse au Chocolat	380	15	33
Potage Creme Crecy (Carrot Soup)	360	18	14
Salade Nicoise (Tuna/Oliv./Veg.)	450	13	14
Veal Cordon Bleu (Veal/Ham/Ch)	650	25	18
Vichyssoise (Pot./Leek Soup), 1 c.	200	9	15

German

	C	F	Cb
Bavarian Bread Dumpling, 3 small	330	10	28
Beef: Goulash with Veges	520	20	46
Black Forest Cake, 1 slice	380	16	30
Bratwurst: Grilled, 1 medium, 6 oz	540	12	58
Chicken: Fried, Viennese-style	530	20	28
Livers w. Apple/On., 6 oz	460	28	10
Herring, Pickled: Rollmops, 4 oz	260	16	3
with Sour Cream, 4 oz	310	20	3
Hot Sausage Curry	300	7	6
Kugelhupf (Yeast Cake), 1 lge sl.	400	58	3
Sauerbraten Pork (Pot Roast)	650	35	15
Torte: Linzer (Alm./Raspb. Jam)	430	18	58
Sacher (Choc./Apricot Jam)	260	12	23
Weiner Schnitzel, 1 med.	750	35	38

Greek

	C	F	Cb
Baklava Pastry, 1 only, 3³/4 oz	400	21	45
Calamari, deep fried, 1 cup	300	13	17
Galactobureko, 1 only (Filo, Custard, Pastry in Syrup)	360	15	48
Kataifi (Filo, Nut, Pastry in Syrup)	350	11	56
Moussaka, 1 serve, 8 oz	350	22	22
Souvlakia (Lamb), each, 2 oz	120	6	1
Stuffed Tomatoes, 2 only	250	2	17
Taramosalata, 1 Tbsp, 1/2 oz	40	3	2
Tyropita (Filo/Egg/Cheese Pastry)	350	26	31
Tzatziki (Cucumber/Yog. Dip), 1 T.	20	1	1
Vine Leaves, stuffed, 3 rolls, 6 oz	200	5	13

Indian & Pakistan

Per Serving
(Meat dishes allow 4 oz meat/serving)

	C	F	Cb
Aloo Samosa, each (Savory Pastries w. Potato fill.)	150	12	12
Alu Gosht Kari (Meat/Pot. Curry)	600	40	23
Ande ki Kari (Egg, Tom Sce), each	250	23	7
Bhona Gosht (Mint Broil Lamb)	560	28	5
Chicken Pilaf (Murgh Biriyani)	700	53	50
Chapati/Roti, 7" diam. piece (Baked Whole Wheat Bread)	60	<1	11
Dal (Lentil Puree), 1 cup, no oil	230	1	37
1 Tbsp Tadka (oil topping)	120	13	0
Dhakla, 1 oz	105	5	13
Dhansak, 1/2 cup	105	3.5	11
Fish Jhol (Fish in Gravy)	230	10	5

Indian & Pakistan (Cont)

	C	F	Cb
Gosht Kari (Meat Curry/Tom./Pot.)	460	25	17
Imli Chatni (Chutney), 1 Tbsp	30	0	7
Lamb Pilaf	520	35	40
Machchi Molee (Fish, C'nut Milk)	690	45	15
Masala Gosht (Beef/Tom./Gravy)	400	25	18
Mulligatawney Soup, average	300	15	8
Murgh Tikka, 1 cup	300	4	7
Naan, 1 oz	75	2	11
Pappadom, 1 large/2 small	50	3	5
Pesrattu, 9" crepe	130	5	15
Pork Vendaloo Curry	620	47	3
Rajmah (Kidney Bean Curry)	400	17	56
Rogan Josh (Lamb/Yoghurt Sce.)	500	30	3
Saag Gosht (Beef/Spinach Sce)	430	26	10
Shahi Korma (Braised Lamb)	430	28	3
Tandoori Chicken: Breast	260	13	5
Leg/Thigh portion	300	17	6

Italian Dishes

	C	F	Cb
Cannelloni, 1 tube, 6 oz	280	15	18
Chicken Cacciatore	370	22	4
Gnocchi, Spinach	300	18	17
Lasagne with meat, 10 oz	400	17	36
Manicotti, cheese/tomato	230	14	18
Minestrone Soup, 1 cup	260	6	28
Osso Buco (Veal/Tom./Mushr.)	550	28	5
Ravioli, 8 oz	300	12	30
Risotto (Chicken)	420	12	70
Spaghetti: Plain, 1 cup, 5 oz	185	1	44
Restaurant: 2 cups, plain	370	2	88
+ Bolognese (Meat Sce)	650	16	90
+ Marinara (Seafoods)	700	20	90
+ Napoletana (Tom. Sce)	540	13	105
Saltimbocca (Veal/Ham/Cheese)	430	28	5
Tortellini, 20 pieces	530	20	74
Veal Marsala	400	20	11
Veal Parmigiana	350	20	5
Pizza: Per 1/2 Pizza (12")			
Vegetarian/Cheese:			
Thin Crust	650	26	63
Thick Crust	850	35	108
Sausage/Pepperoni: Thin Crust	700	32	68
Thick Crust	900	62	135

(Also see Pizza Hut, Domino's, Shakey's, Godfather's Pizza ~ Fast Foods Section.)

Japanese

Sushi

	C	F	Cb
Lunch Menu (Assorted Sushi)			
Regular, 1 serving	330	3	56
Deluxe, 1 serving	430	4	72
Sushi Rice, ckd, 1 Tbsp	25	<1	5
1 cup, 5¼ oz	380	3	82
Nigiri-Zushi: (Fish wrapped Sushi)			
Per 1 oz piece:			
Ebi-zushi (Jumbo Shrimp)	20	<1	3
Kani-zushi (Surimi Crab)	30	<1	5
Maguro-zushi (Tuna)	25	<1	4
Sake-zushi (Salmon)	35	1	4
Suzume-zushi (Baby Snapper)	30	<1	4
Tai-zushi (Red Snapper)	30	<1	4
Nori-Maki-Zushi: *Per Piece*			
(Seaweed-wrapped Sushi Rolls)			
Anago-maki (Conger Eel)	20	1	2
California-maki (Crab/Caviar/Avocado)			
½ roll	70	1	10
Futo-maki (Egg Omelet, Shellfish, Veg.),			
1 piece	70	1	10
Kobana-maki (Egg Om., Cucum.)	35	<1	6
Kappa-maki (Cucumber)	15	0	3
Tekka-maki (Tuna)	20	<1	4
Uni-maki (Sea Urchin)	20	<1	4
Inari-Zushi (Bean Curd Pouches w. Sushi)			
1 pouch, 3 oz	130	2	23
Tamago-Yaki (Omelet-wrapped Sushi)			
1 piece	45	1	5
Sashimi (Slice Raw Seafood/Beef)			
Ika (Squid), 4 oz	105	2	0
Hamachi (Yellowtail), 4 oz	165	6	0
Naguro (Yellowfin Tuna), 4 oz	120	1	0
Niku (Beef), 5 oz	200	10	0
Saba (Mackerel), 4 oz	160	7	0
Suzuki (Sea Bass), 4 oz	110	<1	0
Tako (Octopus), 4 oz	95	1	0
Dipping Sauces: Aver. 2 Tbsp	30	0	7
Ginger Vinegar Dress., 2 Tbsp	20	0	5
Miso Soup w. tofu pces, 1 cup	85	3	11
Sukiyaki (Beef/Tofu/Veg.), 8 oz	400	24	32
Tempura (Batter-fried Shrimp & Veges.)			
3 large shrimp & veges	320	18	25
1 shrimp only	60	4	3
Teppan Yaki (Steak, Seafood & Veges.)			
10 oz serving	470	30	15
Teriyaki Beef, 4 oz serving	350	25	4
Sake Wine (16% alc.), 3 fl.oz	115	0	7

Kosher/Deli Foods

	C	F	Cb
Bagel/Bialy,			
½ small, 1 oz	80	1	16
Beiglach (Cheese Knish)	350	17	35
Blintzes, average, 1 only	120	1	25
w. Sour Crm. & Preserves	370	10	30
Borscht, (no cream), 1 cup	85	3	14
Diet/Reduced Cal., 1 cup	30	1	7
Cabbage Roll (meat/rice), 5 oz	170	6	21
Chicken Broth, 1 cup	80	8	0
with vegetables	100	8	5
with noodles	150	9	16
Lowfat, plain, 1 cup	25	1	0
Cholent, 1 med serve, 1 cup	350	16	48
Chopped Liver: 1 serve, 3 oz	110	6	5
with Egg Salad, ¼ cup	100	7	3
Farfel, dry, ½ cup	90	<1	21
Hallah (Yeast Bread), 1 sl., 1 oz	85	2	14
Gefilte Fish Balls:			
Regular, medium, 2 oz	55	2	4
with jelled broth	80	2	6
Cocktail size, 1 oz	30	1	2
Sweet, medium, 2 oz	65	2	4
with jelled broth	95	2	9
Herring: Smoked, 2 oz	120	8	0
in Sour Cream, 2 oz	150	10	0
Kasha, cooked, ½ cup	90	<1	20
Kipfel (Vanilla/Almd. Cookie), 1 pce.	60	2	7
Knaidlach, 1 ball	40	2	5
Knish: Kasha/Potato, 1 only	130	4	20
Cheese, 1 only	350	17	35
Kreplach, beef, 1 piece	40	1	6
Kugel, potato/noodle, 1 serve	150	7	20
Latkes (Potato Pancake), 2 oz	200	11	22
3 Latkes w. Sour Cr./Apple Sce	750	25	95
Lochshen: Plain, 1 cup	130	2	26
Pudding, 1 cup	380	13	48
Lox (Smoked Salmon), 2 oz	65	2	0
Mandelbrot (Almond Bread), 1 slice,			
¼" thick	45	2	5
Matzo: 1 board, 1 oz	110	<1	21
(Also see Matzoh ~ Page 96)			
Matzo Balls, 2 small, 1 large	90	3	12
Soup, with 1 large ball	180	7	24
New York Cheesecake, 4 oz	350	24	26
Pierogi, potato/cheese, 1 pce	90	4	11
Reuben Sandwich	920	60	28
Schmaltz (Rend'd chick. fat), 1 T.	90	10	0

Lebanese/Middle East

	C	F	Cb
Baba Ghannouj, 2 Tbsp, 1 oz	70	6	2
(Eggplant/Seasame Dip)			
Baklava, 1 pastry, 1³/4 oz	245	18	18
(Pastry, Nuts, Syrup)			
Cabbage Rolls, 1 roll, 3 oz	100	3	12
(Cabbage Leaf, Meat, Rice)			
Cous Cous, 1 serve	400	21	43
(Semolina, Milk, Fruit, Nuts)			
Felafel (Chick Pea Fritter):			
Fried, 1 medium, 1 oz	60	4	4
Hummus, 1/4 cup, 2.2 oz	105	3	5
Fried Kibbi, 1 piece, 3 oz	180	8	15
(Wheat, Meat, Pinenuts)			
Kafta, 1 skewer, 1¹/2 oz	85	5	2
(Ground Lamb Saus. on Skewer)			
Kibbeh Naye, 1 cup, 9 oz	450	18	28
(Raw Lamb, Bulgur & Spices)			
Lebanese Omelet, 1 serving, 4 oz	200	12	13
(Egg, Spinach, Pinenuts, Onion)			
Pilaf, 1 cup	400	11	60
(Rice, Onion, Rais., Apr. Spice)			
Shawourma, 1 serve, 4 oz	280	15	2
(Spit Roast Beef)			
Shish Kabob, 1 stick, 2¹/2 oz	130	7	2
Spinach Pie, 1 piece, 3¹/2 oz	290	21	20
Sweet Almond Sanbusak, 1 pce	200	15	11
(Pastry, Almonds, Spices)			
Tabouli, 1 serve, 4 oz	170	14	7
Tahini Sauce, aver., 1 Tbsp	90	8	2

Mexican

	C	F	Cb
Black Bean Soup, 1 bowl	200	3	34
Bueso Fresco, 1/4 cup	80	4.5	8
Burritos (Taco Bell): Bean	380	12	54
Big Beef Supreme	520	23	51
Chili, plain, 1/4 cup	90	6	4
Chili con Carne, w. Beans, 1 cup	310	17	15
w/out Beans, 1 cup	370	28	10
Corn Chips, 1/2 cup, 1 oz	160	10	17
Empanadas, average, 1 small	230	10	28
Enchilada, average	330	10	49
Fajitas: Chicken (Soft)	200	7	20
Guacamole, 2 Tbsp, 1 oz	120	12	2
Horchata 1 cup, 8 fl. oz	120	0.5	27
Margarita (w. 1¹/2 oz Tequila)	160	0	6
Menudo, 1/2 cup	55	1.5	10

Mexican (Cont)

	C	F	Cb
Nachos:			
Taco Bell, Big Beef	430	24	43
Bellgrande (Taco Bell)	740	39	83
Del Taco: Regular	390	23	39
Macho Nachos	1090	61	110
Quesadilla: Cheese (Taco Bell)	370	20	32
Refried Beans, ³/4 cup, 6 oz	160	3	26
Sopaipillas (flky. pstry.puffs), 1 pc	100	7	10
w. honey & cream	200	14	18
Taco (Taco Bell): Regular	170	10	11
Chicken	180	5	23
Taco Supreme	230	13	13
Big Border Taco	280	16	17
Taco Salad w. Salsa	840	52	85
Taco Sauce, average, 1/4 cup	15	0	3
Taco Shell, regular	50	2	6
Tamales, Van Camp's (can), 1/2 c	150	8	14
Tostada (Taco Bell)	300	14	31
Tortilla, corn, 6" diam.	70	1	14
Tortilla Chips, 1 oz	150	8	18

Extra Listings of Mexican Dishes:
- Frozen Entrees/Meals ~ See Page 55
- Fast Foods Section (Taco Bell, Del Taco).
- Canned Bean/Chili Products ~ See Page 64

Polish

	C	F	Cb
Cabbage Rolls w. Sour Cr., 2 sm.	220	10	30
Chicken Casserole w. Mush., 1 c.	520	27	5
Kielbasa (Sausages, Onions,	350	28	2
fried, 2 large.)			
Meatballs in Sour Cream,	300	16	11
3 x 1¹/2" balls			
Pierogi, Fruit/Veg, 3" ball	80	2	15
Pork Goulash (Pork/Veg. Stew)	550	21	38
Pot Roast with Vegetables	630	21	28

Brooklyn

Soul Foods

	C	F	Cb
Breakfast Sausage, fried, 2 patties	250	17	0
Cornbread, homemade, 3 oz	200	7.5	28
Fatback, raw, 1/4 oz	60	6.5	0
Ham Hock, 1 oz	90	6.5	0
Hog Maw, 1 oz	45	2.5	0
Hominy, 3/4 cup	85	1	17
Hush Puppies, 5 pces, 3 oz	260	12	35
Kale, ckd, 1/2 cup	20	0.5	4
Neck Bones, Pork, 1 oz	65	4	0
Opossum, 1 oz	65	3	0
Oxtail, 1 oz	70	3.5	0
Pig Ear, 1/4 ear	50	3	0
Pig Foot, 1/2 foot	70	4.5	0
Pig Tail, 1/3 tail	115	10	0
Poke Salad, ckd, 1/2 cup	15	0.5	3
Pork Brains, 1 oz	40	2.5	0
Pork Cracklings, 1/2 oz	80	6	0
Pork Chitterlings, simmered, 3 oz	260	25	0
Pork Skin, 1 cup	70	4.5	0
Sousemeat, 1 oz	60	4.5	0
Succotash, 1/2 cup	80	1	17
Sweet Potato Pie, 1/8 of 9" pie	250	12	34
Tongue Pork, 1/3 tongue	75	5.5	0
Tripe, 2 oz	55	2	0
Vienna Sausage, 2 small, 1 oz	90	8	1

Thai Foods

	C	F	Cb
Appetizers: Satay Pork, 1 oz	100	4	2
Spring Roll, 1 1/4 oz	110	6	13
Soups: Tom Yam (Hot & Sour):			
with Seafood, 1 cup	100	3	4
Vegetarian, 1 cup	50	0	11
Mud Crab w. Coconut, 1 cup	400	30	16
Curries: Chick. w. Ginger, 1 cup	390	34	4
Thick Red Curry w. Beef, 1 cup	600	50	7
Thai Chicken Curry, 1 cup	340	23	4
Massaman Curry, 1 cup	680	57	8
Green Curry w. Pork, 1 cup	480	44	5
Stir Fry: Per 1 Cup			
(Combinations include Meat & Seafood)			
Comb. w. Fried Rice Noodles	470	33	30
Comb. w. Steamed Rice Noodles	360	10	42
Comb. Stir Fry & Veges (no rice)	410	15	65
Stir Fry Vegetables	100	2	18
Salads: Thai Chicken, 1 serving	330	9	17
Thai Beef Salad, 1 serving	260	9	15

Spanish

	C	F	Cb
Arroz Abanda (Fish with Rice)	340	8	31
Arroz Con Pollo (Rice/Chick. Sal)	500	23	50
Clams Marinera, 8 clams	330	16	22
Cochifrito (Lamb w. Lemon/Garlic)	650	25	5
Cochinillo Asado, 2 sl. (Rst Suckling Pig)	300	15	3
Cocido Madrileno (Madrid-Style Boiled Dinner)	450	27	18
Flan de Leche (Caramel Custard)	325	9	52
Fritadera de Ternera (Sauteed Veal)	450	27	2
Gazpacho, 1 bowl	60	2	15
Paella a la Valenciana (Chicken & Shellfish Rice)	900	42	70
Pollo a la Espanola (Chicken)	475	30	4
Ternera al Jerez (Veal w. Sherry)	660	29	6
Zarzuela (Fish & Shellfish Medley)	530	27	40

Vietnamese

	C	F	Cb
Bo Xao Dau Phong: Per Whole Dish (Ginger Beef w.Onion, Fish Sce.)	750	30	10
Bo Nuong (Beef Satay), 2 sticks	265	9	4
Ca Chien Gung (Whole Snapper w. Ginger)	600	16	6
Canh Chay (Veg./Tofu Soup)	80	3	13
Cuu Xao Lan (Curried Lamb, Veges in Coconut)	900	40	80
Ga Chien (Crsp. Chick + Plum Sce)	900	40	105
Ga Nuong (Chicken Satay + Sce.)	240	10	4
Ga Xao Rau(Marinated Chicken Braised w.Veg.)	800	26	100
Rau Cai Xao Chay (Stir Fried Vege., Soy Sauce.)	400	15	65
Thit Heo Goi Baup Cai, each (Spicy Cabbage Rolls w.Pork)	200	7	11

Gourmet & Miscellaneous

	C	F	Cb
Ants Eggs/Larvae, 1 Tbsp	20	0	0
Ants, Choc. coated, 3 Tbsp	140	7	2
Bee Maggots, 3 Tbsp	65	2	0
Caviar, black/red, 1 Tbsp	40	3	0
Caterpillars, canned, 2oz	60	2	0
Frogs Legs, fried, 1 pair (large)	125	7	0
Haggis, boiled, 4oz	350	24	22
Locusts, raw, 1oz	35	1	0
Silkworms, raw, 1oz	60	2	0
Snails (Escargots) ~ See French Foods			
Snake, roasted, 4oz	160	6	0

Sandwiches | C | F | Cb

No Spreads Unless Indicated
(Includes 2 Slices Bread ~ 3 oz)

	C	F	Cb
BLT (5 strips Bacon, 2 Tbsp Mayo)	600	40	46
Breaded Chicken & Salad	540	28	46
Chicken (5 oz) Salad w. Mayo.	580	30	49
Chopped Liver, Egg, Mayo.	630	25	44
Corned Beef (5 oz) w. Mustard	560	28	44
Cream Cheese w. Olives (5 large)	340	14	44
Egg Salad w. Mayonnaise	570	29	49
Egg Salad Club w. Bacon, Mayo.	780	53	49
Grilled Cheese (3 oz)	540	30	44
Ham (4 oz); Cheese (4 oz), Mayo.	910	56	44
Lobster Salad (4 oz) w. Mayo.	530	25	45
Overstuffed Tuna Salad (7 oz)	870	39	75
Reuben (6 oz Beef/Pastrami, 2 oz Cheese,			
2 Tbsp Dressing)	920	60	28
Roast Beef (4 oz) w. Mustard	460	12	45
Roast Pork (4 oz) w. Apple Sauce	500	16	55
Shrimp Salad Club w. Bacon, Mayo.	800	57	48
Sloppy Joe w. Sauce (7 oz)	600	30	45
Steak Sandwich (5 oz cooked)	680	32	41
Triple Cheese (4 oz) Melt	720	45	46
Tuna (5 oz) Salad w. Mayo.	610	30	49
Turkey Breast (5 oz) w. Mayo.	460	18	44
Turkey Breast (5 oz) w. Mustard	360	7	44
Turkey Club w. Bacon, Mayo.	830	38	31
Vegetarian w. Avocado, Cheese	820	49	72

Subs: See *Subway* Page 238

Wraps & Roll-Ups

Average All Types
(Meat/Chicken/Fish/Veges)

	C	F	Cb
Regular size, approx. 9 oz	500	25	48
Large, approx. 15 oz	830	40	80
Jumbo, approx. 22 oz	1400	70	134

Au Bon Pain: See Page 164
Long John Silver: Page 208
Taco Bell Fajita Wraps: Page 240
Wendy's Pitas: Page 244

Bagels

	C	F	Cb
Plain, unfilled, 3 oz	240	2	45
w. 2 Tbsp Cream Cheese	340	12	46
w. 2 oz Lox (Smoked Salmon)	320	4	45

Au Bon Pain: Page 164
Einstein Bros Bagels: Page 191

Croissants | C | F | Cb

	C	F	Cb
Unfilled, medium 1 1/2 oz	180	10	20
w. Ham (2 oz), Salad	280	14	24
w. Ham (2 oz), Cheese (2 oz)	470	30	20
w. Chick (2 oz) Cheese (2 oz)	470	30	20
w. Turkey/Ham/Chse (2 oz ea.)	580	36	20
Au Bon Pain: Ham & Cheese	380	20	36
Spinach & Cheese	270	16	27

Vending Machines

	C	F	Cb
Brownie, frosted	180	9	24
Cheese Balls, 1 oz	150	8	16
Choc Chip Cookies, 4	130	7	19
Choc Milk, 8 fl.oz	225	9	26
Coca Cola Classic, 12 fl.oz	140	0	35
Diet Coke, 12 fl.oz	1	0	0
Corn Chips, 1 oz	160	10	15
Danish Pastry, 2 oz	220	10	25
Donut, plain, 1 3/4 oz	210	12	25
Fruit Pie, 4 oz	290	13	46
Granola/Cereal Bars	130	3	26
Hershey's, 1.55 oz	240	14	25
Hot Fries, 1 oz	140	10	11
Kellogg's Rice Krispies Treat	120	1.5	26
Lance: Captain's Wafers, 1 pkg	230	12	26
Big Town, 1 pkg	250	11	38
M & M's: Plain, 1.7 oz	240	10	34
Peanuts, 1.7 oz	250	13	30
Milk, whole, 8 fl.oz	150	8	12
Reduced Fat, 2%, 8 fl.oz	120	5	12
Milky Way, 2 oz	270	10	41
Onion Rings, 1 oz	120	6	16
Orange Juice, 8.75 fl.oz	120	0	28
Peanuts, roasted, 1 oz	165	14	6
Popcorn, plain, 1 oz	160	10	14
Pork Skins, 1 oz	160	10	0
Potato Chips, 1 oz	150	10	15
Reduced Fat, 1 oz	140	7	20
Pretzels, 1 oz	110	2	22
Raisins, 1/2 oz pkg	40	0	9
Reece's Peanut Butter Cups, 1.8 oz	280	17	28
Snickers, 2.1 oz bar	280	14	35
Tortilla Chips, 1 oz	150	8	22

Fast-Food Chains & Restaurants

Cal Calories

Fat Fat (grams)

%Fc Percent Fat Calories

S.Fat Saturated Fat (grams)

Chol Cholesterol (milligrams)

Sod Sodium (milligrams)

Pro Protein (grams)

Carb Carbohydrates (grams)

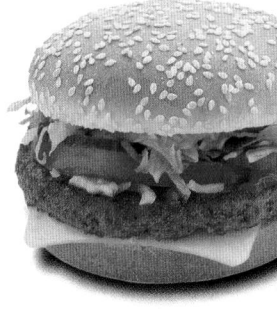

© 2000 ALLAN BORUSHEK

Arby's ®

	Cal	Fat	%FC	S.Fat	Chol	Sod	Pro	Carb
Breakfast Items								
Bacon, 2 strips	90	7	70%	3	15	220	5	0
Biscuit (Plain)	280	15	48%	3	0	730	6	34
Blueberry Muffin	230	9	35%	2	25	290	2	35
Cinnamon Nut Danish	360	11	27%	1	0	105	6	60
Croissant (Plain)	220	12	49%	7	25	230	4	25
Egg	95	8	76%	2	180	55	0.5	0.5
French-Toastix, 6 pieces	430	21	44%	5	0	550	10	52
Ham	45	1	20%	1	20	405	7	0
Sausage	165	15	82%	6	25	320	7	0
Swiss Cheese, 1 slice	45	3	60%	2	12	175	4	0.5
Table Syrup	100	0	0%	0	0	30	0	25
Roast Beef Sandwiches								
Arby's Melt w. Cheddar	370	18	44%	6	31	940	18	36
Arby-Q	430	18	38%	6	37	1320	22	48
Beef 'N Cheddar	490	28	52%	9	50	1215	25	40
Bacon Cheddar Deluxe	540	34	56%	10	44	1140	22	38
Giant Roast Beef	555	28	45%	11	71	1560	35	43
Junior Roast Beef	325	14	39%	5	30	780	17	35
Regular Roast Beef	390	19	44%	7	43	1010	23	33
Super Roast Beef	525	27	46%	9	43	1190	25	50
Chicken Sandwiches								
Breaded Chicken Fillet	535	28	47%	5	45	1015	28	46
Chicken Cordon Bleu	625	33	48%	8	77	1595	38	46
Chicken Fingers (2 Pieces)	290	16	50%	2	32	675	16	20
Grilled Chicken: BBQ	390	13	30%	3	43	1000	23	47
Deluxe	430	20	42%	4	61	850	23	41
Roast Chicken: Club	545	31	51%	9	58	1105	31	37
Deluxe; Santa Fe	435	22	45%	6	54	820	29	35
Sub Shop Sandwiches								
French Dip	475	22	42%	8	55	1410	30	40
Hot Ham 'N Cheese	500	23	41%	7	68	1665	30	43
Italian	675	36	48%	13	83	2090	30	46
Philly Beef 'N Swiss	755	47	56%	15	91	2025	39	48
Roast Beef	700	42	54%	14	84	2035	38	44
Triple Cheese Melt	720	45	44%	16	91	1800	37	46
Turkey	550	27	44%	7	65	2085	31	47
Fish/Ham Sandwiches: Fish Fillet	530	27	46%	7	43	865	23	50
Ham 'N Cheese: Plain	360	14	35%	5	53	1285	24	34
Melt	330	13	35%	4	43	1015	20	34
Light Menu: Garden Salad	60	0.5	7%	0	0	40	3	12
Roast Beef Deluxe	295	10	31%	3	42	825	18	33
Roast Chicken Deluxe	275	6	23%	2	33	775	20	33
Roast Turkey Deluxe	260	7	21%	2	33	1260	20	33
Roast Chicken Salad	150	2	12%	<1	29	420	20	12
Side Salad	25	0.3	12%	0	0	15	1	4
Crouton 1 pkt	60	2	30%	<1	1	155	2	9

	Cal	Fat	%FC	S.Fat	Chol	Sod	Pro	Carb
Potatoes: Curly Fries	300	15	45%	3	0	855	4	38
Cheddar Curly Fries w. Sce	335	18	48%	4	3	1015	5	40
French Fries	245	13	48%	3	0	115	2	30
Potato Cakes	205	12	53%	2	0	400	2	20
Baked Potato (Plain)	355	0.3	0%	0	0	25	7	82
w. Marg/Sour Cream	580	24	37%	9	25	210	9	85
w. Broccoli 'n Cheddar	570	20	32%	5	12	565	14	89
Deluxe Baked Potato	735	36	44%	16	59	500	19	86
Soups: Boston Clam Chowder	190	9	43%	3	25	965	9	18
Cream of Broccoli	160	8	45%	4	25	1005	7	15
Lumberjack Mixed Vegetable	90	4	40%	2	5	1150	2	10
Old-Fashion Chicken Noodle	80	2	22%	0	20	850	6	11
Potato with Bacon	170	7	37%	3	20	905	6	23
Timberline Chili	220	10	41%	4	30	1130	18	17
Wisconsin Cheese	280	18	58%	7	35	1065	10	20
Desserts/Shakes								
Apple Turnover	330	14	38%	7	0	180	4	48
Cherry Turnover	320	13	37%	5	0	190	4	46
Cheesecake (Plain)	320	23	65%	14	95	240	5	23
Chocolate Chip Cookie	125	6	43%	2	10	85	2	16
Chocolate Shake	450	12	24%	3	35	340	15	76
Jamocha Shake	385	10	23%	3	36	260	15	62
Vanilla Shake	360	12	30%	4	36	280	15	50
Polar Swirl: Butterfinger	460	18	35%	8	28	320	15	62
Heath	545	22	36%	5	39	345	15	76
Oreo	480	22	41%	10	35	520	15	66
Peanut Butter Cup	515	24	42%	8	34	385	20	61
Snickers	510	19	33%	7	33	350	15	73
Dressings/Sauces								
Arby's Sauce	15	0.2	12%	0	0	115	0	4
Beef Stock Au Jus	10	0	0%	0	0	440	0	1
Barbeque Sauce	30	0	0%	0	0	185	0	7
Blue Cheese	290	31	96%	6	50	580	2	2
Cheddar Cheese Sauce	35	3	77%	1	4	140	1	1
Honey French	280	23	74%	3	0	400	0	18
Horsey Sauce	60	5	74%	1	5	150	0	2
Mayonnaise	110	12	98%	7	5	80	0	0
Light Cholesterol Free	12	1	75%	0	0	65	0	0.5
Italian Sub Sauce	70	7	90%	1	0	240	0	1
Parmesan Cheese Sauce	70	7	90%	1	5	130	1	2
Red Ranch Dressing	75	6	72%	1	0	115	0	5
Tartar Sauce	140	15	96%	2	30	220	0	0
Thousand Island Dressing	260	26	90%	4	30	420	0	7
Reduced Calorie:								
Honey Mayonnaise	70	7	90%	1	20	135	0	1
Italian	20	1	45%	0	0	1000	0	3
Buttermilk Ranch	50	0	0%	0	0	710	0	12

Au Bon Pain®

	Cal	Fat	%Fc	S.Fat	Chol	Sod	Pro	Carb
Bagels: *Each*								
Plain, 5 oz	350	1.5	3%	0	0	660	14	72
Asiago Cheese, 4.2 oz	380	6	14%	3.5	15	690	17	66
Cheddar & Scallion, 4.2 oz	310	7	20%	4.5	20	650	14	47
Chocolate Chip, 5 oz	380	7	16%	3.5	5	480	12	69
Cinnamon Raisin, 5 oz	360	1.5	3%	0	0	540	12	77
Cranberry Walnut, 5oz	460	4	7%	0.5	0	590	15	93
Dutch Apple w. Walnut Streussel, 5 oz	350	5	13%	0	0	480	11	77
Everything, 4.2 oz	360	2.5	6%	0	0	710	14	72
Honey & Grain, 4.2 oz	360	2	5%	0	0	580	14	72
Jalapeno Double Cheddar, 4.2 oz	290	3.5	10%	2	10	600	12	53
Mocha Chip Swirl, 5 oz	370	3.5	8%	2	0	480	12	72
Onion, 5 oz	370	1.5	3%	0	0	660	14	78
Sesame, 4.2 oz	380	4	9%	0.5	0	540	15	71
Wild Blueberry, 4.5 oz	380	1.5	3%	0	0	570	14	80
Spreads: *Per 2 oz*								
Plain Cream Cheese	180	18	90%	11	50	150	4	2
Lite Bagel: Van. Hazelnut; Strawberry	150	11	66%	7	35	210	5	6
Lite Cream Cheese:	100	8	72%	5	20	280	6	4
Honey Walnut	150	11	66%	7	30	190	4	9
Raspberry	130	10	69%	7	30	200	6	7
Sundried Tomato	120	8	60%	5	20	320	6	6
Veggie	130	11	76%	7	35	230	5	4
Wraps Sandwiches: *Per Sandwich*								
Southwestern Tuna (no dressing)	760	46	54%	14	100	1030	40	48
Chicken Caesar (no dressing)	440	12	25%	5	70	900	37	43
Summer Turkey (no dressing)	430	4.5	9%	0	20	1380	35	62
Sandwiches: Buffalo Chicken	640	19	27%	3.5	85	1650	41	76
Chicken Foca-cha-cha	870	29	30%	5	130	2280	74	80
Fields & Feta	560	17	27%	4	10	850	20	89
For the Love of Olive	570	13	20%	1.5	40	2060	38	80
Fresh Mozzarella, Tomato & Pesto	650	30	42%	12	55	1090	30	69
Honey Dijon Chicken	730	18	22%	6	135	1990	57	85
Hot Roasted Turkey Club	950	50	47%	16	135	2240	50	80
Radically Roasted	620	10	15%	4.5	30	1540	33	69
Steak & Cheese Melt	750	32	38%	8	90	1600	40	79
Thai Chicken	420	6	13%	1	20	1320	20	72
Breads: *Per 1.75 oz Slice*								
French Bread	120	5	38%	0	0	320	4	25
French Parisienne Baguette	110	2	16%	0	0	260	4	22
Multigrain Batard	110	1	8%	0	0	310	5	22
Olive Batard	120	2	15%	0	0	310	5	22
Rye	110	1.5	12%	0	0	310	5	21
Sundried Tomato Batard	110	0	0%	0	0	270	4	22
Tomato Herb; Multigrain Loaf	130	1	6%	0	0	310	5	27
Rolls: Hearth, each	220	1.5	6%	0	0	410	9	43
Petit Pain, each	200	1	5%	0	0	570	7	41

	Cal	Fat	%FC	S.Fat	Chol	Sod	Pro	Carb
Soups: Per 8 oz Serving								
Beef Barley	75	2	24%	0.5	15	660	6	11
Carribean Black Bean	120	1	7%	0	5	770	7	22
Chicken Noodle; Chicken Wild Rice	80	1.5	17%	0	15	670	8	10
Clam Chowder	270	19	63%	9	65	730	11	16
Cream of Broccoli	220	18	74%	9	40	770	5	14
Enchilada w. Tomatilla	170	8	42%	3	20	910	6	14
Garden Vegetable	30	0	0%	0	0	820	2	8
Potato & Cheese w. Ham	150	1	6%	5	25	820	5	14
Summer Asparagus	160	11	62%	6	30	880	5	15
Tomato Florentine	60	1	15%	0.5	5	1030	4	13
Vegetarian Chili	140	2.5	16%	0	0	1070	6	27
Salads: Per Serving								
Chicken Caesar	360	11	28%	6	65	910	36	28
Chicken Tarragon w. Almonds	470	23	44%	4	80	500	32	38
Field Green, Gorgonzola & Walnut	400	34	77%	13	50	800	2	9
Garden Salad: Small	100	1	9%	0	0	150	6	20
Large	160	1.5	8%	0	0	290	7	34
Mozzarella & Rst Red Pepper	340	18	48%	10	60	135	22	26
Oriental Chicken	270	4	13%	0.5	70	700	40	17
Pesto Chicken	230	11	43%	2	45	250	6	11
Tuna	490	27	50%	4.5	45	750	26	40
Salad Dressings: Per 3 oz								
Bleu Cheese	410	41	90%	8	40	910	4	8
Buttermilk Ranch	310	32	93%	4	35	270	3	4
Caesar	380	39	92%	5	25	410	5	3
Carribean Balsamic Lime	170	16	85%	2.5	0	630	0	5
Greek	440	50	100%	1	0	870	0	2
Lemon Basil Vinaigrette	330	32	87%	2	0	460	0	15
Mandarin Orange	380	33	78%	3	0	310	0	23
Sesame French	370	30	73%	4.5	0	1010	1	26
Fat Free: Tomato Basil	70	0	0%	0	0	650	1	17
Lite: Honey Mustard	280	17	55%	2	0	460	0	15
Italian	230	20	78%	5	25	410	5	3
Croissants: Per Croissant								
Hot: Ham & Cheese	380	20	47%	12	70	690	16	36
Spinach & Cheese	270	16	53%	9	40	330	9	27
Dessert: Plain	270	15	50%	9	40	240	6	30
Almond	560	37	59%	15	105	250	12	50
Apple	280	10	32%	6	25	180	4	46
Chocolate	440	23	47%	15	30	230	7	53
Cinnamon Raisin	380	13	31%	8	35	290	7	51
Raspberry Cheese	380	19	45%	11	60	300	6	47
Muffins: Per Muffin								
Lowfat: Chocolate Cake	290	3	9%	0.5	20	630	4	68
Triple Berry	270	4	10%	0.5	25	560	5	60
Gourmet Muffins~ Next Page								

	Cal	Fat	%Fc	S.Fat	Chol	Sod	Pro	Carb
Muffins: Per Muffin								
Gourmet: Blueberry	410	15	33%	2.5	85	380	8	64
Carrot Pecan	480	23	43%	5	55	650	8	61
Chocolate Chip	490	20	37%	7	35	560	8	70
Corn	470	18	34%	2.5	65	570	8	70
Pumpkin w. Streussel Topping	470	18	34%	3	60	550	8	74
Raisin Bran	390	11	25%	4	45	1030	9	65
Cookies: Per Cookie								
Almond Biscotti	200	10	45%	3.5	35	45	4	24
Chocolate Almond Biscotti	240	13	49%	6	35	50	5	28
Chocolate Chip	280	13	42%	8	40	85	3	40
Cranberry Almond Macaroon	160	8	45%	5	0	115	2	22
English Toffee	220	12	49%	7	45	110	2	28
Ginger Pecan	260	15	52%	6	40	115	5	30
Oatmeal Raisin	250	10	36%	3.5	30	240	3	40
Shortbread	390	25	58%	15	65	190	3	39
Desserts: Per Piece								
Apple Coffee Cake	480	24	45%	12	100	285	6	60
Apple Strudel	440	26	53%	8	0	780	5	48
Cherry Strudel	450	29	58%	12	0	730	5	45
Caramel Apple Bar	370	18	44%	3	25	200	4	54
Key Lime Blueberry Bar	340	15	40%	5	110	290	5	45
Mochaccino Bar	405	24	53%	10	37	295	5	44
Pear Ginger Tea Cake	380	20	47%	3	0	200	3	47
Southern Pecan Bar	560	35	56%	11	50	300	1	60
Walnut Fudge Brownie	380	18	43%	11	100	150	5	56
Specialties: Per Piece								
Pecan Roll, 6.8 oz roll	900	48	48%	15	50	480	1	111
Drinks: Per 16 oz								
Blast: Malt Shoppe	370	4.5	11%	2.5	15	220	11	71
Strawberry Banana Split	380	2	5%	1.5	10	125	7	82
Hot Hazelnut; Str'berry/ Van. Choc.	310	6	17%	3.5	25	180	11	57
Hot Caramel/Raspberry Mocha	330	6	17%	3.5	25	180	11	57
Frozen Blast: Original; Mocha	320	3	8%	2	10	150	9	64
Wilch Blast: Malt Shoppe	450	9	18%	6	35	350	19	74
Original Frozen Mocha	350	7	18%	4.5	30	240	16	56
Strawberry Banana Split	280	5	16%	3.5	25	190	13	45
Iced Cappuccino: Small, 9 fl.oz	110	4	33%	2.5	15	110	7	10
Medium, 12 fl.oz	150	6	36%	3.5	25	150	10	15
Large, 20 fl.oz	270	10	33%	6	40	270	18	26
Iced Tea: Peach, Small, 8 fl.oz	90	0	0%	0	0	15	0	22
Medium, 12 fl.oz	130	0	0%	0	0	20	0	33
Large, 16 fl.oz	170	0	0%	0	0	30	0	44

Deluxe: Per Regular Scoop	Cal	Fat	%Fc	S.Fat	Chol	Sod	Pro	Carb
Banana Nut	260	17	58%	8	50	70	4	26
Banana Strawberry	240	12	45%	8	50	75	3	30
Baseball Nut	280	16	51%	8	50	95	4	31
Black Walnut	280	19	61%	10	55	85	5	23
Blueberry Cheesecake	260	12	42%	7	45	140	3.5	35
Butterfinger	300	15	45%	7	31	120	4	39
Caramel Choc. Crunch	290	17	53%	11	50	150	4	33
Cherry Cheesecake	260	12	42%	7	25	45	4	35
Cherries Jubilee	240	13	9%	8	50	75	3	29
Chewy Babe Ruth	300	17	51%	11	55	115	4	32
Choc O The Irish	280	17	55%	11	55	105	4	30
Chocoholic's Resolution	300	16	48%	10	50	115	4	37
Chocolate	270	16	53%	10	55	110	4	30
Chocolate Almond	310	20	58%	10	50	100	6	30
Chocolate Chip	270	18	60%	11	60	85	4	26
Chocolate Chip Cookie Dough	300	17	51%	10	60	125	4	35
Chocolate Fudge	290	15	47%	8	41	180	4	34
Chocolate Mousse Royale	310	18	52%	9	50	105	4	35
Chocolate Raspberry Truffle	280	14	45%	9	50	95	4	36
Chocolate Ribbon	250	13	47%	9	50	80	3	30
Chunka Cherry Burn Love	250	13	47%	8	50	80	3	29
Chunky Heath Bar	300	18	54%	11	50	125	3	33
Cinnamon Tax Crunch	280	14	45%	7	45	125	4	35
Cookies 'n Cream	300	19	57%	12	55	140	4	29
Coconut	280	19	61%	13	60	85	4	24
Decorating Vanilla	250	16	58%	10	65	85	3	24
English Toffee	290	16	50%	10	55	125	3	34
French Vanilla	280	18	58%	10	90	90	4	25
Fudge Brownie	310	19	55%	11	50	130	5	35
German Choc Cake	310	15	44%	7	32	100	5	39
Gold Medal Ribbon	270	13	42%	8	50	170	3	35
Here Comes The Judge	270	13	42%	9	36	100	4	36
Jamoca	250	15	54%	10	60	85	3	25
Jamoca Almond Fudge	280	16	51%	8	45	70	4	30
Kahlua & Choc. Cream	270	14	48%	9	55	90	4	29
Lemon Custard	260	15	52%	9	80	100	4	29
Martian Mint	260	15	52%	9	40	140	3	30
Mint Choc Chip	270	18	60%	11	60	85	4	26
Naughty New Year's Resolution	310	20	58%	9	45	125	6	40
New York Cheesecake	270	16	54%	11	45	135	4	30
Nutty Coconut	310	21	61%	10	50	85	4	27
Nutty or Nice	290	16	50%	9	54	130	3	36
Old Fashion Butter Pecan	290	20	62%	10	60	90	4	23
Oregan Blackberry	230	12	47%	8	51	69	4	25
Peach	240	12	45%	8	50	70	3	28
Peanut Butter 'n Cookie	330	22	60%	10	50	170	6	29

	Cal	Fat	%Fc	S.Fat	Chol	Sod	Pro	Carb
Deluxe (Cont)								
Per Regular Scoop								
Peppermint	270	14	47%	9	55	80	3	33
Pink Bubblegum	270	14	47%	9	55	75	3	34
Pistachio-Almond	300	21	63%	10	55	80	6	23
Pralines 'n Cream	290	16	50%	8	50	135	3	34
Pumpkin Patch	250	13	47%	8	45	90	3	31
Quarterback Crunch	290	17	53%	12	50	135	3	32
Red, White & Boo	260	12	42%	12	45	80	3	36
Reeses Peanut Butter	310	19	55%	11	55	125	5	30
Rocky Road	300	17	51%	9	50	105	5	34
Rudolph's Red Raspberry Sorbet	140	0	0%	0	0	10	0	36
Rum Raisin	250	13	47%	8	50	70	3	36
S'Crunch Ous Crunch	310	16	46%	10	45	110	4	40
S'Mores	300	13	39%	8	29	100	4	41
Snickidy Doo Dah	300	16	48%	9	50	160	4	35
Strawberry Cheesecake	270	14	47%	9	45	130	3	34
Strawberry Shortcake	280	16	51%	10	50	125	3	32
Triple Chocolate Passion	290	18	56%	10	55	110	5	34
Vanilla	240	14	52%	9	52	115	4	24
Very Berry Strawberry	220	10	41%	5	30	95	3	30
Winter White Chocolate	270	16	53%	11	45	90	3	33
Winter Wondermint	270	14	47%	9	55	80	3	33
World Class Chocolate	280	16	51%	9	55	105	4	32
Light Icecream: Regular Serving								
Almond Butterscotch	260	9	30%	4.5	22	120	9	39
Choc Caramel Nut	260	6	21%	4.5	11	165	9	44
Double Raspberry	200	5	20%	2	22	90	6	35
Espresso 'n Cream	220	6	25%	2	11	135	6	39
Pistachio Creme Chip	265	9	30%	5	22	120	9	37
Praline Dream	240	6	23%	4.5	11	160	6	39
Rocky Path	290	9	28%	3	22	120	9	42
Non Fat Icecream: Regular Serving								
Average all flavors	240	0	0%	0	0	210	6	50
No Sugar Added: Regular Serving								
Average all flavors	220	5	20%	3	10	120	6	40
Soft Serving Icecream: Regular Serving								
Caramel Praline	260	0	0%	0	6	190	9	55
Vanilla	260	0	0%	0	6	190	11	55
Ices, Sherbets, Sorbets: Regular Serving								
Ices: Daquiri	240	0	0%	0	0	20	0	59
Grape	220	0	0%	0	0	20	0	59
Margarita	240	0	0%	0	0	20	0	61
Sherbets: Rainbow/Orange	260	5	17%	2	11	55	2	57
Sorbets:								
Pink Raspberry Lemonade	260	0	0%	0	0	20	0	64
Red Raspberry	260	0	0%	0	0	20	0	66

	Cal	Fat	%FC	S.Fat	Chol	Sod	Pro	Carb
Yogurt Gone Crazy								
For Heaven's Cake	260	5	17%	3	20	165	6	53
Have Your Cake	240	5	19%	2	11	220	9	48
Maui Brownie Madness	310	6	17%	2	11	220	9	48
Perils of Praline	310	6	17%	4	11	230	9	55
Raspberry Cheese Louse	290	6	19%	4	20	200	9	53
Frozen Yogurt: Regular Scoop								
Low Fat: All flavors, aver.	260	4	14%	2	15	165	9	50
Non Fat: All flavors, aver.	240	0	0%	0	0	120	6	50
Truly Free; average	200	0	0%	0	11	180	9	40
Novelties: Per Serving								
Chillyburger, all types	220	11	45%	7	25	100	4	27
Sundae Bars: Per Serving								
Jamoca Almond Fudge	280	17	55%	9	20	60	5	28
Peanut Butter Choc	340	27	71%	11	20	115	7	22
Pralines 'n Cream	280	17	55%	10	10	105	4	28
Tiny Toon Bars								
All varieties, 1 serving	240	17	64%	11	25	40	3	20
Cappy Blast Bars								
All varieties, average	120	4	30%	3	15	35	2	20
Fountain Drinks								
Cappy Blast	290	10	31%	7	50	105	6	42
w. Whipped Cream, 2 tsp	320	13	37%	9	55	105	0	43
Mocha Cappy Blast	330	11	30%	7	50	130	6	55
w. Whipped Cream, 2 tsp	360	14	35%	9	55	130	0	56
Paradise Blast/Pina Colada	330	9	25%	5	40	55	3	55
Paradise Blast/Stawberry	300	6	18%	4	25	775	2	56
Malt Shake/Vanilla IC	660	31	42%	19	145	250	15	84
Malt Powder	110	1.5	12%	1	0	80	2	23
Toppings								
Butterscotch, 2 oz	200	2	9%	na	6	160	1	47
Hot Fudge, 1 oz	100	3	27%	na	0	45	1	17
No Sug.Add/Fat Free	90	0	0%	0	2	95	2	20
Praline Caramel, 1 oz	90	0	0%	0	0	105	0	19
Strawberry, 1 oz	60	0	0%	0	0	5	0	14
Whipped Cream, 2 tsp	30	3	90%	2	5	0	0	1
White & Colored Sprinkles	20	0.5	22%	0	0	0	0	3
Baby Gummy Bears, 75 pieces	130	0	0%	0	0	15	3	30
Cones								
Sugar	60	3	45%	0	0	50	1	7
Cake	25	0.5	18%	0	0	55	1	4
Waffle Cone., large	120	1.5	11%	0	0	55	0	14
Fresh Baked	145	2	12%	0.5	13	5	2	30
Smoothies: Per 8 fl.oz								
Blueberry Strawberry	150	0	0%	0	0	70	4	31
Orange Banana	120	0	0%	0	5	75	5	25
Strawberry Banana	170	0	0%	0	5	75	4	39

Big Boy

Sandwiches	Cal	Fat	%Fc	S.Fat	Chol	Sod	Pro	Carb
Turkey	225	5	20%	2	75	835	22	24
Chicken w. Mozzarella	405	13	29%	6	76	420	42	26
Dinners (w.Bread; No Dressing)								
Chicken Breast: w.Salad	350	13	34%	3	65	340	38	20
w.Mozzarella & Salad	370	12	29%	4	76	355	42	24
Cajun & Salad	350	13	34%	4	65	610	38	20
Chckn. & Veg. stir-fry (no bread)	560	14	22%	4	68	750	43	68
Fish:Cod Baked; Dijon, Salad	430	18	38%	4	68	570	44	21
Cod, Cajun, Salad	365	12	30%	4	68	460	43	20
Spaghetti Marinara & Salad	450	6	12%	3	8	760	15	87
Soup: Cabbage, 1 bowl	45	1	21%	2	1	730	2	9
1 cup	40	0	0%	0	1	625	2	8
Vegetables								
Vegetable Stir-fry	410	10	22%	2	0	705	9	74
Beans, green	30	0	0%	0	0	0	2	6
Carrots	35	0	0%	0	0	40	1	8
Corn	90	1	10%	0	0	0	3	21
Mixed Vegetables	30	0	0%	0	0	40	2	5
Peas	80	0	0%	0	0	130	6	13
Potato, Baked	165	0	0%	0	0	10	5	37
Rice	115	0	0%	0	0	640	3	25
Roll	140	0	0%	0	2	185	3	30
Salad: Chicken Breast, Dijon	390	11	25%	2	65	415	42	31
Dinner, without Dressing	20	0	0%	0	0	10	1	4
Dressing: Buttermilk	35	2	50%	1	10	150	0	4
Desserts: 'No-No' frozen dessert	75	0	0%	0	0	35	2	17
Yogurt, frozen, regular	70	0	0%	0	2	30	2	16
Shake	185	0	0%	0	2	130	8	36

Blimpie ®

Subs *Per 6" Sub*	Cal	Fat	%Fc	S.Fat	Chol	Sod	Pro	Carb
Blimpie Best	410	13	29%	5	50	1480	26	47
Cheese Trio	510	23	41%	13	60	1060	26	51
Club	450	13	26%	6	40	1350	30	53
Grilled Chicken	400	9	20%	2	30	950	28	52
5 Meatball	500	22	40%	8	25	970	23	52
Ham & Swiss	400	13	29%	7	35	970	25	47
Ham, Salami, Provolone	590	28	43%	11	70	1880	32	52
Roast Beef	340	4.5	13%	1	20	870	27	47
Steak & Cheese	550	26	42%	4	70	1080	27	51
Tuna	570	32	50%	5	50	790	21	50
Turkey	320	4.5	14%	1	10	890	19	51
Salad: Grilled Chicken, no dressing	350	12	31%	0	140	1190	47	13

Bojangles'®

	Cal	Fat	%Fc	S.Fat	Chol	Sod	Pro	Carb
Cajun Spiced Chicken								
Breast	280	17	55%	3	75	565	18	12
Leg	265	16	55%	3	96	530	19	11
Thigh	310	23	67%	5	67	465	15	11
Wing	355	25	63%	5	94	630	21	11
Cajun Roast Chicken								
Breast, without skin	145	5	31%	1	84	560	24	<1
Leg, without skin	160	8	45%	2	125	565	23	<1
Thigh, without skin	215	15	63%	3	95	430	20	<1
Wing, without skin	230	15	59%	3	117	620	22	3
Southern Style Chicken								
Breast	260	16	55%	3	76	700	16	12
Leg	260	15	52%	4	94	445	19	11
Thigh	310	21	61%	5	78	630	16	14
Wing	340	21	56%	5	86	685	17	19
Sandwiches/Nuggets								
Buffalo Bites	180	5	25%	2	105	720	27	5
Cajun Fillet, no dressing	340	11	29%	5	435	400	22	41
Chicken Supremes	340	16	42%	6	58	630	21	26
Grilled Fillet, no dressing	235	5	19%	3	51	540	23	25
Biscuit Sandwiches								
Biscuit (plain)	245	12	44%	3	2	665	4	30
Bacon	290	17	53%	5	10	810	8	26
Bacon, Egg & Cheese	550	42	69%	14	160	1250	17	27
Cajun Fillet	455	21	61%	6	41	950	20	46
Country Ham	270	15	49%	4	20	1010	9	26
Egg	400	30	66%	6	120	630	8	26
Sausage	350	23	64%	7	20	810	9	26
Smoked Sausage	380	23	60%	9	20	940	10	27
Steak	650	49	68%	13	34	1125	14	37
Fixins'								
Bo Rounds	235	11	42%	4	13	330	3	31
Cajun Pintos	110	0	1%	10	0	480	6	18
Marinated Cole Slaw	135	3	20%	0	0	455	1	26
Corn on the Cob	140	2	13%	0	0	20	5	34
Dirty Rice	165	6	33%	2	10	760	5	24
Green Beans	25	0	0%	0	0	710	1	6
Macaroni & Cheese	200	14	63%	4	26	420	7	12
Potatoes, no Gravy	80	1	11%	0	0	380	2	16
Seasoned Fries	345	19	49%	5	13	480	5	40

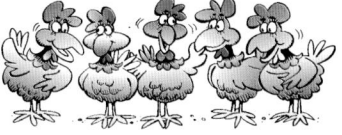

171

	Cal	Fat	%Fc	S.Fat	Chol	Sod	Pro	Carb
Entrees								
Chicken: 1/4 white meat w. skin	330	17	46%	5	175	530	43	2
No skin or wing	160	4	20%	1	95	350	31	0
1/4 dark meat w. skin	330	22	60%	6	180	460	31	2
No skin	210	10	43%	2.5	150	320	28	1
1/2 chicken w. skin	630	37	53%	19	370	960	74	2
Original Chicken Pot Pie, 1 pie	750	34	41%	9	115	2380	34	78
Ham w. Cinnamon Apples	350	13	33%	5	75	1750	25	35
Meat Loaf & Tom Sauce	370	18	44%	8	120	1170	30	22
Meat Loaf & Gravy	390	22	51%	8	120	1040	30	19
Turkey Breast, no skin	170	1	5%	0.5	100	850	36	1
Soup								
Chicken, 3/4 cup	80	3	34%	1	25	470	9	4
Chicken Tortilla, 1 cup	220	11	45%	4	35	1410	10	19
Salads								
Caesar Entree, 10 oz	520	43	74%	12	40	1420	20	16
no dressing, 8 oz	240	13	49%	7	25	780	19	14
Chicken Caesar, 13 oz	670	47	63%	13	120	1860	45	16
Chunky Chicken Salad	370	27	66%	5	120	800	28	3
Mediterranean Pasta, 3/4 cup	170	10	53%	3	10	490	4	16
Tortellini Salad, 3/4 cup	380	24	57%	5	90	530	14	29
Sandwiches								
Chicken Salad	680	30	39%	4	145	1350	38	63
Chicken w. Cheese & Sauce	750	33	38%	12	135	1860	41	72
No Cheese or Sauce	430	5	10%	1	65	910	34	62
Ham w. Cheese & Sauce	760	35	41%	13	100	1880	38	71
No Cheese or Sauce	450	9	18%	3	45	1600	25	66
Meat Loaf w. Cheese	860	33	35%	16	165	2270	46	95
No Cheese	690	21	27%	7	120	1610	40	85
Ham & Turkey Club w. Chse & Sce	890	44	43%	20	150	2350	48	76
No Cheese or Sauce	430	6	13%	2	55	1330	29	64
Turkey w. Cheese & Sauce	710	28	35%	10	110	1390	45	68
No Cheese or Sauce	400	4	8%	1	60	1070	32	51
Side Dishes								
Corn, 3/4 cup	190	4	19%	1	0	130	5	39
Coleslaw, 3/4 cup	280	16	51%	2.5	25	520	2	32
Hot Cinnamon Apples, 3/4 cup	250	4.5	16%	0.5	0	45	0	56
Macaroni Cheese, 3/4 cup	280	10	32%	6	20	760	12	36
Mash Potatoes & Gravy, 3/4 cup	200	9	40%	5	25	560	3	27
Rice Pilaf, 2/3 cup	180	5	25%	1	0	600	5	32
Stuffing, 3/4 cup	310	12	35%	2	0	1140	5	44
Baked Goods								
Brownie	450	27	54%	7	80	190	6	47
Corn Bread, 1 loaf	200	6	27%	1.5	25	390	3	33
Choc Chip Cookie	340	17	45%	6	25	240	4	43
Oatmeal Raisin Cookie	320	13	37%	3	25	260	4	48

	Cal	Fat	%FC	S.Fat	Chol	Sod	Pro	Carb
Breakfast								
Biscuit, 3 oz	300	15	45%	3	0	830	6	35
Biscuit with Egg	380	21	50%	5	140	1010	11	37
Biscuit with Sausage	490	33	60%	10	35	1240	13	36
Biscuit w. Sausage, Egg, Cheese	620	43	62%	14	185	1650	20	37
Croissan'wich®: w. Sausage/Cheese	450	35	70%	12	45	940	13	21
w. Sausage/Egg/Cheese	550	42	69%	14	250	1110	20	22
French Toast Sticks (5), 4 oz	440	23	47%	5	2	490	7	51
Hash Brown Rounds: Small	240	15	56%	6	0	440	2	25
Large, 4 1/2 oz	410	26	57%	10	0	50	3	42
Cini-Minis: 4 Rolls w. Icing	550	26	47%	7	25	750	6	71
Vanilla Icing only, 1 oz	110	3	25%	1	0	40	0	20
A.M. Express® Grape/Strawb. Jam	30	0	0%	0	0	0	0	7
Burgers								
Whopper® Sandwich	660	40	54%	12	85	900	29	47
without Mayonnaise	510	23	40%	10	70	750	29	46
Whopper® w. Cheese Sandwich	760	48	57%	17	110	1380	35	47
Double Whopper® Sandwich	920	59	58%	21	155	980	49	47
w. Cheese Sandwich	1010	67	60%	26	180	1960	55	47
Whopper JR® Sandwich	400	24	54%	8	55	530	19	29
without Mayonnaise	320	15	44%	7	45	460	19	27
Whopper® w. Cheese Sandwich	450	28	56%	10	65	770	22	28
Big King™ Sandwich	640	42	59%	18	125	980	38	28
Hamburger	320	15	42%	6	50	530	20	27
Cheeseburger	360	19	45%	9	60	770	21	27
Bacon Cheeseburger	400	22	50%	10	70	1240	24	27
Bacon Double Cheeseburger	620	38	55%	18	125	1230	41	28
Double Cheeseburger	580	36	56%	17	120	1060	38	27
Chicken & Fish Sandwiches								
BK Big Fish® Sandwich	720	43	54%	9	80	1180	23	59
BK Broiler® Chicken Sandwich	530	26	43%	5	105	1060	29	45
without Mayonnaise	370	9	22%	4	80	900	29	45
Chicken Sandwich	710	43	55%	9	60	1400	26	54
Chick'N Crisp Sandwich	460	27	53%	6	35	890	16	37
Chicken Tenders®: 4 pieces	180	11	56%	3	30	470	11	9
5 pieces	230	14	56%	4	40	590	14	11
8 pieces	350	22	56%	7	65	940	22	17
French Fries (Salted): Small, 2 3/4 oz	250	13	47%	5	0	550	2	32
Medium, 4 oz	400	21	47%	8	0	820	3	50
King Size, 6 oz	590	30	46%	12	0	1180	5	74
Onion Rings: Medium, 3 1/2 oz	380	19	45%	2	0	550	5	46
King Size, 5 1/2 oz	600	30	45%	7	4	880	8	74
Dipping Sauces (1 oz): Barbecue	35	0	0%	0	0	400	0	9
Honey Flavored	90	0	0%	0	0	10	0	23
Honey Mustard	90	6	60%	1	10	150	0	10
Ranch	170	17	90%	3	0	200	0	2
Sweet & Sour	45	0	0%	0	0	50	0	11

Burger King® (Cont)

	Cal	Fat	%Fc	S.Fat	Chol	Sod	Pro	Carb
Dutch Apple Pie, 4 oz	300	15	45%	3	0	230	3	39
Shakes: Vanilla, medium	400	9	20%	5	30	330	13	73
Chocolate: Small	330	7	0%	4	25	250	9	58
Medium	440	10	20%	6	30	330	12	75
Medium, syrup added	570	10	16%	6	30	520	14	105
Strawberry, medium	550	9	13%	5	30	350	13	104
Coca-Cola® (¹/4 ice): Small, 16 fl.oz	150	0	0%	0	0	15	0	37
Medium, 22 fl.oz	210	0	0%	0	0	20	0	58
Sprite (¹/4 ice), medium, 22 fl.oz	200	0	0%	0	0	50	0	50
Tropicana® Orange Juice, 10 fl.oz	140	0	0%	0	0	0	2	33
Reduced Fat Milk - 2% Fat, 8 fl.oz	130	5	35%	3	20	120	8	12
Condiments/Toppings								
American Cheese, 2 slices, 25g	90	8	80%	5	25	420	6	0
Bacon, 3 pieces, 8g	40	3	60%	1	10	170	3	0
Bull's Eye BBQ Sauce, ¹/2 oz	20	0	0%	0	0	140	0	5
Ketchup, ¹/2 oz	15	0	0%	0	0	180	0	4
King Sauce, ¹/2 oz	70	7	90%	1	4	70	0	2
Land O'Lakes Whipped Blend, 10g	65	7	97%	1	0	75	0	0

Carvel® Ice Cream

	Cal	Fat	%Fc	S.Fat	Chol	Sod	Pro	Carb
Soft Serving								
Chocolate: Small	300	16	47%	10	40	160	6.5	35
Regular	420	22	47%	13	55	220	9	48
Large	530	28	47%	17	70	280	11	62
No Fat: Small	190	0	0%	0	0	65	3	45
Regular	265	0	0%	0	0	90	4.5	62
Large	335	0	0%	0	0	120	5.5	78
Vanilla: Small	320	16	45%	10	65	175	8	34
Regular	440	22	45%	13	90	240	11	46
Large	560	28	45%	17	120	310	14	59
No Fat: Small	190	0	0%	0	0	90	6	40
Regular	265	0	0%	0	0	120	9	55
Large	335	0	0%	0	0	155	11	70
Sherbet, all flavors: Small	220	1.5	6%	1	8	70	3.5	50
Regular	310	2	5%	1	11	100	4.5	68
Large	390	3	7%	1.5	14	125	5.5	87
Novelties: Flying Saucers	240	10	37%	5	30	180	5	33
Reduced Fat	180	2.5	23%	0.5	0	140	4	36
Chipsters	380	18	43%	9	30	240	6	50
Reduced Fat	320	11	31%	4.5	0	200	5	53
Brown Bonnet Cone: regular	380	21	50%	15	40	150	6	43
Reduced Fat	300	11	33%	9	0	95	5	47
Piece of Cake, all types, 4 oz	270	14	47%	9	30	160	5	33
Sinful Love Bar, 4 oz	460	29	57%	14	20	240	8	48

	Cal	Fat	%FC	S.Fat	Chol	Sod	Pro	Carb
Platters								
Broiled Shrimp	720	8	10%	1	155	1760	32	131
Broiled Chicken	802	10	11%	2	82	1650	46	131
Broiled Fish	734	7	8%	1	49	1645	36	131
Fish & Chicken	777	10	12%	1	66	1650	41	131
Lunches								
Broiled Shrimp	421	7	15%	1	155	1725	25	64
Broiled Chicken	503	9	16%	2	82	1615	39	65
Broiled Fish	435	7	14%	1	49	1610	28	65
Broiled Fish & Chicken	478	8	15%	1	66	1610	34	68
Stuffed Crab	91	7	46%	na	na	250	8	16
Sandwiches								
Broiled Chicken	450	19	38%	na	105	860	40	29
Side Items								
Baked Potato	280	0	0%	0	0	20	6	64
Breadstick	110	4	33%	0	0	210	3	16
Cole Slaw	160	12	68%	na	16	245	3	1
Corn on the Cob	250	2	7%	na	0	15	9	60
Cheese, 1 oz	54	5	83%	na	14	205	3	<1
Crackers (4)	50	1	18%	na	3	150	1	8
Cracklins, 1 oz	220	17	70%	na	0	740	1	16
Dinner Salad	20	0	0%	0	0	15	1	4
French Fries	300	10	30%	na	0	150	3	50
Fried Okra	300	16	48%	na	0	445	7	34
Green Beans	45	2	39%	na	4	750	2	5
Hushpuppy	125	4	29%	na	0	465	2	20
Rice	124	0	0%	0	0	9	3	28
Vegetable Medley	35	1	25%	na	0	115	1	4
White Beans	125	0.2	1%	na	2	100	8	22
Salad Dressings: Per Serving								
Blue Cheese	110	12	98%	na	14	100	<1	<1
French	110	11	89%	na	7	190	<1	4
Ranch	90	10	98%	na	15	230	<1	<1
Sour Cream, Imitation	30	3	90%	3	0	na	0	1
Sauces: Cocktail	35	0.4	8%	0	0	250	<1	8
Sweet & Sour	50	0	0%	0	0	5	0	13
Tartar	75	7	84%	na	10	160	<1	3
Desserts								
Carrot Cake	435	23	48%	na	32	415	8	49
Cheesecake	420	31	66%	na	141	480	7	30
Chocolate Cake	305	10	30%	na	20	260	4	49
Pecan Pie	460	20	39%	na	4	375	5	64

Carl's Jr®

	Cal	Fat	%Fc	S.Fat	Chol	Sod	Pro	Carb
Breakfast								
French Toast Dips; No Syrup	410	25	55%	6	0	380	6	40
Sunrise Swch; No Bacon/Saus.	370	21	51%	6	225	710	14	31
Breakfast Burrito	430	26	54%	12	460	810	22	29
Scrambled Eggs	160	11	62%	4	425	125	13	1
English Muffin w. Marg.	230	10	39%	2	0	330	5	30
Breakfast Quesadilla	300	14	42%	6	225	750	14	27
Bacon, 2 Strips	40	4	90%	2	10	125	3	0
Sausage, 1 Patty	200	18	81%	7	35	530	7	0
Sandwiches								
Famous Big Star Hamburger	610	38	56%	11	70	890	26	42
Super Star Hamburger	820	53	58%	20	120	1030	43	41
1/3 lb Classic Dbl. Cheeseburger	660	42	57%	16	110	1060	34	37
Western Bacon Cheeseburger:	870	35	46%	16	90	1490	34	59
Double	970	57	53%	27	145	1810	56	58
Big Burger	470	20	38%	8	55	810	25	46
Hamburger	200	8	36%	4	25	500	11	23
BBQ Chicken Sandwich	310	6	17%	2	55	830	31	34
Chicken Club Sandwich	550	29	47%	8	85	1160	35	37
Santa Fe Chicken	530	30	51%	7	85	1230	30	36
Hot & Crispy Sandwich	400	22	49%	5	45	980	14	35
Carl's Catch Fish Sandwich	560	30	48%	7	60	1220	17	54
Great Stuff Potatoes: Plain	290	0	0%	0	0	40	6	68
Broccoli & Cheese	530	22	37%	5	15	930	11	76
Bacon & Cheese	630	29	41%	7	40	1720	20	76
Sour Cream & Chive	430	14	29%	3	10	160	8	70
Muffins/Desserts								
Per Serving								
Blueberry Muffin	340	14	37%	2	40	340	5	49
Bran Muffin	370	13	32%	2	45	410	7	61
Cheese Danish	400	22	49%	5	15	390	5	49
Chocolate Chip Cookie	370	19	46%	8	25	350	3	49
Chocolate Cake	300	10	30%	3	23	260	3	49
Cinnamon Roll	420	13	28%	4	15	570	9	68
Strawberry Swirl Cheesecake	300	17	51%	9	55	220	6	31
Side Orders								
Breadstick, 1 serving	35	<1	7%	0	0	60	1	7
Chicken Stars, 6 pieces	230	14	55%	3	85	450	13	11
CrissCut Fries, large	550	34	56%	9	0	1280	7	55
French Fries, regular	370	20	49%	7	0	240	4	44
Hash Brown Nuggets, 1 serving	270	17	57%	4	0	410	3	27
Onion Rings, 1 serving	520	26	45%	6	0	840	8	63
Zucchini, 1 serving	380	23	54%	6	0	1040	7	38
Salads-To-Go								
Charbroiled Chicken, 1 serving								
No Dressing	260	9	31%	5	70	530	28	11
Garden Salad, 1 serving	50	3	50%	2	5	75	3	4

	Cal	Fat	%Fc	S.Fat	Chol	Sod	Pro	Carb
Dressings: Blue Cheese	310	34	99%	6	25	360	2	1
Fat Free French	70	0	0%	0	0	760	0	18
Fat Free Italian	15	0	0%	0	0	800	0	4
House	220	22	90%	4	20	440	1	3
1000 Island	250	24	86%	4	20	540	<1	7
Sauces: BBQ	50	0	0%	0	0	270	<1	11
Honey	90	0	0%	0	0	5	0	23
Mustard	45	<1	10%	0	0	150	0	10
Salsa	10	0	0%	0	0	160	0	2
Sweet 'n Sour	50	0	0%	0	0	60	0	11
Shakes: Chocolate, small	390	7	16%	5	30	280	9	74
Strawberry, small	400	7	16%	5	30	240	9	77
Vanilla, small	330	8	22%	5	35	250	11	54

Chick-Fil-A®

	Cal	Fat	%Fc	S.Fat	Chol	Sod	Pro	Carb
Chick-Fil-A Sandwiches								
Chicken	290	9	27%	2	50	870	24	29
Chicken Deluxe	300	9	27%	2	50	870	25	31
Chicken (no bun/pickles)	160	8	44%	2	45	690	21	1
Chargrilled Chicken:	280	3	11%	1	40	640	27	36
Deluxe	290	3	10%	1	40	640	28	38
No bun, no pickles	130	3	23%	1	30	630	27	0
Club (no dressing)	390	12	28%	5	70	980	33	38
Chick. Salad (on whole wheat)	320	5	12%	2	10	810	25	42
Soup								
Hearty Breast of Chicken	110	1	8%	0	45	760	16	10
Strips, Nuggets								
Chick-n-Strips (4-count)	230	8	30%	2	20	380	29	10
Nuggets (8-pack)	290	14	52%	3	60	770	28	12
Salads								
Chick-n-Strips Salad	290	9	28%	2	20	430	32	21
Chargrilled Chicken Garden	170	3	18%	1	25	650	26	10
Chicken Salad Plate	290	5	14%	0	35	570	21	40
Side Orders								
Coleslaw (small)	130	6	38%	1	15	430	6	11
Carrot & Raisin Salad (small)	150	2	13%	0	6	650	5	28
Waffle Potato Fries (salted)	290	10	31%	4	5	960	1	49
(unsalted)	290	10	31%	4	5	80	1	49
Desserts/Beverages								
Icedream (small cup)	350	10	26%	3	70	390	16	50
Icedream (small cone)	140	4	25%	1	40	240	11	16
Lemon Pie (slice)	280	22	71%	6	5	550	1	19
Fudge Nut Brownie	350	16	40%	3	30	650	10	41
Cheesecake: with Topping	290	23	72%	10	10	550	14	9

Church's® Fried Chicken

	Cal	Fat	%Fc	S.Fat	Chol	Sod	Pro	Carb
Fried Chicken: Breast	200	12	54%	3	65	510	19	4
Leg	140	9	58%	2	45	160	13	2
Thigh	230	16	63%	4	80	520	16	5
Wing	250	16	58%	4	60	540	19	8
Tender Strip	80	4	45%	1	15	140	6	5
Side Items: Apple Pie	280	12	39%	3	5	340	2	41
Biscuit	250	16	58%	3	5	640	2	26
Cajun Rice	130	7	48%	2	5	260	1	16
Cole Slaw	92	6	59%	1	0	230	4	8
Corn on the Cob	140	3	19%	1	0	15	4.5	24
French Fries	210	11	47%	3	0	60	3	29
Okra	210	16	69%	3	0	520	3	19
Potatoes & Gravy	90	3	30%	1	0	520	1	14

Cousins Subs®

	Cal	Fat	%Fc	S.Fat	Chol	Sod	Pro	Carb
Bread: Italian, 1 oz	65	2	28%	0.5	1	410	4	12
Cold Italian Subs								
Regular	620	40	58%	12	79	2010	35	30
Cousins Special	730	49	60%	15	111	2490	40	30
Genoa & Cheese	670	45	60%	15	75	2005	37	30
Cappocolla & Cheese/Genoa	570	34	54%	11	70	1850	35	30
Cold Subs (No extra mayonnaise)								
BLT	360	14	35%	5	18	1420	20	34
Cheese Sub	430	20	42%	14	57	1635	31	30
Club Sub	495	19	35%	9	143	2830	50	30
Cold Veggie	360	14	35%	7	36	1590	26	33
Ham Sub	310	8	23%	3	55	1440	29	30
Ham & Cheese	385	14	33%	6.5	77	1750	35	30
Roast Beef	360	9	23%	3.5	24	1570	41	30
Seafood with Crabn	555	34	55%	11	35	1750	25	38
Tuna Sub	520	28	48%	7	65	1450	30	32
Turkey Sub	325	8.5	24%	3	72	2020	32	30
Hot Sub								
Cheese Steak	470	17	32%	11	40	840	33	46
Double	550	26	36%	16	64	640	44	35
Chicken Breast (no Mayo)	320	6	17%	2	3	1390	37	30
Gyro: Regular	550	23	38%	8	36	650	28	57
w. Tzatziki Sauce	600	27	41%	10	56	760	29	58
Hot Veggie	380	11	26%	0	0	320	21	48
Italian Sausage	815	58	64%	19	35	5200	45	30
Meatball & Cheese	680	43	57%	18	104	3610	44	30
Pepperoni Melt (no mayo)	465	20	39%	9	101	1910	41	30
Philly Cheese Steak	510	23	41%	15	45	430	32	43
Steak Sub	425	12	25%	8	40	360	28	51

For mayonnaise add: 235 Cals; 26g Fat; 9g Sat.Fat; 30mg Cholesterol

	Cal	Fat	%FC	S.Fat	Chol	Sod	Pro	Carb
Mini Sub: Cousins Special	290	14	43%	6	6	680	13	26
Cheese (no mayonnaise)	230	11	43%	7.5	30	870	17	16
Ham (no mayonnaise)	170	4	21%	1.5	29	765	16	16
Ham & Cheese (no mayo)	205	7.5	33%	3.5	41	930	17	16
Meatball & Cheese	365	23	57%	10	55	1930	23	16
Seafood w. Crab	300	18	54%	6	19	935	13	21
Tuna	480	37	69%	10	56	670	14	22
Turkey (no mayonnaise)	170	4.5	24%	1.5	38	1080	17	16
For mayonnaise add: 125 Cals; 14gFat; 4.5g Sat.Fat; 16mg Cholesterol								
Kids Subs: Cheeseburger	290	17	53%	6	41	460	14	22
Hot Dog	275	16	52%	6	24	770	10	22
PBJ	360	12	30%	3	0	930	13	50
French Fries: Small	275	13	43%	5.5	11	240	3.5	38
Medium	400	17	38%	8	16	355	8.5	55
Large	525	25	43%	11	21	465	9	72
Chips: 1 1/2 oz	230	15	59%	4	0	270	3	22
w. Sour Cream, 1 1/2 oz	230	14	55%	4	0	270	3	22
Soups: Chicken Noodle, Regular	105	2.5	21%	1	18	920	6	13
Clam Chowder, Regular	160	5.5	30%	2	13	640	8	19
Salads: Chef	195	8	37%	3.5	109	1000	24	6
Garden	135	6	40%	2.5	65	385	15	6
Italian	290	17	53%	6.5	106	1065	26	6
Seafood	175	6	31%	2.5	65	1045	21	12
Side	70	4	51%	2.5	39	200	8.5	0
Tuna	305	20	59%	4	85	465	26	6
Cookies: Choc Chip	210	11	47%	4	20	190	2	25
Cranberry Walnut	190	8.5	40%	2.5	na	65	2.5	24

Dairy Queen®/Brazier®

	Cal	Fat	%FC	S.Fat	Chol	Sod	Pro	Carb
Burgers								
DQ® Homestyle: Hamburger	290	12	37%	5	45	630	17	29
Cheeseburger	340	17	45%	8	55	850	20	29
Double Cheeseburger	540	31	52%	16	115	1130	35	30
Bacon Dble Cheeseburger	610	36	53%	18	130	1380	41	31
Ultimate Burger	670	43	58%	19	135	1210	40	29
Hot Dogs: Regular	240	14	52%	5	25	730	9	19
Chili 'n' Cheese Dog	330	21	57%	9	45	1090	14	22
Sandwiches: Chicken Breast Fillet	430	20	42%	4	55	760	24	37
Grilled	310	10	29%	2.5	50	1040	24	30
with Cheese	480	25	47%	7	70	980	27	38
Chicken Strip Basket: w. Gravy	1000	50	45%	13	55	2260	35	102
French Fries: Medium	350	18	46%	3.5	0	630	4	42
Large	440	23	47%	4.5	0	790	5	53
Onion Rings	320	16	45%	4	0	180	5	39

Continued Next Page

	Cal	Fat	%FC	S.Fat	Chol	Sod	Pro	Carb
Ice Cream & Desserts								
Cones/Soft Serve:								
DQ® Vanilla Soft Serv., 1/2 cup	140	4	26%	3	15	70	3	22
DQ® Choc. Soft Serv., 1/2 cup	150	5	30%	3.5	15	75	4	22
Vanilla Cone: Small	230	7	27%	4.5	20	115	6	38
Medium	330	9	25%	6	30	160	8	53
Large	410	12	26%	8	40	200	10	65
Chocolate Cone: Small	240	8	30%	5	20	115	6	37
Medium	340	11	27%	7	30	160	8	53
Dipped Cone: Small	340	17	45%	9	20	130	6	42
Regular	510	25	44%	13	30	190	8	59
Novelties/Treats: Banana Split	510	12	21%	8	30	180	8	96
Buster Bar®	450	28	56%	12	15	280	10	41
Choc. Chip Cookie Dough Blizzard®:								
Small	660	24	33%	13	55	440	12	99
Medium	950	36	34%	19	75	660	17	143
Choc. Sand. Cookie Blizzard®:								
Small	520	18	31%	9	40	380	79	10
Regular	640	23	32%	11	45	500	97	12
Chocolate Sundae: Small	280	7	22%	4	20	140	5	49
Medium	400	10	22%	6	30	210	8	71
Dilly® Bar: Chocolate	210	13	56%	7	10	75	3	21
DQ® 8" Round Cake, 1/8 Cake	340	12	32%	7	25	250	7	53
DQ® Fudge Bar	50	0	0%	0	0	70	4	12
DQ® Sandwich	150	5	30%	2	5	115	3	23
DQ® Treatzza Pizza™, 1/8 pizza:								
Heath®	180	7	35%	3.5	5	160	3	28
M & M's®	190	7	33%	4	5	160	3	29
DQ® Vanilla Orange Bar	60	0	0%	0	0	40	2	17
Fudge Cake Supreme™	890	38	30%	22	65	960	11	124
Lemon DQ Freez'r®, 1/2 cup	80	0	0%	0	0	10	0	20
Peanut Buster® Parfait	730	31	38%	17	35	400	16	99
Starkiss®	80	0	0%	0	0	10	0	21
Strawberry Shortcake	430	14	29%	9	60	360	7	70
Frozen Yogurt								
Cup of Yogurt: Regular	230	0.5	2%	0	5	150	8	48
DQ® Nonfat F frozen Yogurt, 1/2 cup	100	0	0%	0	0	70	3	21
Yogurt Cone: Medium	260	1	5%	<1	9	160	9	56
Yogurt Strawb. Sundae: Medium	280	0.5	2%	0	5	160	8	61
Heath® Breeze®: Small	470	10	19%	6	10	380	11	85
Regular	710	18	23%	11	20	580	15	123
Strawberry Breeze®: Small	320	0.5	31%	0.5	5	190	10	68
Medium	460	1	31%	1	10	270	13	99
Malts, Shakes, Slushes								
Chocolate Malt: Medium	880	22	22%	14	70	500	19	153
Chocolate Shake: Medium	770	20	23%	13	70	420	17	130
Misty® Slush: Medium	290	0	0%	0	0	30	0	74

	Cal	Fat	%Fc	S.Fat	Chol	Sod	Pro	Carb
Tacos: Regular	140	8	51%	3	16	100	6	10
Double Beef: Regular	170	10	53%	3	25	150	8	12
Deluxe	205	13	57%	5	35	160	9	13
Soft Taco: Regular	145	6	37%	3	16	225	5	17
Double Beef	180	8	40%	3	25	275	7	18
Chicken Taco	185	13	63%	3	35	275	8	10
Chicken Soft Taco	200	11	49%	3	35	400	7	16
Kid's Meal - Taco	530	17	29%	6	16	375	18	87
Tostada: Regular	140	8	51%	3	15	335	6	12
Burritos: Red, Regular	340	12	32%	5	26	1035	15	46
Green, Regular	330	11	30%	3	22	1150	14	46
Chicken	265	10	34%	4	36	770	13	32
Deluxe	550	34	56%	10	83	980	21	40
Combination	415	17	37%	7	49	1035	21	46
Deluxe Combo	455	20	40%	9	59	1050	22	49
"The Works"	450	18	36%	6	27	1250	15	60
Macho Combo	775	31	36%	15	100	2180	38	87
Del BeefN	440	20	41%	9	63	880	23	43
Macho Beef	895	41	41%	18	139	1970	49	84
Steak & Egg Burrito	500	25	45%	9	337	1070	30	41
Breakfast Burrito	256	11	39%	4	90	410	9	30
Salads: Taco	235	19	73%	6	31	270	9	9
Taco Deluxe	740	49	60%	16	83	1280	26	57
Chicken	255	19	67%	6	58	475	12	8
Burgers: Hamburger	230	8	31%	3	29	650	11	26
Del Burger	385	20	47%	6	42	1065	14	35
Cheeseburger	285	13	41%	6	42	850	14	26
Del Cheeseburger	440	25	51%	9	55	1270	18	35
Kid's Meal - Hamburger	620	20	29%	7	29	800	14	96
Quesadilla: Regular	485	27	50%	6	75	870	23	37
Chicken	545	31	51%	16	113	1150	30	38
Spicy Jack: Regular	475	27	51%	16	76	940	23	37
Chicken	540	30	50%	17	114	1215	31	38
Nachos: Regular	390	23	53%	4	2	505	6	39
Macho Nachos	1090	61	50%	13	46	1740	26	110
Side Dishes: Beans & Cheese	120	3	22%	2	9	890	7	17
French Fries (Small):	240	11	41%	4	0	135	3	32
Regular	400	19	43%	6	0	230	5	54
Large	570	26	41%	9	0	320	8	76
Nacho Fries	670	34	45%	11	2	925	10	80
Chili Cheese Fries	560	30	48%	13	38	845	15	58
Dressings: Sour Cream, 1 oz	60	6	90%	4	20	15	0	0
Guacamole, 1 oz	60	6	90%	0	0	130	1	2
Salsa - Side, 2 oz	14	0	0%	0	0	308	0	3
Hot Sauce - Pouch	2	0	0%	0	0	38	0	0
Salsa Dressing, 1 oz	35	3	77%	2	10	85	0	1
Nacho Cheese Sauce	100	8	72%	2	2	401	2	4

Denny's®

	Cal	Fat	%Fc	S.Fat	Chol	Sod	Pro	Carb
Breakfast: All American Slam	1030	87	76%	21	725	1925	48	24
w.Toast, 1 slice	1120	88	71%	21	725	2090	51	41
w.Bagel	1265	88	63%	21	725	2420	57	70
w.Biscuit, plain	1405	109	70%	26	725	2675	53	64
French Slam	1030	71	62%	20	777	1430	44	58
w.Toast, 1 slice	1120	71	58%	0	777	1595	47	75
w.Bagel	1265	72	51%	20	777	1925	53	104
w.Biscuit, plain	1405	93	60%	25	777	2180	49	98
Original Grand Slam	795	50	57%	14	460	2240	34	65
w.Syrup & Margarine	1030	60	52%	16	460	2385	34	101
Scram Slam	975	80	74%	18	700	1750	42	30
w.Toast, 1 slice	1065	81	68%	23	700	1915	45	47
w.Bagel	1210	81	60%	23	700	2245	51	76
w.Biscuit, plain	1350	102	68%	28	700	2500	82	70
Slim Slam (w.Syrup/Topping)	640	12	17%	3	34	1770	34	98
Southern Slam	1065	84	71%	23	484	2450	37	47
Super/Play It Again Slam	1190	75	57%	21	690	3555	51	98
Omelette (no extras): Ultimate	780	62	72%	14	640	1360	31	29
Eggs Benedict	860	55	57%	23	525	1945	35	45
Farmer's Omelette	915	70	72%	20	635	955	29	29
Ham 'n Cheddar	745	55	66%	10	660	1520	36	24
Veggie-Cheese	715	53	66%	10	645	955	29	29
Steak & Eggs (no extras)								
Chicken Fried	725	55	68%	18	450	1505	28	31
Porterhouse	1225	95	68%	32	570	1370	70	21
Sirloin	810	64	71%	18	476	950	37	21
T-Bone	1045	82	71%	26	530	1190	56	21
Pork Chop and Eggs	555	36	58%	9	470	970	33	21
Moons Over My Hammy	810	48	53%	8	430	2250	44	46
Waffles: Plain	305	21	63%	3	146	200	7	23
w. Syrup & Butter	540	31	52%	5	146	345	7	59
Hot Cakes: Plain (3)	490	7	13%	1	0	1820	12	95
w. Syrup & Butter	725	17	21%	3	0	1965	12	130
French Toast: w. Syrup & Butter	725	37	46%	6	317	430	19	80
Breakfast Sides: Applesauce	60	0	0%	0	0	15	0	15
Bacon, 4 slices	160	18	98%	5	36	640	12	1
Bagel, 1 only	235	1	4%	0	0	495	9	46
Biscuit; Plain	375	22	53%	5	0	750	5	40
w. Sausage & Gravy	570	38	60%	10	24	1475	11	45
Cream Cheese, 1 oz	100	10	90%	6	31	90	2	1
Egg: 1 only	135	12	80%	3	205	60	6	1
Egg Beaters (Egg Substitute)	70	5	64%	1	1	140	5	1
Grits, 4 oz	80	0	0%	0	0	520	2	18
Ham, 3 oz	95	3	28%	1	23	760	15	2
Hashed Browns, 4 oz	220	14	57%	2	0	425	2	2
Covered, 6 oz	320	23	65%	7	30	605	9	2
Covered & Smothered, 8 oz	360	26	65%	7	30	790	9	26

	Cal	Fat	%FC	S.Fat	Chol	Sod	Pro	Carb
Breakfast Sides (Cont)								
Muffins: English, each	125	1	7%	0	0	200	5	24
Blueberry, each	310	14	41%	0	0	190	4	42
Oatmeal, 4 oz	100	2	18%	0	0	175	5	18
Sausage, 4 links	355	32	81%	2	64	945	16	0
Syrup, 3 Tbsp	145	0	0%	0	0	25	0	36
Reduced Calorie	25	0	0%	0	0	70	0	9
Toppings: 3 oz	105	0	0%	0	0	15	0	26
Toast, 1 slice dry	90	1	10%	0	0	165	3	17
Whipped Margarine; 1/2 oz	90	10	100%	2	0	120	0	0
Whipped Cream, 2 oz	25	2	72%	0	7	5	0	2
Soup: Cheese	295	23	10%	13	20	895	6	13
Chicken Noodle	60	2	30%	0	10	640	2	8
Clam Chowder	215	11	46%	9	5	905	5	22
Cream of Brocoli	195	12	55%	9	0	820	4	15
Cream of Potato	220	12	49%	9	0	760	4	23
Split Pea	145	6	37%	2	5	820	8	18
Vegetable Beef	80	1	11%	1	5	820	6	11
Salads (no dressing/bread)								
Buffalo Chicken	615	37	54%	8	88	1260	40	36
Fried Chicken	505	31	55%	8	94	1175	38	30
Garden Chicken Delite	277	5	16%	1	67	785	30	30
Grilled Chick. Caesar w. Dressing	655	47	65%	9	86	1730	37	23
Oriental Chicken w. Dressing	570	26	41%	5	67	1655	33	49
Side Caesar w. Dressing	340	25	66%	4	5	725	8	20
Side Garden	115	4	31%	1	0	150	3	16
Sandwiches (no fries/sides): BLT	635	46	65%	8	55	1115	18	37
Bacon Cheddar Burger	935	63	61%	25	165	1730	53	43
Big Texas BBQ	930	58	56%	24	163	2270	53	53
Charleston Chicken	635	32	45%	5	66	1240	29	53
Chicken Melt	520	30	50%	5	40	1195	26	43
Classic Burger	675	40	53%	15	105	1140	37	42
w. Cheese	835	55	59%	20	137	1595	47	43
Club Sandwich	720	38	47%	7	75	1665	32	62
Delidinger	850	45	48%	6	80	3240	56	62
Deluxe Grilled Cheese	480	26	49%	2	1	1135	18	44
Fisherman's Choice	905	56	55%	8	70	1705	30	74
French Dip w. Horseradish	530	16	39%	3	75	1895	41	53
Fried Fish	905	56	55%	8	70	1705	29	74
Garden Burger	655	32	44%	6	26	1020	21	72
Patty Only	160	3	17%	0	10	390	11	22
Grilled Chicken	510	20	35%	5	83	1810	34	52
Ham & Swiss on Rye	535	31	52%	4	36	1710	23	40
Patty Melt	695	44	57%	13	115	1010	38	40
Prime Rib	660	37	50%	5	80	1745	33	47
Super Bird	620	32	46%	5	60	1180	35	48
Turkey Breast	475	26	49%	3	57	1180	23	39

Denny's® (Cont)

	Cal	Fat	%FC	S.Fat	Chol	Sod	Pro	Carb
Dressings: BBQ Sauce	50	1	18%	0	0	595	0	11
Blue Cheese, 1 oz	125	12	86%	4	20	405	4	4
Caesar	140	15	96%	2	2	340	1	1
French: Regular	105	10	86%	2	7	275	0	3
Reduced Calorie	75	5	60%	1	0	265	0	8
Honey Mustard Fat-Free	40	0	0%	0	0	120	0	9
Horseradish Sauce, 1 oz	170	20	99%	3	45	230	1	3
Italian Dressing: Creamy	105	10	86%	2	0	305	0	4
Reduced Calorie	23	1	39%	0	0	515	0	3
Oriental Peanut Dressing	105	8	69%	1	0	400	1	6
Ranch	100	11	99%	2	8	215	1	1
Sour Cream, 1 1/2 oz	90	9	90%	6	20	25	1	2
Thousand Island, 1 oz	105	10	86%	2	20	210	0	2
Appetizers: Buffalo Chicken Strips	735	42	51%	4	96	1675	48	43
Buffalo Wings (12)	855	54	57%	17	500	5550	92	1
Chicken Quesadilla	830	55	60%	23	181	1980	50	43
Chicken Strips (5)	720	33	41%	4	95	1665	47	56
Mozzarella Sticks w. Sauce (8)	755	43	51%	24	48	5425	37	56
Onion Ring Basket (7)	440	27	55%	7	0	1160	6	44
Sampler	1120	59	47%	19	70	3430	44	104
Entrees: Battered Cod w. Sce	730	47	58%	7	105	1335	30	48
Charleston Chicken	330	18	49%	4	65	995	25	16
Chicken Fried Steak	265	17	58%	8	27	670	15	14
Chicken Strip w. Dressing	635	25	35%	1	95	1510	47	55
Fried Shrimp Dinner	560	32	51%	6	135	1115	19	49
Grilled Alaskan Salmon	295	14	43%	2	102	260	43	1
Grilled Chicken Dinner	130	4	28%	1	65	560	24	0
Grilled Chopped Steak	400	26	58%	11	90	450	30	12
Pork Chop Dinner	385	24	56%	8	120	845	40	0
Porterhouse Steak	710	54	61%	24	160	715	56	0
Pot Roast Dinner	260	11	38%	4	140	1085	40	5
Roast Turkey & Stuffing	700	27	35%	1	100	2345	47	63
Sirloin Steak Dinner	270	21	70%	9	62	275	22	0
Steak & Shrimp	645	42	59%	14	150	1145	36	31
T-Bone Steak Dinner	530	40	68%	18	120	535	42	0
Skillets: Sausage Supreme	1170	96	74%	31	620	2370	40	36
Meat Lover's	1345	108	72%	37	675	3065	60	34
Big Texas Chicken Fajita	1185	88	67%	33	680	2405	60	43
Canadian Scramble	840	62	66%	25	640	2185	50	34
Kids Meals: Frenchtastic Slam	450	32	66%	10	310	665	20	22
Smiley Face Hotcakes w. Meat	465	22	42%	7	38	1410	14	63
Wacky Waffles	215	12	50%	3	78	100	4	23
Pigs in a Blanket	480	21	40%	7	32	1685	16	63
Burgerlicious w. Cheese	340	20	53%	6	40	580	15	24
Pizza Party	400	15	34%	3	10	1090	18	47
The Big Cheese	334	20	54%	2	24	830	10	28
Dennysaur Chicken Nuggets	190	13	61%	4	30	340	10	10

	Cal	Fat	%Fc	S.Fat	Chol	Sod	Pro	Carb
Sides								
Broccoli in Butter Sauce	50	2	36%	2	2	280	3	7
Carrots in Honey Glaze	80	3	34%	1	0	220	1	12
Corn in Butter Sauce	120	4	30%	2	5	260	3	19
Cornbread Stuffing	180	9	45%	0	0	405	4	20
French Fries, unsalted	325	14	39%	3	0	130	5	44
seasoned	260	12	42%	3	0	555	5	35
Gravy, all types, average	15	0.5	30%	0	0	120	0	2
Green Beans w. Bacon	60	4	60%	2	5	390	1	6
Green Peas in Butter Sauce	100	2	18%	2	5	360	5	14
Potato: Baked, plain	185	0	0%	0	0	15	4	43
Mashed	105	1	8%	0	0	380	3	21
Rice Pilaf	110	2	16%	0	0	330	2	21
Desserts: Banana Royale	548	25	41%	15	64	185	6	80
Chocolate Cake	370	17	41%	4	29	375	4	53
Ice Cream Cake	280	10	32%	6	40	110	3	47
Lowfat Choc Chip Yogurt	110	2	16%	0.5	5	60	4	20
Malt Shake, average	580	27	42%	17	108	240	12	77
Rainbow Sorbet	110	1.5	11%	1	5	30	1	25
Pies, 1/6 slice: Apple	430	20	42%	5	<5	390	3	59
Apple w. Equal	370	20	49%	5	<5	360	3	43
Cheesecake	470	27	52%	13	90	280	8	48
Cherry	540	21	35%	5	<5	430	5	83
Chocolate Pecan	790	37	42%	9	70	460	6	107
Coconut Cream	480	26	49%	16	15	440	5	58
Dutch Apple	440	19	39%	5	0	290	3	65
French Silk	650	43	59%	26	165	220	6	60
German Chocolate	580	33	51%	18	15	460	7	66
Key Lime	600	27	41%	15	35	300	10	79
Lemon Meringue	460	17	33%	4	95	310	5	71
Pecan	600	28	42%	4	50	430	5	81
Dessert Toppings: Blueberry	70	0	0%	0	0	10	0	17
Chocolate, 2 oz	320	25	70%	0	0	85	2	27
Fudge, 2 oz	200	10	45%	7	3	95	1	30
Strawberry, 2 oz	80	1	11%	0	0	10	1	17
Sundaes								
Single Scoop, no topping	190	14	66%	6	37	40	3	14
Double Scoop, no topping	375	27	65%	12	75	85	6	29
Banana Split	895	43	43%	19	75	175	15	121
Hot Fudge Cake	690	38	50%	11	60	485	9	83
Flavored Coffee: Average	70	1	13%	1	2	5	0	16

 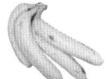 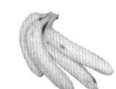

Domino's® Pizza

	Cal	Fat	%Fc	S.Fat	Chol	Sod	Pro	Carb
14" Hand Tossed: *Per 2 Slices*								
Beef	365	14	35%	6	26	745	16	44
Cheese	320	10	28%	4	18	620	14	44
Italian Sausage & Mushroom	365	13	32%	6	27	755	16	46
Pepperoni	375	15	36%	6	32	870	17	49
X-tra Cheese & Pepperoni	425	19	40%	8	39	910	19	45
Ham	335	11	30%	4.5	19	775	16	44
Veggie	345	11	29%	4	18	845	14	47
14" Thin Crust: *Per Slice ($^1/_6$)*								
Beef	300	15	45%	7	26	835	13	28
Cheese	255	11	39%	5	18	710	11	28
Pepperoni	310	16	46%	7	29	885	13	28
X-tra Cheese & Pepperoni	355	20	55%	9	38	1000	16	28
Ham	270	12	40%	5.5	25	865	13	28
Italian Sausage & Mushroom	300	15	45%	6	27	845	13	30
Veggie	280	12	39%	5	18	985	11	31
14" Deep Dish: *Per 2 Slices*								
Beef	505	24	43%	9	31	1105	20	55
Cheese	460	20	39%	7	23	980	18	55
Pepperoni	515	25	44%	9	35	1155	20	55
X-tra Cheese & Pepperoni	560	29	46%	11	44	1270	23	55
Ham	475	21	40%	7.5	30	1135	20	55
Italian Sausage & Mushroom	510	24	42%	8.5	32	1165	20	57
Veggie	485	21	39%	7	23	1205	18	59
12" Hand Tossed: *Per 2 Slices*								
Beef	405	16	36%	7	30	825	18	49
Cheese	350	11	28%	5	19	670	15	49
Pepperoni	410	16	35%	7	32	870	17	49
X-tra Cheese & Pepperoni	460	20	39%	9	42	1000	21	49
Ham	370	11	27%	5	26	835	17	49
Italian Sausage & Mushroom	365	13	32%	6	27	755	16	49
Veggie	370	12	29%	5	19	745	15	52
12" Thin Crust: *Per Slice ($^1/_4$)*								
Beef	325	17	47%	7	30	915	14	30
Cheese	270	12	40%	5	19	760	12	30
Pepperoni	335	17	46%	7	32	960	15	30
X-tra Cheese & Pepperoni	385	21	49%	9	42	1080	18	31
Ham	290	12	37%	5	26	920	15	30
Italian Sausage & Mushroom	330	16	44%	6	31	930	15	32
Veggie	300	13	39%	5	19	830	13	33
12" Deep Dish: *Per 2 Slices*								
Beef	525	26	45%	10	36	1155	21	52
Cheese	470	21	40%	8	25	1000	18	52
Pepperoni	530	27	46%	10	38	1200	21	52
Ham	480	22	41%	8	32	1160	21	52
Italian Sausage & Mushroom	525	26	45%	10	36	1170	21	54
Veggie	490	23	42%	8	25	1070	19	54

	Cal	Fat	%FC	S.Fat	Chol	Sod	Pro	Carb
6" Deep Dish: *Per 2 Slices*								
Beef	635	31	44%	12	39	2000	25	65
Cheese	590	27	41%	10	31	1210	23	65
Pepperoni	640	32	45%	12	41	1370	25	66
Ham	610	28	41%	10	38	1370	25	66
Italian Sausage & Mushroom	440	31	63%	11	40	1345	25	67
Vegge	610	28	41%	10	31	1265	23	67
Toppings: Cheddar Cheese	55	4.5	74%	3	14	80	3	0.5
Bacon	80	6.5	73%	2	10	180	4	0
Green Peppers, Onions, Mushrooms	5	0	0%	0	0	1	0	1
Canned Mushrooms	5	0	0%	0	0	65	0	1
Olives: Green	12	1	75%	0	0	245	0	0.5
Ripe	13	1	69%	0	0	65	0	0.5
Anchovies	25	1	36%	0	9	395	2	0.5
Extra Cheese	45	4	71%	2	9	115	3	0
Sides: Breadstick, 1 stk	80	3	34%	0.5	0	160	2	11
Cheesy Bread, 1 piece	105	5	43%	2	6	180	3	11
Barbeque Wings, each	50	2	36%	0.5	26	175	6	2
Hot Wings, each	45	2	40%	0.5	26	355	5	0.5
Garden Salad: Small, no dressing	20	0.3	13%	0	0	15	1	4
Large, no dressing	40	0.5	11%	0	0	25	2	8
Dressings: Blue Cheese, 1½ oz	220	24	98%	4	40	440	2	2
Creamy Caesar, 1½ oz	200	22	99%	3	10	470	1	2
Honey French, 1½ oz	210	18	77%	3	0	300	0	14
House Italian, 1½ oz	220	24	98%	3	0	440	0	1
Lite Italian, 1½ oz	20	1	45%	0	0	0	0	2
Ranch, 1½ oz	260	29	100%	4	5	380	0	0.5
Fat Free Ranch, 1½ oz	40	0	0%	0	0	560	0	10
1000 Island, 1½ oz	200	20	90%	3	25	320	0	5

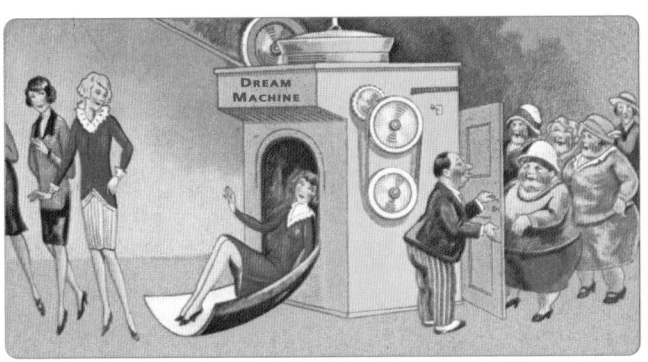

Dunkin' Donuts®

	Cal	Fat	%Fc	S.Fat	Chol	Sod	Pro	Carb
Cake Donuts: *Each*								
Blueberry	290	16	50%	3.5	10	400	3	35
Butternut	300	16	48%	4.5	0	360	3	36
Chocolate	300	16	48%	3	0	370	3	38
Chocolate Coconut	290	16	50%	3.5	0	370	4	33
Chocolate Glazed	250	14	48%	3	0	280	3	29
Cinnamon	270	15	57%	3	0	360	3	31
Coconut	290	17	53%	5	0	360	3	33
Double Chocolate	310	17	50%	3.5	0	370	3	37
Dunkin' Donut	240	15	56%	3	0	390	3	25
Glazed	270	15	57%	3	0	360	3	33
Jelly Stick	290	12	37%	2.5	0	390	3	44
Old Fashioned	250	15	54%	3	0	360	3	26
Powdered	270	15	50%	3	0	350	3	32
Sugared	310	20	58%	4	0	380	4	28
Toasted Coconut	320	19	53%	5	0	360	3	33
Whole Wheat Glazed	310	19	55%	4	0	380	4	32
Yeast Donuts: *Each*								
Apple Crumb	230	10	40%	3	0	270	3	34
Apple N' Spice	200	8	36%	1.5	0	270	3	29
Bavarian Kreme	210	9	38%	2	0	270	3	30
Black Raspberry	210	8	34%	1.5	0	360	3	32
Blueberry Crumb	240	10	37%	3	0	260	3	36
Boston Kreme	240	9	33%	2	0	280	3	36
Chocolate Frosted	200	9	40%	2	0	260	3	29
Chocolate/Vanilla Kreme Filled	270	13	43%	3	0	260	3	35
Glazed	180	8	40%	1.5	0	250	3	25
Jelly Filled	210	8	34%	1.5	0	280	3	32
Lemon	200	9	40%	2	0	270	3	28
Maple/Marble Frosted	210	9	38%	2	0	260	3	30
Strawberry	210	8	34%	1.5	0	260	3	32
Strawberry/Vanilla Frosted	210	9	33%	2	0	260	3	30
Sugar Raised	170	8	42%	1.5	0	250	3	22
Muffins: *Each*								
Apple n' Spice: Regular	350	12	30%	2.5	35	390	4	57
Lowfat	240	1.5	5%	0	0	460	4	54
Banana Nut: Regular	360	15	37%	3	35	490	7	52
Lowfat	250	1.5	90%	0	0	430	4	57
Blueberry: Regular	320	12	29%	3	35	480	6	49
Lowfat	250	1.5	5%	0	0	430	4	55
Bran Lowfat	240	1	4%	0	0	430	4	57
Cherry: Regular	340	12	32%	3	40	510	6	53
Lowfat	250	1.5	5%	0	0	430	4	56
Chocolate Chip: Regular	400	17	38%	6	35	440	6	58
Lowfat	250	2.5	90%	1	0	470	4	53
Corn: Regular	390	15	36%	2.5	55	590	6	57
Lowfat	240	2.5	7%	1	45	480	3	52

	Cal	Fat	%Fc	S.Fat	Chol	Sod	Pro	Carb
Muffins (Cont): *Each*								
Cranberry Orange Nut: Regular	350	15	38%	3	35	500	6	52
Lowfat	240	1.5	5%	0	0	430	4	55
Honey Raisin Bran	390	12	27%	2	20	620	11	60
Lemon Poppy Seed	360	13	32%	2.5	35	530	5	56
Oat Bran	370	13	31%	2	20	620	11	55
French Roll: Baked	140	1	6%	0	0	220	3	27
Cake Munchkins								
Butternut (3)	200	11	49%	3	0	240	2	25
Chocolate Glazed (3)	200	10	45%	2	0	250	2	26
Cinnamon (4)	240	13	49%	3	0	290	3	29
Coconut (3)	200	12	49%	3.5	0	240	2	23
Glazed (3)	200	10	45%	2	0	250	2	27
Glazed Raised (4)	210	7	30%	2	0	170	3	36
Jelly (3)	170	5	26%	1	0	170	2	28
Lemon (3)	160	6	24%	1	0	160	2	23
Plain (4)	220	14	57%	3	0	310	2	22
Powdered Sugar (4)	250	14	50%	3	0	310	2	29
Sugar Raised (6)	220	12	49%	2.5	0	290	4	26
Toasted Coconut (3)	200	11	47%	3	0	250	2	24
Crullers/Sticks								
Glazed	290	15	46%	3	0	350	3	37
Glazed Chocolate	280	15	48%	3	0	360	3	35
Plain	240	15	56%	3	0	340	3	25
Powdered	270	15	50%	3	0	340	3	30
Sugar	250	15	54%	3	0	340	3	27
Fancies: Apple Fritter	300	14	42%	3	0	360	4	41
Apple Tart	290	10	31%	3	0	330	5	45
Apple Turnover	350	15	39%	4	0	340	5	49
Bismark	340	15	39%	3.5	0	340	3	50
Blueberry Tart	300	10	30%	3	0	320	5	48
Blueberry Turnover	370	15	36%	4	0	330	5	54
Bow Tie	300	17	50%	3.5	0	340	4	34
Cinnamon Raisin	330	13	35%	3	0	300	5	48
Coffee Roll	270	14	46%	3	0	340	4	38
Choc./Maple/Vanilla Frosted	290	15	46%	3	0	340	4	36
Eclair	270	11	36%	2.5	0	290	3	39
Glazed Fritter	260	14	48%	3	0	330	4	31
Lemon Tart	280	11	35%	3	0	340	5	43
Lemon Turnover	350	15	39%	4	0	360	5	48
Raspberry Tart	310	10	29%	3	0	350	5	51
Raspberry/Strawberry Turnover	380	15	36%	4	0	370	5	57
Strawberry Tart	310	10	29%	3	0	340	5	51
Cookies: Chocolate varieties	230	12	46%	6	35	110	3	27
Oatmeal Raisin Pecan	220	10	40%	5	25	110	3	29
Peanut Butter varieties	240	14	51%	6	30	150	5	24
Bagels ~ Next Page								

	Cal	Fat	%FC	S.Fat	Chol	Sod	Pro	Carb
Bagels								
Blueberry	340	1	3%	0	0	670	10	75
Cinnamon Raisin	340	1	3%	0	0	480	10	74
Egg	350	1.5	2.5%	0	25	610	11	72
Everything; Poppyseed	360	2	5%	0	0	710	11	74
Garlic	360	1	2.5%	0	0	720	11	76
Onion	330	1	3%	0	0	660	10	70
Plain	340	1	3%	0	0	710	10	73
Pumpernickel	350	1.5	2.5%	0	0	560	11	75
Salt	340	1	3%	0	0	3030	10	73
Sesame	380	4.5	10%	0.5	0	720	12	74
Cream Cheese, (per packet): Lite	130	11	76%	7	30	250	5	3
Average other flavors	180	17	85%	11	50	310	3	3
Croissants: Almond	200	22	99%	5	5	270	6	34
Chocolate	400	25	56%	9	5	240	5	37
Cheese	240	15	56%	3	5	260	6	28
Plain	290	18	55%	6	5	270	5	26
Lunch Sandwiches								
Broccoli & Cheese	370	21	51%	6	20	680	10	36
Ham & Cheese	710	32	41%	13	85	1840	33	29
Roast Beef & Cheese	490	27	50%	8	30	680	31	28
Tuna Salad	540	30	50%	6	50	1140	30	39
Chicken Salad	540	31	52%	7	75	710	27	37
Seafod Salad	480	26	49%	6	50	1020	16	45
Soup								
Chicken Noodle	80	1.5	17%	0	15	890	6	12
Minestrone	100	1	9%	0	0	900	5	16
Harvest Vegetable	80	2	23%	0	0	1120	4	12
Chile Con Carne w. Beans	300	15	45%	0	45	690	17	25
New England Clam Chowder	200	10	45%	3	30	1050	10	16
Beef Noodle	90	1	10%	0	20	980	8	12
Cream of Broccoli	200	11	50%	6	25	1050	8	17
Manhattan Clam Chowder	70	0.5	6%	0	5	890	5	11
Split Pea w. Ham	190	9	43%	3	15	830	8	20
Coffee (No Cream or Sugar)								
Decaf (10 oz)	0	0	0%	0	0	0	0	0
Hazelnut (10 oz)	5	0	0%	0	0	10	0	1
Other varieties (10 oz)	5	0	0%	0	0	5	0	1
Cream, 1 oz	60	5	75%	3	20	10	1	1
Coolatta: Per 16 oz								
Chocolate	370	4	10%	0	0	115	0	77
Coffee: w. Cream	410	22	48%	14	75	65	3	51
w. Milk	260	4	7.5%	2.5	15	75	4	52
w. 2% Milk	240	2	7.5%	1.5	10	80	4	52
w. Skim Milk	230	0	0%	0	0	60	4	52
Pink Lemonade; Strawberry	350	5	13%	0	0	30	0	88
Orange Mango Fruit	350	4	10%	0	0	115	0	86

	Cal	Fat	%Fc	S.Fat	Chol	Sod	Pro	Carb
Bagels								
Average all types, 4 oz	330	1	3%	0	0	500	11	70
Chocolate Chip Bagel, 4 oz	370	3	8%	2	0	500	11	76
Egg Bagel, 3 1/2 oz	340	3	8%	1	35	500	11	69
Sesame Dip/Sunflower	350	5	13%	1	0	700	12	70
Cream Cheese								
Plain, 2 Tbsp	100	10	90%	7	30	100	2	2
Plain Lite, 2 Tbsp	60	5	70%	3	15	110	2	2
Smoked Salmon, 2 Tbsp	90	8	80%	6	25	200	2	2
Flavors, average, 2 Tbsp	100	8	80%	6	25	100	2	4
Veggie Lite, 2 Tbsp	60	5	75%	4	15	150	2	2
Spreads								
Butter, 1 Tbsp	100	11	100%	8	30	110	0	0
Carrot & Houmous, 4 Tbsp	65	2	35%	0	0	260	2	9
Fruit Spreads, 2 Tbsp	75	0	0%	0	0	0	0	19
Hummus, 2 Tbsp	60	4	35%	0.5	0	60	1	6
Peanut Butter, 2 Tbsp	190	16	70%	2	0	110	8	3
Sandwiches								
Carrot Hummus	420	3.5	7%	0	0	780	15	83
Classic NY Lox & Bagel	630	24	35%	13	75	1240	26	77
Deli Melt, Ham	620	17	25%	10	0	1700	37	78
Reuben	790	33	35%	12	100	1900	42	82
Smoked Turkey	590	16	25%	9	45	1500	35	75
Turkey Pastrami	790	34	40%	19	0	1800	45	77
Garden Tomato Pizza Melt	610	18	25%	10	55	1200	32	80
Grilled Cheese Melt	500	12	20%	7	35	970	25	74
Ham & Cheese	570	15	20%	6	80	1400	32	79
Hummus Sandwich	480	8	15%	1	0	650	15	86
Lowfat Chicken Salad	570	9	14%	7	45	1060	28	79
Lowfat Tuna Salad	510	8	14%	1.5	30	1100	31	78
Pepperoni Pizza Melt	740	30	36%	15	85	1800	38	79
Tuna Melt	840	36	38%	19	120	1600	52	78
Veg-Out	420	6	13%	3	20	700	14	78
Soups: Per Regular Cup								
Amish Corn Chowder	180	6	30%	1.5	5	670	5	25
Chicken & Rice	180	10	50%	2.5	15	1070	7	15
Chicken Noodle	100	2.5	23%	1	15	900	6	13
Farmer's Market Veg.	40	0.5	11%	0	0	400	2	7
Irish Potato	170	8	41%	2.5	5	650	5	19
Jamaican Black Bean	70	1	63%	0	0	460	3	11
Louisiana Turkey Chili	80	2.5	28%	0	20	320	6	9
Monterey White Bean	120	2	15%	0	0	650	5	19
New England Clam Chowder	170	9	48%	2.5	25	800	9	15
Pasta	60	1	15%	0	0	450	2	11
Santa Fe Vegetarian	170	2	10%	0	0	730	3	23
Tomato Florentine	80	1.5	19%	1	0	870	2	14
Wisconsin Cheddar & Broccoli	170	19	99%	15	15	770	5	14

	Cal	Fat	%Fc	S.Fat	Chol	Sod	Pro	Carb
Bagel Chips								
Plain, 1 oz serving	90	0	0%	0	0	140	3	18
Flavors, average, 1 oz	90	1	10%	0	0	130	3	16
Cookies & Muffins								
Chocolate Choc Chip Brownie	340	15	40%	4	10	200	3	51
Ice Cinnamon Bun, 5 oz	550	16	25%	5	20	650	11	70
Cookies:								
Black & White, 4 oz	400	12	28%	3	15	260	3	70
Chocolate Chunk, 4 oz	500	24	40%	9	35	390	6	68
Oatmeal Raisin, 4 oz	430	18	34%	4	40	360	7	70
Peanut Butter, 4 oz	540	31	50%	6	40	620	10	55
Sugar, 4 oz	530	28	50%	7	45	420	6	64
Muffins:								
Banana Nut	220	12	50%	2	40	170	3	25
Blueberry	200	10	45%	2	40	120	3	25
Chocolate Chip	240	13	45%	3	40	120	3	28
Fat Free Cranberry Orange	130	0.5	0%	0	0	260	4	27
Lowfat Apple Date	160	2	10%	0	0	200	3	35
Lowfat Lemon Poppyseed	150	3	15%	0	0	220	3	28
Scones								
Cheddar Chive	310	15	45%	8	35	670	8	37
Cinnamon	325	11	30%	6	15	535	6	50
Garden Salads								
Bagel Croutons, 1/4 bag	25	1	20%	0	0	75	1	4
Broccoli & Pasta	200	11	50%	2	0	350	4	20
Caesar Salad: Regular	210	13	56%	4	15	500	5	7
Large	390	35	80%	7	25	900	9	14
Chicken Salad: Regular	150	7	42%	1.5	45	540	16	4
Fruit Salad	110	0.5	4%	0	0	10	1	25
Fruit & Yogurt Cup	160	1	5%	0	0	15	1	32
Fusilli w. Black Olive	360	23	58%	3	0	400	6	33
Greek Pasta Salad	450	30	60%	9	45	950	12	35
Grilled Chicken Caesar	480	37	69%	3	75	1100	26	11
Idaho Potato Salad	150	7	42%	1.5	5	200	2	19
Lowfat: Homestyle Coleslaw	90	3.5	35%	0.5	5	300	1	13
Potato & Dill	150	3.5	21%	0	0	750	2	20
Potato & Mustard	110	2.5	20%	0	0	350	2	19
Southwestern	150	1	6%	0	0	700	6	29
Coffee & Tea: Per 12 fl.oz								
Almond Delight	190	4	19%	3	20	150	8	29
Non Fat	150	0	0%	0	5	130	8	29
Cafe Au Lait	100	3.5	31%	2	15	100	6	9
Non Fat	70	0	0%	0	5	100	6	10
Cappuccino	90	3.5	25%	2	15	100	6	9
Mocha	230	6	23%	4.5	15	135	8	34

Other Coffees and Teas ~ See Pages 146-148

	Cal	Fat	%FC	S.Fat	Chol	Sod	Pro	Carb
Chicken								
Breast	160	6	34%	2	110	390	26	0
Leg	90	5	50%	2	75	150	11	0
Thigh	180	12	60%	4	130	230	16	0
Wing	110	6	49%	2	80	220	12	0
Tortillas								
Corn, each, 6"	70	1	13%	0	0	35	1	14
Flour, each, 6"	90	3	30%	0	0	225	3	13
Side Dishes: Per Serving								
Coleslaw	205	16	70%	3	11	360	2	12
Corn on the Cob, 5 1/2"	145	2	12%	0	0	20	5	33
French Fries	325	14	39%	3	0	330	5	44
Pinto Beans	185	4	19%	0	0	745	11	29
Potato Salad	255	14	49%	2	15	530	3	30
Smokey Black Beans	255	13	46%	5	11	610	6	29
Spanish Rice	130	3	21%	1	0	400	2	24
Specialities: (no dressing)								
Flame-Broiled Chicken Salad	170	5	26%	0	56	765	27	11
Garden Salad	30	0	0%	0	0	20	3	6
Chicken (no Tostada/Cream)	330	14	38%	5	80	1280	35	26
Steak (no Tostada/Sr.Cream)	525	31	53%	14	100	1205	40	26
Tostada Shell	440	27	55%	4	0	610	7	42
Burritos								
Bean, Rice & Cheese	480	15	28%	5	15	1250	16	72
Classic/Spicy Hot Chicken	560	22	35%	7	117	1500	30	61
Grilled Steak	705	32	41%	13	77	1690	39	68
Loco Grande Chicken	630	26	37%	7	129	1650	33	67
Smokey Black Bean	565	22	35%	8	22	1340	16	78
Whole Wheat Chicken	590	26	40%	9	146	1200	31	60
Tacos								
Chicken Soft	225	12	48%	4	66	585	16	15
Chicken Al Carbon	265	12	41%	2	28	225	10	30
Steak Al Carbon	400	22	49%	7	46	470	20	30
Pollo Bowl	505	13	23%	2	56	2070	37	69
Taquito	370	17	41%	4	25	690	15	43
Condiments								
Guacamole, 1 3/4 oz	50	3	54%	0	0	280	0	5
Lite Sour Cream, 1 oz	45	3	60%	0	12	25	2	2
Salsa; Jalepeno Hot Sauce	5	0	0%	0	0	100	0	1
Dressings								
Bleu Cheese	300	32	96%	6	50	590	2	2
Light Italian	25	1	36%	0	0	990	0	3
Ranch	350	39	100%	6	5	500	1	2
Thousand Island	270	27	90%	4	30	460	1	9
Desserts								
Flan	220	2	8%	2	5	140	6	46
Churro	150	8	48%	2	4	160	2	18

Fazoli's® Italian Food

	Cal	Fat	%Fc	S.Fat	Chol	Sod	Pro	Carb
Soup; Bread								
Minestrone Soup	90	1	10%	<1	0	1040	5	16
Bean & Pasta Soup	175	7	37%	1	4	1080	7	20
Breadstick	130	4	28%	<1	0	330	3	20
Dinners: Per Serving								
Baked Spaghetti Parmesan	565	21	34%	10	51	590	32	65
Baked Ziti: Regular	330	13	35%	5	30	350	20	38
Large	570	20	32%	8	109	520	32	68
Chicken Parmesan	480	14	26%	5	132	370	55	34
Chicken Cacciatore	425	7	15%	1	50	655	28	63
Fettucine: Alfredo	400	13	29%	5	20	710	12	58
Broccoli	430	13	27%	5	20	730	13	62
Carbonara	620	30	43%	14	148	215	22	64
w. Sausage & Mushroom	515	11	19%	2	8	365	17	91
Lasagna: Regular	530	24	41%	10	120	1150	33	47
Broccoli	570	27	43%	10	120	1445	34	50
Meatball Sub	650	30	42%	10	87	1535	28	62
Peppery Chicken	540	16	26%	6	144	765	36	63
Ravioli: w. Tomato Sauce	330	15	41%	1	27	715	16	36
w. Meat Sauce	360	16	40%	2	45	700	22	34
Sampler Platter	610	20	30%	4	74	905	27	80
Shrimp: Pasta	550	19	31%	<1	242	1120	37	58
& Scallop Fettucine	520	14	24%	5	181	1095	36	63
Spaghetti: w. Tomato Sauce	340	7	19%	1	2	175	11	62
w. Meat Sauce	370	8	19%	2	20	160	19	60
w. Meatballs	580	25	39%	6	59	870	24	67
w. Spicy Mediterranean	350	8	20%	1	2	320	10	60
Pizza: Per Serving								
Cheese	360	11	27%	6	33	620	10	45
Pepperoni	430	17	36%	7	33	910	12	45
Combination	485	21	39%	9	44	1040	13	47
Salads: No Dressing								
Italian Chef Salad	390	30	69%	5	65	1310	22	10
Pasta Salad	400	20	45%	0	14	1030	9	46
Garden Salad	30	0	0%	0	0	20	2	5
Dressings: Per 1 oz								
Honey French	160	14	79%	2	0	230	0	11
House Italian	140	14	90%	<1	0	225	0	3
Reduced Calorie	70	4	51%	1	0	110	0	2
Ranch	180	20	100%	3	8	250	0	1
1000 Island	140	14	90%	2	15	230	0	4
Desserts: Per Serving								
Lemon Ice	140	0	0%	0	0	10	0	36
Cheesecake: Plain	270	21	70%	14	88	210	7	16
Choc. Choc. Chip	300	22	66%	14	83	200	8	22
Strawberry Topping	40	0	0%	0	0	1	0	10

Godfather's™ Pizza

	Cal	Fat	%Fc	S.Fat	Chol	Sod	Pro	Carb
Original Crust: Per Slice								
Cheese Pizza: Mini, 1/4 pizza	130	3	26%	na	8	180	7	20
Medium, 1/8 pizza	230	5	26%	na	14	340	13	35
Large, 1/10 pizza	260	6	27%	na	18	395	15	36
Jumbo, 1/10 pizza	380	9	26%	na	27	580	22	53
Combo Pizza: Mini, 1/4 pizza	175	7	27%	na	16	380	10	21
Medium, 1/8 pizza	310	11	34%	na	27	660	17	36
Large, 1/10 pizza	340	12	33%	na	30	740	20	38
Jumbo, 1/10 pizza	505	18	26%	na	47	1095	30	56
Golden Crust: Per Slice								
Cheese Pizza: Medium, 1/8 pizza	210	10	31%	na	12	310	10	26
Large, 1/10 pizza	240	12	38%	na	14	365	12	28
Combo Pizza: Medium, 1/8 pizza	270	12	42%	na	22	560	13	28
Large, 1/10 pizza	305	14	42%	na	25	675	16	31

Golden Corral®

	Cal	Fat	%Fc	S.Fat	Chol	Sod	Pro	Carb
Chicken								
Grilled	170	5	26%	na	100	520	32	0
Fried	370	19	46%	na	85	570	37	14
Shrimp, fried	250	12	43%	na	90	470	12	24
Steak: Ribeye, 6 oz	450	35	70%	na	120	220	34	0
Sirloin, 5 oz	230	14	55%	na	90	270	27	0
Chopped, 4 oz	320	23	65%	na	100	160	28	0
Tips w. Onions	290	13	40%	na	120	260	30	8
Baked Potato	225	2	8%	na	0	60	5	46
Texas Toast	170	6	32%	na	0	230	5	26

Haagen-Dazs®

	Cal	Fat	%Fc	S.Fat	Chol	Sod	Pro	Carb
Ice Cream: Per 1/2 Cup								
Baileys Irish Cream	270	17	56%	10	38	85	5	23
Belgian Chocolate Chocolate	330	21	57%	12	85	60	5	29
Brownies a la Mode	280	18	58%	11	100	115	4	26
Butter Pecan	310	23	67%	11	110	160	5	20
Capppucino Commotion	310	21	61%	12	100	105	5	25
Caramel Cone Explosion	310	20	58%	12	95	130	5	27
Cherry Vanilla	240	15	60%	10	100	75	4	23
Chocolate	270	18	60%	11	115	75	5	22
Chocolate Chocolate Chip/Mint	300	20	60%	12	100	70	5	26
Coffee	270	18	60%	11	120	85	5	21
Coffee Chip	290	19	59%	12	100	75	5	25
Cookie Dough Dynamo	300	19	57%	12	95	140	4	29

Continued Next Page

	Cal	Fat	%FC	S.Fat	Chol	Sod	Pro	Carb
Ice Cream: *Per ¹/2 Cup (Cont)*								
Cookies & Cream	270	17	57%	11	110	115	5	23
Deep Chocolate Peanut Butter	350	24	62%	11	80	100	8	28
Dulce De Lache Caramel	290	17	53%	10	100	110	5	28
French Vanilla Coffee	270	18	60%	11	120	85	5	21
Macadamia Brittle	300	20	60%	11	110	120	4	25
Macadamia Nut	320	24	68%	12	110	115	5	20
Midnight Cookies & Cream	300	18	54%	11	90	140	5	29
Mint Chip	290	19	58%	12	105	105	4	26
Pralines & Cream	290	18	56%	9	95	180	4	27
Rum Raisin	270	17	57%	10	110	75	4	22
Strawberry	250	16	58%	10	95	80	4	23
Strawberry Cheesecake Craze	270	16	53%	9	100	140	4	27
Swiss Chocolate Almond	300	20	60%	11	100	65	6	23
Vanilla	270	16	53%	11	120	85	5	21
Vanilla Chocolate Chip	310	20	58%	12	105	90	5	28
Vanilla Swiss Almond	310	21	61%	11	105	80	6	23
Lowfat Ice Cream: *Per ¹/2 Cup*								
Chocolate Fudge Brownie	190	2.5	12%	1.5	30	110	7	34
Coffee Fudge	170	2.5	13%	1.5	25	95	5	32
Strawberry	150	2	60%	1	15	40	5	28
Vanilla Caramel	180	2.5	68%	1.5	20	120	6	32
Ice Cream Sandwich								
Vanilla	260	15	52%	9	65	125	4	32
Vanilla & Chocolate	270	14	46%	8	65	120	4	32
Ice Cream Bars: *Single Pack*								
Chocolate & Dark Chocolate	350	24	62%	15	85	60	5	28
Coffee Almond Crunch	360	26	65%	15	100	85	5	27
Strawberry White Chocolate	320	23	64%	14	70	75	4	24
Vanilla & Almonds	370	27	66%	14	90	80	6	26
Vanilla & Milk Chocolate	330	24	65%	14	90	75	5	24
Sorbet: *Per ¹/2 Cup*								
Tropical Passionfruit	120	0	0%	0	0	0	0	28
Chocolate	120	0	0%	0	0	70	2	28
Mango; Raspberry; Zesty Lemon	120	0	0%	0	0	0	0	31
Margarita; Strawberry	130	0	0%	0	0	0	0	32
Soft Serve: Mango; Raspberry	100	0	0%	0	0	0	0	25
Frozen Yogurt: *Per ¹/2 Cup*								
Vanilla; Cherry Vanilla	140	0	0%	0	<5	45	6	30
Vanilla Fudge	160	0	0%	0	<5	100	6	34
Vanilla Raspberry Swirl	130	0	0%	0	<5	30	4	28
Soft Serve								
Coffee	140	4	26%	2.5	35	75	5	20
Nonfat Chocolate/Vanilla	110	0	0%	0	0	65	4	23
Nonfat Chocolate Mousse	80	0	0%	0	0	65	5	24

	Cal	Fat	%Fc	S.Fat	Chol	Sod	Pro	Carb
Breakfast Items								
Biscuits: Rise 'N' Shine	390	21	48%	6	0	1000	6	44
Apple Cinnamon 'N' Raisin	200	8	36%	2	0	350	2	30
Sausage	510	31	55%	10	25	1360	14	44
Sausage & Egg	630	40	57%	22	285	1480	23	45
Bacon & Egg	570	33	52%	11	275	1400	22	45
Bacon, Egg & Cheese	610	37	55%	13	280	1630	24	45
Ham	400	20	45%	6	15	1340	9	47
Ham, Egg & Cheese	540	30	50%	11	285	1660	20	48
Country Ham	430	22	46%	6	25	1930	15	45
Ultimate Omelet	570	33	52%	12	290	1370	22	45
Big Country:								
Sausage	1000	66	59%	38	570	2310	41	62
Bacon	820	49	54%	15	535	1870	33	62
Frisco Breakfast Sandwich (Ham)	500	25	.45%	9	290	1370	24	46
Hash Rounds	230	14	55%	3	0	560	3	24
Biscuit 'N' Gravy	510	28	49%	9	15	1500	10	55
Pancakes: Three Pancakes	280	2	6%	1	15	890	8	56
w. 1 Sausage Pattie	430	16	33%	6	40	1290	16	56
w. 2 Bacon Strips	350	9	23%	3	25	1130	13	56
Hamburgers & Sandwiches								
Hamburger	270	11	37%	3	35	670	14	29
Cheeseburger	310	14	41%	6	40	890	16	30
Mushroom 'N' Swiss	490	25	46%	12	80	1100	28	39
Cravin' Bacon Cheeseburger	690	46	60%	15	95	1150	30	38
1/4 Pound Double Cheeseburger	470	27	52%	11	80	1290	27	31
Frisco Burger	720	46	57%	16	95	1340	33	43
Roast Beef: Regular	320	16	45%	6	43	820	17	26
Big	460	24	47%	9	70	1280	26	35
The Boss	570	33	52%	12	85	910	·27	42
The Works	530	30	51%	12	80	1030	25	41
Mesquite Bacon Cheeseburger	370	18	44%	7	45	970	19	32
Chicken Fillet Sandwich	480	18	44%)	3	55	1280	26	54
Grilled Chicken Sandwich	350	11	28%	2	65	950	25	38
Hot Ham 'N' Cheese	310	12	35%	6	50	1410	16	34
Fisherman's Fillet	560	27	43%	7	65	1330	26	54
Fried Chicken								
Breast, each	370	15	36%	4	75	1190	29	29
Wing, each	200	8	36%	2	30	740	10	23
Thigh, each	330	15	41%	4	60	1000	19	30
Leg, each	170	7	37%	2	45	570	13	15
French Fries: Small	240	10	37%	3	0	100	4	33
Medium	350	15	39%	4	0	150	5	49
Large	430	18	38%	5	0	190	6	59
Mashed Potatoes, 4 oz	70	0.5	6%	0.5	0	330	2	14
Gravy, 1.5 oz	20	0.5	22%	0	0	260	1	3
Baked Beans, 5 oz	170	1	5%	0	0	600	8	32

Hardee's® (Cont)

	Cal	Fat	%FC	S.Fat	Chol	Sod	Pro	Carb
Salads & Dressings: ColeSlaw	240	20	75%	3	10	340	2	13
Side Salad; no dressing	25	0.5	18%	0	0	45	1	4
Garden Salad; no dressing	220	13	53%	9	40	350	12	11
Grilled Chicken Salad; no dressing	150	3	18%	1	60	610	20	11
Fat Free French Dressing	70	0	0%	0	0	580	0	17
Ranch Dressing	290	29	90%	4	25	510	1	6
Thousand Island Dressing	250	23	83%	3	35	540	1	9
Shakes & Desserts								
Vanilla	350	5	13%	3	20	300	12	65
Chocolate	370	5	12%	3	30	270	13	67
Strawberry	420	4	9%	3	20	270	11	83
Peach	390	4	9%	3	25	290	10	77
Cool Twist: Vanilla Cone	170	22	11%	1	10	130	4	34
Chocolate Cone	180	2	1%	1	5	110	5	34
Sundaes: Hot Fudge	290	6	19%	3	20	310	7	51
Strawberry	210	2	9%	1	10	140	5	43
Big Cookie	280	12	39%	4	15	150	4	41
Peach Cobbler: Small	310	7	20%	1	0	360	2	60

Harveys®

	Cal	Fat	%FC	S.Fat	Chol	Sod	Pro	Carb
Breakfast Items								
Pancakes	90	1	10%	na	8	na	2	17
Sausage	170	14	75%	na	12	na	9	3
Toast, plain	250	3	11%	na	1	na	8	48
Burgers								
Hamburger: Regular	360	14	35%	na	17	na	12	40
Double	530	26	44%	na	34	na	31	44
Super	480	19	36%	na	112	na	37	38
Cheeseburger	420	18	39%	na	30	na	22	41
Chicken Fingers, 1 serving	240	12	45%	na	57	na	15	18
Sandwiches: Chicken	420	16	34%	na	110	na	19	46
Western	350	10	26%	na	265	na	15	58
Sides: French Fries	480	24	45%	na	5	na	10	56
Hash Browns	150	9	55%	na	2	na	2	15
Hot Dog	330	15	41%	na	50	na	12	32
Onion Rings	290	14	44%	na	5	na	4	36
Muffins								
Blueberry	260	6	21%	na	1	na	4	45
Bran	300	13	39%	na	1	na	5	42
Apple Turnover, each	180	7	35%	na	7	na	1	28
Drinks: Apple Juice	80	2	23%	na	0	na	2	20
Orange Juice	80	1	12%	na	0	na	1	18
Shakes: Chocolate	320	11	31%	na	36	na	12	74
Strawberry; Vanilla	300	10	30%	na	36	na	11	69

I Can't Believe It's Yogurt ®

	Cal	Fat	%Fc	S.Fat	Chol	Sod	Pro	Carb
Original Frozen Yogurt								
Per Regular Serving (9 fl.oz)								
Awesome Amaretto	280	6	19%	4	20	230	6	51
Cookies 'N Cream	260	3	10%	1	5	200	7	54
French Vanilla	260	6	20%	4	45	200	7	47
Peanut Butter Bliss	310	12	46%	4	15	200	7	46
White Chocolate Mousse	280	7	22%	4	15	200	7	49
Nonfat Frozen Yogurt								
Average all flavors: Regular	220	0.5	2%	0	5	150	6	48
Small, 6.2 fl.oz	160	0	0%	0	0	100	4	32
Nonfat (w. NutraSweet)								
Average all flavors: Regular	190	0.5	2%	0	5	160	6	40
Small, 6.2 fl.oz	140	0.5	3%	0	5	110	4	29

In–N–Out Burger ®

	Cal	Fat	%Fc	S.Fat	Chol	Sod	Pro	Carb
Burgers								
Hamburger	340	16	24%	5	50	570	18	32
Cheeseburger	410	21	33%	9	55	940	21	35
Double Double (2 patties/2 sl. chse)	600	34	52%	15	130	1420	34	39
French Fries, 125g	400	18	27%	5	0	45	7	54
Shakes (15 oz)								
Chocolate	690	36	55%	24	95	350	9	83
Vanilla	680	37	57%	25	90	390	9	78
Strawberry	690	33	51%	22	85	280	8	91

Int'l House of Pancakes~ IHOP ®

	Cal	Fat	%Fc	S.Fat	Chol	Sod	Pro	Carb
Pancakes: (Syrup/Butter extra)								
Buttermilk, 1 (2 oz)	105	3	25%	1	30	460	3	17
Short Stack, 3	315	9	25%	3	90	1380	9	51
Full Stack, 5	525	15	25%	5	150	2300	15	85
Buckwheat, 1 (2$^1/2$ oz)	135	5	33%	1	60	370	4	19
Country Griddle, 1 (2$^1/4$ oz)	135	4	26%	1	38	500	4	22
Harvest Grain 'N Nut, 1	160	8	45%	1.5	38	390	4.5	18
Crepes (Egg Pancakes), 1 (2 oz)	100	5	45%	1	66	210	2	12
Syrup: 1 Tbsp	50	0	0%	0	0	0	0	12
Whipped Butter, 1 Tbsp	70	7	90%	4.5	20	70	0	0
Waffles (Plain): Regular, 1 (4 oz)	300	15	45%	3.5	70	470	6	37
Belgian: Regular, 1 (6 oz)	410	20	44%	11	145	880	4	49
Harvest Grain 'N Nut, 1	450	28	56%	12	145	870	10	40

Jack in the Box®

	Cal	Fat	%Fc	S.Fat	Chol	Sod	Pro	Carb
Breakfast								
Breakfast Jack	300	12	36%	5	185	890	18	30
Pancake Platter	400	12	27%	3	30	980	13	59
Sausage Croissant	670	48	64%	19	250	940	21	39
Sourdough Breakfast Sandwich	380	21	47%	8	355	1120	21	31
Supreme Croissant	570	36	57%	15	245	1240	21	39
Ultimate Breakfast Sandwich	620	36	51%	15	245	1800	36	39
Hash Browns	160	11	62%	3	0	310	1	14
Country Crock Spread	25	3	100%	0.5	0	40	0	0
Grape Jelly, 1 packet	40	0	0%	0	0	5	0	9
Pancake Syrup, 1 packet	120	0	0%	0	0	5	0	30
Burgers								
Hamburger	280	12	35%	4	45	560	13	32
Cheeseburger	330	15	41%	6	60	760	15	32
Double	450	24	48%	12	75	970	24	35
Ultimate	1030	79	69%	26	205	1200	50	30
Bacon Ultimate	1150	89	69%	30	230	1770	57	31
Jumbo Jack: Regular	560	36	57%	12	80	680	28	31
w. Cheese	650	43	59%	16	105	1090	32	32
Sourdough Jack	670	43	58%	16	110	1180	32	39
1/4 lb. Burger	510	27	48%	10	65	1080	26	39
Sandwiches								
Chicken Caesar	520	26	45%	6	55	1050	27	44
Chicken Fajita Pita	280	9	25%	4	75	840	24	25
Chicken Sandwich	450	26	52%	5	45	1030	16	38
Chicken Supreme	680	45	59%	11	85	1500	23	46
Grilled Chicken Fillet	520	26	45%	6	140	1240	27	42
Philly Cheesesteak	520	25	44%	9	155	1980	33	41
Spicy Crispy Chicken	560	27	43%	5	50	1020	24	55
Finger Foods								
Egg Rolls - 3 piece	440	24	49%	7	30	960	3	54
5 piece	750	41	49%	12	50	1640	5	92
Chicken Breast Pieces - 5 piece	360	17	43%	3	80	970	27	24
Stuffed Jalapenos - 7 piece	470	28	58%	11	50	1560	14	41
10 piece	680	40	58%	15	75	2220	20	59
Bacon/Cheddar Potato Wedges	800	58	65%	16	55	1470	20	49
Mexican Food								
Taco	190	11	52%	4	20	410	7	15
Monster Taco	290	18	55%	6	40	550	11	21
Salsa	10	0	0%	0	0	200	0	2
Teriyaki Bowls								
Chicken	670	4	5%	1	15	1620	29	128
Soy Sauce	5	0	0%	0	0	480	<1	<1
Salads: No Dressing								
Garden Chicken	200	9	40%	4	65	420	23	8
Side	50	3	51%	2	10	75	2	3

	Cal	Fat	%FC	S.Fat	Chol	Sod	Pro	Carb
Salad Dressings								
Blue Cheese	210	18	77%	4	15	750	1	11
Buttermilk House	290	30	93%	11	20	560	1	6
Low Calorie Italian	25	1.5	54%	0	0	670	0	2
Thousand Island	250	24	86%	4	20	570	1	10
Croutons	50	2	36%	0.5	0	105	1	8
Curly Fries								
Seasoned	420	24	51%	5	0	1070	5	39
Chili Cheese	650	41	57%	12	25	1640	12	60
French Fries								
Regular	360	17	44%	4	0	740	4	48
Jumbo Fries	430	20	43%	5	0	890	4	58
Onion Rings	460	25	49%	5	0	780	7	50
Condiments								
Cheese: American, 1 slice	45	4	70%	2.5	10	200	2	0
Swiss-style, 1 slice	40	3	67%	2	10	190	3	0
Packet: Hot Sauce	5	0	0%	0	0	110	<1	1
Ketchup	10	0	0%	0	0	100	0	3
Mayonnaise	150	17	100%	2.5	15	120	0	0
Mustard	5	0	0%	0	0	55	0	0
Chinese Hot Mustard	10	0	0%	0	0	50	0	1
Dipping Sauce: Tartar	220	23	90%	4	20	240	1	2
Barbecue	45	0	0%	0	0	300	1	11
Buttermilk House	130	13	90%	5	10	240	<1	3
Sweet & Sour	40	0	0%	0	0	160	<1	11
Sour Cream	60	6	90%	4	20	30	1	1
Desserts								
Carrot Cake	370	16	36%	3	35	340	3	54
Cheesecake	310	18	52%	9	65	210	8	29
Double Fudge Cake	300	10	30%	3	50	320	3	50
Hot Apple Turnover	340	18	49%	4	0	510	4	41
Ice Cream Shakes								
Chocolate, regular	630	27	39%	16	85	330	11	85
Cappuccino, regular	630	29	41%	17	90	320	11	80
Oreo Cookie Classic, regular	790	36	41%	19	95	490	13	91
Strawberry, regular	640	28	39%	15	85	300	10	85
Vanilla, regular	610	31	46%	18	95	320	12	73
Drinks								
Orange Juice	80	0	0%	0	0	0	1	20
Lowfat Milk (2%)	120	5	38%	3	20	120	8	12
Coca Cola, small	190	0	0%	0	0	20	0	51
Ramblin Root Beer	240	0	0%	0	0	45	0	61
Sprite, small	190	0	0%	0	0	60	0	48
Dr Pepper	190	0	0%	0	0	25	0	49

Jamba Juice®

Smoothies: Per 24 fl.oz	Cal	Fat	%Fc	S.Fat	Chol	Sod	Pro	Carb
Banana Berry	520	1.5	3%	0	0	30	6	120
Boysenberry Bliss	500	1	1%	0	0	40	9	117
Citrus Squeeze	450	2.5	5%	0	0	30	5	105
Coffee Colossus	420	0	0%	0	0	100	7	99
Coldbuster	460	2.5	5%	0	0	100	6	105
Cranberry Craze	430	2	4%	0	0	50	6	99
Femme Phenom	500	1.5	3%	0	0	50	9	110
Ghirardelli Chocolossus	420	1.5	3%	0	0	80	9	93
Hawaiian Lust	480	5	9%	2	0	20	4	105
Jamba Powerboost	440	1.5	3%	0	0	30	11	96
Lo-Cal Motion	280	1	3%	0	0	20	4	66
Orange Oasis	430	1	2%	0	0	50	9	96
Orange Zinger	410	2.5	5%	1	10	30	5	90
Pacific Passion	450	1.5	3%	0	0	30	5	105
Papaya Paradise	550	6	10%	2	0	30	5	120
Peach Pleasure	480	2	3%	0	0	30	4	114
Raspberry Rage	530	1	2%	0	0	40	9	123
Razzmatazz	490	1	2%	0	0	30	9	123
Soymilk Splash	380	1	2%	0	0	50	12	81
Strawberries Wild	470	0.5	1%	0	0	40	7	111

Note: Figures for saturated fat, cholesterol and sodium are author estimates.

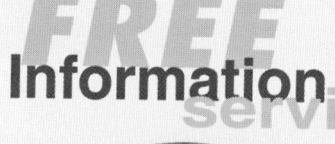

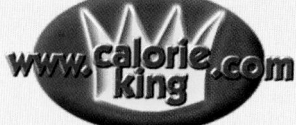

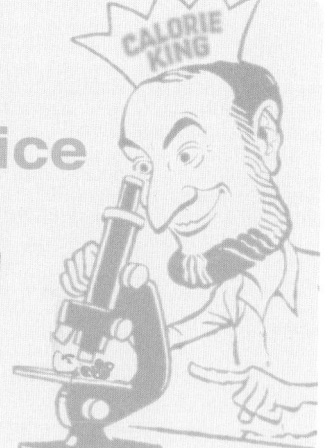

Check out nutritional data for the latest food products.

Extra Details ~ See Inside Back Cover

Kenny Roger's Roasters®

	Cal	Fat	%Fc	S.Fat	Chol	Sod	Pro	Carb
Chicken								
1/4 White Meat: w. Skin	245	11	39%	3	136	605	35	1
no Skin or Wing	145	2	13%	0.5	92	420	31	<1
1/4 Dark Meat: w. Skin	270	17	57%	4	165	525	29	<1
no Skin	170	7	37%	2	130	455	25	<1
1/2 Chicken: w. Skin	515	28	49%	7	300	1130	65	2
no Skin or Wing	315	10	29%	3	220	880	56	<1
Turkey: Sliced Breast	160	2	11%	0.5	78	590	34	0
Sandwiches, Pitas, Pies								
Turkey Sandwich	385	12	28%	2	88	920	39	30
BBQ Chicken Pita	400	7	16%	1	112	1310	33	51
Chicken Caesar Pita	605	35	52%	3	122	830	36	34
Roasted Chicken Pita	685	35	46%	3	159	1620	47	42
Chicken Pot Pie	710	33	42%	11	69	1500	26	78
Soup								
Chicken Noodle, 1 cup	55	1	16%	0.5	13	560	4	7
1 bowl	90	2	20%	0.5	22	930	7	12
Salads: No Dressing								
Chicken Caesar	285	9	28%	3	122	700	34	18
Pasta Salad	230	12	47%	2	40	300	6	28
Roasted Chicken	290	10	31%	2	218	575	35	19
Side Salad	25	0	0%	0	0	15	1	5
Sour Cream & Dill Pasta	230	16	63%	3	16	430	4	20
Tomato Cucumber	125	2	14%	1	0	795	1	10
Side Dishes: Per Serving								
Cinnamon Apples	200	5	22%	3	13	5	0	41
Cole Slaw	225	16	64%	3	13	290	1	18
Corn: Muffin	175	8	41%	1	0	210	2	24
On the Cob	70	0.5	6%	0.5	0	10	2	14
Sweet Corn Niblets	115	0.5	3%	0.5	0	385	3	28
Cornbread Stuffing	325	19	53%	3	5	765	7	34
Creamy Parmesan Spinach	120	6	45%	3	12	550	10	10
Honey Baked Beans	150	1	6%	0.5	0	790	6	32
Italian Green Beans	115	8	63%	1	0	375	2	10
Macaroni & Cheese	200	6	27%	3	26	660	6	24
Potatoes: Baked Sweet	265	0	0%	0	0	25	4	62
Garlic Parsley	260	12	42%	5	16	870	3	37
Real Mashed	295	14	43%	3	2	480	4	39
Potato Salad	390	27	62%	3	0	630	3	34
Rice Pilaf	175	5	26%	0.5	0	145	3	43
Steamed Vegetables	50	0	0%	0	0	60	3	8
Zucchini & Squash Santa Fe	70	5	64%	0.5	0	210	<1	8

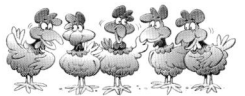

KFC®

Original Recipe®	Cal	Fat	%FC	S.Fat	Chol	Sod	Pro	Carb
Breast	400	24	54%	6	135	1115	29	16
Drumstick	140	9	58%	2	75	420	13	4
Thigh	250	18	65%	4.5	95	750	16	6
Whole Wing	140	10	64%	2.5	55	415	9	5
Extra Crispy™ : Breast	470	28	54%	8	160	874	39	17
Drumstick	195	12	52%	3	77	375	15	7
Thigh	380	27	61%	7	118	625	21	14
Whole Wing	220	15	58%	4	55	415	10	10
Hot & Spicy Chicken: Breast	505	29	52%	8	162	1170	38	23
Drumstick	175	10	51%	3	77	360	13	9
Thigh	355	26	66%	7	126	630	19	13
Whole Wing	210	15	64%	4	55	350	10	9
Other Entrees: Chunky Pot Pie	770	42	49%	13	70	2160	29	69
Crispy Strips: Colonels, 3 pieces	300	16	48%	4	56	1105	26	18
Spicy, 3 pieces	335	15	40%	4	70	1140	25	23
Popcorn Chicken: Small, 3.5 oz	362	23	57%	6	43	610	17	21
Large, 6 oz	620	40	58%	10	73	1046	30	38
Wings: Hot Wings, 6 pieces	470	33	63%	8	150	1230	27	18
Honey BBQ Wings, 6 pces	607	38	56%	10	193	1145	33	33
Sandwiches								
Original Recipe Chicken: w. Sauce	450	22	44%	5	70	940	29	39
without Sauce	360	13	33%	3.5	60	890	36	28
Honey BBQ Flavored Chicken, w. Sce	310	6	17%	2	125	560	28	37
Triple Crunch Chicken: w. Sauce	490	29	53%	6	70	710	26	39
without Sauce	390	15	34%	4.5	50	650	25	29
Triple Crunch Zinger: w. Sauce	550	32	52%	7	65	630	26	39
without Sauce	390	15	34%	4.5	50	650	36	25
Tender Roast Chicken: w. Sauce	350	15	38%	3	75	880	32	26
without Sauce	270	5	16%	1.5	65	690	31	23
Side Dishes: Per Serving								
BBQ Baked Beans, 5.5 oz	190	3	14%	1	5	760	6	33
Biscuit, 2 oz	180	10	50%	2.5	0	560	4	20
Coleslaw, 5 oz	232	13	52%	2	8	284	2	26
Corn on the Cob, 5.7 oz	150	1.5	14%	0.5	0	20	5	35
Macaroni & Cheese, 5.4 oz	180	8	40%	3	10	860	7	21
Mashed Potatoes w. Gravy, 4.8 oz	120	6	45%	1	<1	440	1	17
Potato Salad, 5.6 oz	230	14	55%	2	15	540	4	23
Potato Wedges, 4.8 oz	280	13	42%	4	5	750	5	28
Desserts: Dble Choc Chip Cake, 2.7 oz	320	16	45%	4	65	230	4	41
Little Bucket Parfaits: Chocolate Crm	290	18	56%	11	15	330	3	37
Fudge Brownie	280	10	32%	3.5	145	190	3	44
Lemon Creme	410	14	30%	8	20	290	7	62
Strawberry Shortcake	200	7	31%	8	10	220	1	33
Colonels Pies: Apple Pie Slice, 4 oz	310	14	40%	3	0	280	23	44
Pecan Pie Slice, 4 oz	490	23	42%	5	85	510	5	68
Strawberry Creme Pie Slice, 2.7 oz	280	15	48%	8	10	130	4	32

	Cal	Fat	%Fc	S.Fat	Chol	Sod	Pro	Carb
Original Skinless Flame Broiled Chicken								
Leg & Thigh	175	8	41%	2	54	365	21	3
Breast & Wing (skin on wing)	220	8	33%	2	27	495	34	3
Original Breast Meat	160	4	32%	1	23	400	28	2
Half Original Chicken (skin on wing)	390	16	37%	4	81	860	55	6
Rotisserie Chicken: Leg & Thigh	300	18	54%	5	114	515	31	1
Breast & Wing	355	16	40%	4	140	675	50	1
Half Rotisserie Chicken	655	34	46%	9	254	1190	80	2
Fresh Roasted Carved Turkey								
Turkey Breast Sandwich	540	7	11%	0	118	800	50	1
1/2 Turkey Breast Sandwich	270	4	13%	0	60	400	25	34
1/4 lb Sliced White Meat	155	1	6%	0	95	60	34	0
1/4 lb Sliced Dark Meat	210	8	34%	0	96	90	32	0
Open-Faced Turkey S'wich: w. extras	670	21	28%	10	161	1395	51	70
Hand-Carved Turkey Dinner: w. extras	905	45	45%	12	165	1380	42	83
Turkey Pot Pie, 1/4 pie, 5.5 oz	220	8	33%	2	27	495	34	3
Salads: Per Regular (no dressing)								
BBQ Chicken Salad, 15 1/2 oz	465	21	40%	8	121	740	40	30
Caesar Salad, 9 1/2 oz	170	8	42%	4	11	485	10	16
Chicken Caesar Salad, 12 oz	310	11	32%	4	83	545	36	16
Chinese Chicken Salad, 17 oz	295	8	24%	2	71	170	31	23
Koo Koo Roo House Salad, 16 oz	165	6	32%	2	7	360	9	21
Koo Koo Roo Slaw (side)	55	2	32%	0	0	230	1	10
Pesto Pasta Salad	170	5	26%	1	16	250	10	21
12 Vegetable Chopped Salad, 13 oz	80	1	11%	0	0	65	5	16
Soup: Ten Vegetable, 8 oz	120	3	22%	0	0	620	3	21
Sandwiches: BBQ Chicken	570	14	22%	7	115	1540	43	70
Original Chicken Breast	750	47	56%	10	128	1075	35	50
Chicken Caesar	730	37	45%	12	144	2140	51	50
Turkey Breast	540	7	11%	0	118	800	50	68
Dressings: Balsamic Viniagrette, 2 T.	90	9	90%	1	0	240	0	3
BBQ, 2 Tbsp	40	0	0%	0	0	280	0	10
Caesar, 2 Tbsp	160	17	95%	4	14	180	0	1
Chinese Chicken Salad, 2 Tbsp	110	8	65%	2	0	110	0	8
Chopped Salad, 2 Tbsp	100	7	63%	5	0	350	0	8
Cranberry Sauce, 1 oz	45	0	0%	0	0	15	0	11
Gravy, 2oz	25	1	36%	0	0	310	1	3
Lahvash (flatbread), each	95	0	0%	0	0	145	4	20
Hot Sides								
Baked Yam	360	0	0%	0	0	25	5	86
Black Beans	140	2	13%	0	0	570	8	23
Confetti Rice	130	0	0%	0	0	165	3	30
Creamed Spinach	140	12	77%	6	38	395	3	10
Hand-Mashed Potatoes	185	5	24%	3	15	360	3	32
Italian Vegetables	35	2	50%	1	5	125	1	4
Macaroni & Cheese	270	11	36%	6	31	245	11	28
Roasted Garlic Potatoes	115	2	15%	1	3	165	2	22

Krystal®

Breakfast	Cal	Fat	%Fc	S.Fat	Chol	Sod	Pro	Carb
Biscuit: Country Ham	335	17	46%	4	23	1150	14	31
Sausage	440	30	61%	8	49	670	10	31
Bacon, Egg & Cheese	420	26	56%	8	153	900	14	33
Pancakes	250	12	43%	2	0	210	5	31
Sunriser	260	17	59%	5	162	545	14	17
Sandwiches: Big K	540	35	58%	14	93	1280	29	29
Krystal: Regular	160	7	39%	2	22	32	10	16
Double	280	14	45%	4	43	585	18	24
Cheese	190	10	48%	4	29	450	11	16
Double Cheese	340	19	50%	8	57	815	21	25
Bacon, Egg & Cheeseburger	520	34	59%	14	89	1080	26	29
Burger Plus	415	26	56%	10	63	620	20	28
w. Cheese	475	31	59%	13	77	870	23	28
Crispy Crunchy Chicken	470	24	46%	7	56	950	16	48
Plain Pup	160	9	50%	5	20	470	6	12
Chili Pup	180	10	50%	6	24	600	7	13
Chili Cheese Pup	210	13	56%	7	31	640	9	14
Chili: Regular	220	8	33%	3	19	855	11	27
Large	330	12	33%	5	28	1285	16	41
French Fries: Small	260	13	45%	4	9	115	3	33
Regular	360	18	45%	6	12	160	4	45
Large	460	23	45%	8	16	205	5	59
Kriss Kross Fries: Regular	485	29	53%	11	31	605	5	52
w. Cheese	515	31	54%	12	31	805	5	54
Chili Cheese	625	39	56%	16	61	1110	12	57
Chocolate Shake	275	10	33%	5	32	180	8	44
Pies: Apple Pie	300	10	30%	4	0	420	3	49
Lemon Meringue Pie	340	9	24%	3	50	190	7	57
Pecan Pie	450	23	46%	6	55	290	5	56

La Salsa Fresh Mexican Grill®

Estimates Only	Cal	Fat	%Fc	S.Fat	Chol	Sod	Pro	Carb
Taco: Mexico City Taco, Chicken	250	7	20%	2	50	130	17	27
Fish Taco (Sonora)	225	9	36%	4	45	440	15	21
La Salsa, Chicken w. Cheese	300	10	30%	4	55	220	17	35
Vegetarian w. Cheese	290	8	25%	3	5	285	12	39
Burrito: Bean & Cheese	535	14	24%	6	10	920	16	27
Californian 'Veggie'	600	19	29%	8	20	800	20	87
El Champion Burrito (12", 2lbs)	1100	52	43%	18	200	1200	60	100
Burrito Grande	550	26	43%	9	95	530	30	50
Sides: Cheese, 0.5 oz	60	5	75%	3	20	150	3	30
Black Beans (no cheese), 5 oz	290	1	3%	1	0	110	15	38
Rice, 3.5 oz	170	3	16%	0	0	230	3	30
1/2 Rice & 1/2 Beans (no cheese)	310	3	10%	0	9	250	9	44
Salsa, 2 Tbsp	15	0	0%	0	0	300	0	3

Little Caesars® Pizza

Pizza: Per Slice	Cal	Fat	%FC	S.Fat	Chol	Sod	Pro	Carb
12" Round: Cheese	170	6	32%	3	15	330	9	22
Pepperoni	190	8	38%	3.5	20	410	9	22
12" Single Slice: Cheese	350	13	33%	5.5	35	670	17	45
Pepperoni	390	16	37%	7	40	830	19	45
14" Round: Cheese	200	7	32%	3	20	360	10	25
Pepperoni	220	9	37%	4	25	460	11	25
Meatsa	250	12	43%	4.5	30	610	12	25
Supreme	230	10	39%	4	25	480	11	26
Veggie	190	7	33%	3	15	470	9	25
Stuffed Crust: Cheese	240	11	41%	4.5	20	470	11	25
Pepperoni	280	13	42%	5.5	30	580	13	58
16" Round: Cheese	210	7	30%	3	20	390	10	27
Pepperoni	230	10	39%	4	25	500	11	27
18" Round: Cheese	220	8	33%	3.5	20	410	11	29
Pepperoni	250	11	40%	4.5	25	530	12	29
Pan! Pan!: Cheese, medium	160	6	34%	2.5	15	410	7	21
Pepperoni, medium	170	7	37%	3	20	480	8	21
Cheese, large	170	7	37%	3	15	430	8	21
Pepperoni, large	190	9	43%	3.5	20	490	8	21
Crazy Bread: 1 stick, 1.4 oz	100	2.5	22%	0.5	0	105	3	16
Crazy Sauce: 4 oz	60	0	0%	0	0	260	2	11

Long John Silver's®

	Cal	Fat	%FC	S.Fat	Chol	Sod	Pro	Carb
Flavorbaked								
Fish, 1 piece	90	2.5	26%	1	35	320	14	1
Chicken	110	3	24%	1	55	600	19	0
Crispy Fry: Fish & Chips	710	42	53%	10	30	na	16	66
Lemon Crumb Baked: Fish, 1 piece	195	2	9%	na	145	635	35	10
Sandwiches								
Batter-Dipped Fish (no sauce)	320	13	37%	4	30	800	17	40
Ultimate Fish	430	21	44%	7	35	1340	18	44
Flavorbaked Fish	320	14	39%	7	55	930	23	28
Flavorbaked Chicken	290	10	31%	2	60	970	24	27
Grab n Go: Battered Chicken, 1 serve	320	12	34%	3	20	850	14	41
w. Cheese	370	17	41%	8	35	1090	17	41
Battered Fish, 1 serve	300	11	33%	3	20	770	11	39
w. Cheese	350	16	41%	8	35	1010	14	39
Popcorn Munchers: Chicken, 4 oz	380	23	55%	4	35	1030	23	20
Fish/Shrimp, 4 oz	310	15	44%	3	75	1310	15	31
Batter-Dipped: Shrimp, 1 serve	35	2.5	64%	0.5	10	95	1	2
Chicken	120	6	45%	2	15	400	8	11
Fish	170	11	58%	2.5	30	470	11	12
Breaded: Chicken Strips/Fish	105	5	43%	1	15	350	6	11
Clams	300	17	51%	4	40	670	11	31

Wraps	Cal	Fat	%Fc	S.Fat	Chol	Sod	Pro	Carb
Chicken: Salsa, Regular, 11 oz	690	32	40%	7	20	1690	18	81
Large, 22 oz	1370	64	40%	13	35	3370	36	162
Cajun/Ranch/Tartar: Average								
Regular, 11 oz	730	36	45%	7	25	1830	18	82
Large, 22 oz	1450	72	45%	14	50	3650	36	165
Fish: Salsa, Regular, 11.5 oz	690	32	40%	7	25	1640	18	84
Large, 23 oz	1380	64	40%	14	45	3280	35	167
Cajun/Ranch/Tartar: Average								
Regular, 11.5 oz	730	36	45%	8	25	1780	18	85
Large, 23 oz	1450	72	45%	15	58	3550	35	170
Popcorn Shrimp:								
Salsa, Regular, 11 oz	690	32	40%	9	40	1660	16	84
Large, 22 oz	1380	64	40%	17	85	3310	32	170
Cajun/Ranch/Tartar: Average								
Regular, 11 oz	730	36	45%	9	45	1810	16	86
Large, 22 oz	1450	72	45%	18	95	3600	32	172
Side Items: Fries, regular	250	15	54%	3	0	500	3	28
Fries, large, 5 oz	420	24	51%	4	0	830	5	46
Cheese Sticks	160	9	50%	4	10	360	6	12
Hushpuppy, 1 piece	60	2.5	37%	0	0	25	1	9
Corn Cobbette:	140	8	51%	2	0	0	3	19
without Butter	80	0.5	6%	0	0	0	3	19
Green Beans	30	0.5	15%	0	<5	310	2	5
Rice	140	3	19%	1	0	210	3	26
Slaw	140	6	39%	na	0	260	1	20
Soup: Broccoli Cheese, 8 oz	180	12	60%	4.5	15	1240	5	13
Salads: Side Salad, no dressing	25	0	0%	0	0	15	1	4
Grilled Chicken Salad	140	2.5	16%	0.5	45	260	20	10
Garden Salad	45	0	0%	0	0	25	3	9
Ocean Chef Salad	130	2	14%	0	60	540	14	13

Mrs Winner's Chicken®

Chicken:	Cal	Fat	%Fc	S.Fat	Chol	Sod	Pro	Carb
Baked Fillet	120	2	15%	na	35	360	10	<1
Breaded Chicken Sandwich	205	10	44%	na	35	1000	19	12
Chicken Fillet Sandwich	380	7	17%	na	30	540	12	45
Chicken Salad	585	8	12%	na	5	875	9	39
Chicken Salad Sandwich	315	6	17%	na	<5	600	10	33
Biscuit	245	5	18%	na	<1	500	4	45
Cole Slaw	190	16	76%	na	<5	560	1	9
Potato Fries	225	9	36%	na	<5	220	6	27
Seafood Salad	555	9	15%	na	5	760	5	41
Steak Sandwich	540	11	18%	na	20	650	11	43

Mrs Fields' Cookies®

	Cal	Fat	%FC	S.Fat	Chol	Sod	Pro	Carb
Per 1 Cookie, 2.5 oz								
Butter; Butter Toffee	290	12	37%	9	50	250	3	40
Chewy Fudge	300	14	42%	9	35	80	3	40
Coconut Macadamia	280	13	42%	5	20	220	2	39
Debra's Special; Milk Choc	280	12	38%	8	40	180	4	39
Milk Choc w. Walnuts	320	17	48%	9	40	180	4	37
Milk Choc Macadamia	320	18	50%	9	40	180	4	38
Oatmeal Raisin	240	9	34%	5	30	220	2	39
Peanut Butter	310	16	46%	8	45	250	3	34
Pumpkin Harvest	270	14	46%	7	40	280	4	31
Semi-Sweet Chocolate	280	14	45%	6	30	150	2	40
with Pecans	300	16	48%	8	30	180	3	37
with Walnuts	310	16	46%	8	35	170	3	38
Triple Chocolate	300	14	42%	9	35	180	3	41
White Chunk Macadamia	310	17	50%	9	35	170	4	37
Nibblers: Per 2 Cookies, 1 oz								
Debra's Special	100	4.5	40%	2	10	80	1	13
Milk Choc w. Walnuts	120	6	45%	3	10	65	1	14
Milk Chocolate	110	5	40%	3	10	60	1	15
Peanut Butter	110	6	49%	2.5	16	95	2	13
White Chunk Macadamia	120	7	53%	3.5	10	80	1	13

Mazzio's Pizza®

	Cal	Fat	%FC	S.Fat	Chol	Sod	Pro	Carb
Appetizers: Per Serving								
Garlic Bread w. Cheese, 2 slices	700	35	45%	7	15	1280	21	74
Meat Nachos	500	37	67%	17	15	1200	21	21
Sandwiches: Ham & Cheese	790	39	44%	13	85	1900	40	71
BBQ Beef & Cheddar	580	24	37%	11	95	1260	39	51
Chicken & Cheddar	570	24	38%	8	70	1350	33	56
Deluxe Submarine	810	43	48%	13	75	2240	39	68
Pizza: Per Medium Slice								
Original Crust: Cheese	260	8	28%	4	10	450	14	33
Combo	320	13	36%	6	25	780	17	34
Pepperoni	280	11	35%	5	30	600	16	30
Sausage	350	16	41%	7	20	890	18	34
Deep Pan: Cheese	350	13	33%	5	15	620	17	42
Combo	410	18	40%	6	20	930	19	42
Pepperoni	380	17	40%	5	25	740	18	38
Sausage	430	21	44%	8	25	1040	21	41
Thin Crust: Cheese	220	9	37%	4	15	440	13	22
Pasta: Chicken Parmesan	600	19	29%	3	50	1600	39	68
Fettuccine Alfredo, small	440	28	57%	16	55	680	14	34
Meat Lasagna, small	460	25	49%	10	85	1370	24	36
Spaghetti, small	290	10	31%	3	5	800	11	39

McDonald's®

	Cal	Fat	%FC	S.Fat	Chol	Sod	Pro	Carb
Breakfast Menu								
Bacon, Egg & Cheese Biscuit	540	34	56%	10	250	1550	21	38
Biscuit, 2.7 oz	290	15	46%	3	0	780	5	34
Breakfast Burrito	320	20	56%	7	195	660	13	23
Egg McMuffin®	290	12	37%	4.5	235	790	17	27
English Muffin, 2 oz	140	2	13%	0	0	210	4	25
Hash Browns, 2 oz	130	8	55%	1.5	0	330	1	14
Hotcakes (3): Plain, 5.3 oz	310	7	20%	1.5	15	610	9	53
w. Margarine. 2 pats & Syrup	500	17	25%	3	20	770	9	66
Sausage, 1½ oz	170	16	85%	5	35	290	6	0
Sausage McMuffin®	360	23	58%	8	45	740	13	18
with Egg	440	28	57%	10	255	890	19	27
Sausage Biscuit	470	31	59%	9	35	1080	11	40
with Egg	550	37	60%	10	245	1180	18	53
Scrambled Eggs (2), 3½ oz	160	11	62%	3.5	425	170	13	1
Spanish Omelete Bagel	590	38	58%	14	275	1560	27	60
Steak, Egg & Cheese Bagel	660	31	58%	11	285	1300	36	60
Sandwiches								
Arch Deluxe™	550	31	51%	11	90	1010	28	39
with Bacon	590	34	52%	12	100	1150	32	39
Big Mac®	570	32	50%	10	85	1100	26	45
Filet-O-Fish™	470	26	49%	5	50	890	15	44
Crispy Chicken Deluxe™	500	25	45%	4	55	1100	26	43
Grilled Chicken Deluxe, w Mayo	440	20	41%	3	60	1040	27	38
Plain (no mayo)	300	5	15%	1	50	930	27	38
Hamburger	270	9	32%	3.5	30	600	13	34
Cheeseburger	320	13	36%	6	40	830	16	35
Quarter Pounder®	430	21	44%	8	70	840	23	37
with Cheese	530	30	51%	13	95	1310	28	38
French Fries								
Small, 2.4 oz	210	10	43%	1.5	0	135	3	26
Medium	450	22	44%	4	0	290	6	57
Large	540	26	43%	4.5	0	350	8	68
Super Size, 6.2 oz	610	29	43%	5	0	390	9	79
Chicken McNuggets/Sauces								
Chick McNuggets®4 Pces	190	11	52%	2.5	35	360	10	13
6 Pieces	290	17	52%	3.5	55	540	15	20
9 Pieces	430	25	52%	5	80	810	23	28
Hot Mustard Sauce (1 pkg), 1 oz	60	3.5	0%	0	5	240	1	7
Barbeque Sauce (1 pkg), 1 oz	45	0	0%	0	0	250	0	10
Sweet 'N' Sour Sauce (1 pkg), 1 oz	50	0	0%	0	0	140	0	11
Honey (1 pkg), ½ oz	45	0	0%	0	0	0	0	12
Honey Mustard (1 pkg), ½ oz	50	4.5	81%	0.5	10	85	0	3
Light Mayonnaise (1 pkg)	40	4	90%	0.5	5	80	0	<1

	Cal	Fat	%Fc	S.Fat	Chol	Sod	Pro	Carb
Salads/Salad Dressings								
Garden Salad, 6 1/4 oz	35	0	0%	0	0	20	2	7
Grilled Chicken Salad Deluxe	120	1.5	11%	0	45	240	21	7
Croutons (1 pkg)	50	1.5	27%	0	0	105	1	8
Caesar Dressing (1 pkg), 2 oz	160	14	79%	3	20	450	2	7
Fat-Free Herb Vinaigrette (1 pkg), 2 oz	50	0	0%	0	0	330	0	11
Ranch Dressing (1 pkg), 2 oz	230	21	82%	3	20	550	1	10
Red French Reduced Calorie, 2 oz	160	8	34%	1	0	490	0	23
Muffins/Danish								
Lowfat Apple Bran Muffin, 4 oz	300	3	9%	0.5	0	380	6	62
Apple Danish, 3.7 oz	340	15	40%	3	20	340	5	46
Cheese Danish, 3.7 oz	400	21	47%	5	40	400	7	46
Cinnamon Roll, 3.4 oz	390	18	42%	5	65	310	8	50
Desserts/Sundaes/Cookies/McFlurry™								
Baked Apple Pie, 2 3/4 oz	260	13	45%	3.5	0	200	3	34
Chocolate Chip Cookie, 2 3/4 oz	170	10	53%	6	20	120	2	22
McDonaldland ® Cookies, 1 pkg	180	5	25%	1	0	190	3	32
McFlurry™: Butterfinger ®	620	22	32%	14	70	260	16	90
M&Ms ®	630	23	33%	15	75	210	16	90
Nestle Crunch ®	630	24	34%	16	75	230	16	88
Oreo ® Cookie	570	20	31%	12	70	280	15	83
Nuts (Sundae/Topping), 1/4 oz	40	3.5	79%	0	0	55	2	2
Sundaes: Hot Caramel, 6.3 oz	360	10	16%	6	35	180	7	74
Hot Fudge, 6.3 oz	340	12	16%	9	30	170	8	52
Strawberry, 6.3 oz	290	7	16%	5	30	95	7	50
Vanilla Reduced Fat Icecream Cone	150	4.5	27%	3	20	75	4	23
Shakes (Lowfat)								
Choc./Vanilla, small, 14 fl.oz	360	9	23%	6	40	250	11	60
Strawberry, small, 14 fl.oz	360	9	23%	6	40	180	11	60
Drinks								
1% Lowfat Milk, 8 fl.oz ctn	100	2.5	23%	1.5	10	115	8	13
Orange Juice, 6 fl.oz	80	0	0%	0	0	20	1	20
Coca-Cola Classic: (25% ice)								
Small,16 fl.oz	150	0	0%	0	0	15	0	40
Medium, 21 fl.oz	210	0	0%	0	0	20	0	58
Large, 32 fl.oz	310	0	0%	0	0	30	0	86
Diet Coke: Small,16 fl.oz	0	0	0%	0	0	30	0	0
Medium, 21 fl.oz	0	0	0%	0	0	40	0	0
Large, 32 fl. oz	0	0	0%	0	0	60	0	0
Sprite: Small, 16 fl.oz	150	0	0%	0	0	55	0	39
Medium, 21 fl.oz	210	0	0%	0	0	80	0	56
Large, 32 fl. oz	310	0	0%	0	0	115	0	83
Hi-C Orange Drink: Small, 16 fl.oz	160	0	0%	0	0	30	0	44
Medium, 21 fl.oz	240	0	0%	0	0	40	0	64
Large, 32 fl. oz	350	0	0%	0	0	60	0	94

Nathan's® Famous

	Cal	Fat	%FC	S.Fat	Chol	Sod	Pro	Carb
Hamburgers: Regular	435	23	48%	10	77	280	25	32
Double Burger	670	41	55%	18	154	460	44	32
Super Burger	535	32	54%	9	86	525	27	34
Sandwiches								
Breaded Chicken Sandwich	510	25	44%	4	56	930	23	48
Charbroiled Chicken S'wich	290	6	19%	1	53	860	35	24
Cheese Steak Sandwich	485	26	48%	10	73	580	26	37
Chicken Salad	155	4	23%	1	49	345	35	9
Fillet of Fish S'wich	405	15	33%	2	32	715	20	46
Pastrami Sandwich	325	12	33%	4	48	1015	21	34
Turkey Sandwich	270	2	7%	0	27	1460	28	34
Platters								
Chicken, 2 piece	1095	66	54%	14	212	1420	54	72
4 pieces	1790	109	55%	23	425	2370	102	99
Fillet of Fish	1455	74	46%	10	147	1840	60	137
Fried Clam	1025	51	45%	7	49	1825	23	119
Fried Shrimp	795	34	38%	5	83	1435	22	100
French Fries	515	26	45%	0	0	60	8	62
Frank Nuggets (7)	360	24	60%	6	46	740	9	25
Frankfurter	310	19	55%	8	45	820	13	22

Olive Garden®

	Cal	Fat	%FC	S.Fat	Chol	Sod	Pro	Carb
Lunch Entrees								
Capellini Pomodora, 12 oz	380	10	23%	2	5	1030	13	60
Capellini Primavera: Reg, 13 oz	350	7	19%	3	10	820	14	58
with Chicken, 16 oz	510	13	23%	4.5	45	1550	39	59
Chicken Giardino, 13 oz	360	9	22%	3.5	50	900	23	47
Linguine alla Marinara, 10.5 oz	330	6	17%	0.5	0	710	10	57
Shrimp Primavera, 16 oz	400	6	14%	2.5	125	820	26	61
Dinner Entrees								
Capellini Pomodora, 19.5 oz	620	16	23%	4	10	1620	22	98
Capellini Primavera: Reg., 24 oz	600	12	18%	4	10	1450	23	99
with Chicken, 27 oz	760	18	21%	6	50	2190	48	101
Chicken Giardino, 21 oz	550	11	18%	4	85	1000	42	71
Grilled Chicken Capri, 21 oz	550	12	19%	3.5	70	1660	58	52
Linguine alla Marinara, 17 oz	530	9	15%	1	0	1100	17	94
Shrimp Primavera, 30 oz	730	12	15%	4.5	255	1580	50	105
Soup & Breadstick								
Minestrone Soup, 6 fl.oz	100	1	10%	0	0	550	4	17
Breadstick, plain, 1 stick	140	1.5	10%	0	0	270	5	26
Dessert								
Apple Caramellina, 12 oz	560	2	3%	1	5	190	6	131

	Cal	Fat	%FC	S.Fat	Chol	Sod	Pro	Carb
Per Baked Potato (No Skin)								
Ultra-Lites: Chicken Stir-Fry	330	3	8%	1	21	1290	16	62
Chicken Fajita; Carribean Chicken	270	1.5	5%	0.5	21	555	16	50
Chick, Mushroom, Rst Red Pepper	245	2	7%	0.5	21	715	13	45
Crab & Broccoli DeLite	335	2.5	6%	1	35	740	19	55
Vegie & Herb Cheese	240	1.5	5%	1	5	425	13	44
Lite: Chicken Caesar & Broccoli	375	12	29%	3	31	845	19	50
Herb Roasted Vegetable	260	6	20%	1	1	210	6	47
Fresh Mex Chicken; Spinach Souffle	320	9	26%	4	60	570	15	44
Gourmet: Bacon & Cheese	660	47	64%	18	61	920	20	39
Bacon Double Cheeseburger	765	54	63%	21	88	1290	30	40
BBQ Chick, Cheddar, Bacon	685	43	57%	17	90	1765	32	44
Broccoli & Cheese	545	36	59%	14	42	575	16	42
Chicken Broccoli & Chedd.; 3 Cheese	590	37	56%	15	63	820	23	43
Chicken Caesar & Broccoli	710	51	65%	10	36	1375	16	50
Crab, Broccoli & Cheese	595	35	53%	14	55	1230	25	46
Mexican	670	46	62%	14	70	1070	18	48
Philly Steak & Cheese	675	40	53%	15	69	1410	34	46
Potato Skins (with Sour Cream)								
Bacon 'n Cheddar, 9 oz	975	53	50%	25	98	1340	27	100
Southwestern, 11 oz	910	46	45%	22	84	1425	23	105
Fresh Cut Fries: Small, 13 oz	615	39	57%	7	0	320	5	63
Medium, 16 oz	765	49	58%	8	0	400	7	79
Large, 25 oz	1225	78	57%	13	0	640	11	126
Topped Fries: Nacho Cheese	840	54	58%	11	13	625	10	81
Fresh Fries 'n Chicken Tenders	920	50	49%	9	48	895	26	93
Soups: Baked Potato Soup, 13 oz	640	26	36%	11	52	1630	20	81
Broccoli & Chse Potato Soup, 13 oz	665	29	40%	13	58	1435	21	80
Country Skillets: Idaho "Nachos"	1010	61	54%	20	82	840	30	89
BBQ Chick, Cheddar & Bacon	890	57	58%	16	63	760	24	74
Bacon, Ranch & Cheddar	1090	74	61%	20	71	940	22	87

Papa John's Pizza

	Cal	Fat	%FC	S.Fat	Chol	Sod	Pro	Carb
Per Slice: 1/8 Large Pizza (14")								
Original: All the Meats	410	18	40%	7	35	1040	21	42
Cheese; Garden	300	11	28%	3	20	550	14	37
Pepperoni	310	13	38%	5	25	760	15	35
Sausage	340	13	35%	6	25	810	15	40
The Works	370	17	41%	6	29	840	18	37
Thin Crust: All the Meats	330	20	54%	9	39	920	15	23
Cheese; Garden Special	240	12	46%	6	19	540	9	23
Pepperoni	270	15	50%	7	24	580	11	22
Sausage	270	15	50%	7	29	730	12	22
The Works	320	19	52%	8	35	760	14	24
Cheese Sticks, (2)	160	6	34%	1.5	10	290	7	21

Perkins® Family Restaurant

	Cal	Fat	%FC	S.Fat	Chol	Sod	Pro	Carb
Entrees								
Chicken Dinner	620	13	18%	na	136	1360	60	60
Fish Dinner	470	7	13%	na	133	1390	33	60
Fruit Cup	50	0.5	6%	na	0	10	1	12
'Lite & Healthy'	105	2	18%	na	0	495	3.5	15
Omelette								
Country Club	930	79	76%	na	1154	1135	47	6
Deli Ham & Cheese	960	79	74%	na	864	1830	53	8
'Denver' w. Fruit Cup	235	6.5	25%	na	154	795	23	22
'Everything'	695	54	69%	na	814	870	45	9
Granny's Country	940	82	78%	na	810	785	43	7
w. 9oz Hash Browns	1245	90	64%	na	810	870	48	57
Ham & Cheese	645	51	72%	na	743	830	41	2.5
Mushroom & Cheese	685	60	78%	na	744	925	32	5
Seafood w. Fruit Cup	270	5.5	19%	na	197	595	29	28
Hash Browns, 3 oz	100	2.5	23%	na	na	30	1.5	17
Pita Stir-fry:	310	9	27%	na	26	750	44	41
w. Coleslaw	440	18	36%	na	36	880	45	54
& Pasta Salad	625	33	47%	na	37	1395	49	63
w. Pasta Salad	490	24	44%	na	27	1270	48	50
Salads: Chef's, Mini	215	11	46%	na	55	645	23	7
Muffins: Apple	545	24	40%	na	95	730	9	76
Banana Nut	585	29	45%	na	92	700	9	75
Blueberry	505	23	41%	na	88	670	7	71
Bran	475	17	32%	na	0	570	9	83
Carrot	560	23	37%	na	81	780	7	88
Choc Choc Chip	545	26	43%	na	83	630	10	73
Corn	680	17	22%	na	33	1550	12	121
Cranberry Nut	560	28	45%	na	88	670	9	71
Oat Bran: Regular	515	16	28%	na	0	590	10	87
Plain	585	26	40%	na	104	795	9	81
98% fat-free	495	1	2%	na	5	800	12	111
Pancakes								
Buttermilk, (3)	440	12	24%	na	24	990	13	70
Harvest Grain:								
w. Low-Cal Syrup (5)	475	3.5	6%	na	0	1640	11	93
Short Stack (3)	270	2	7%	na	0	1020	7	56
Syrup, low cal: 1.5 oz	25	0	0%	na	na	0	0	7
Pies (Per Slice): Apple Pie	520	26	45%	na	0	460	3	72
made w. *Equal*	420	24	51%	na	0	370	3	55
Cherry Pie	570	26	41%	na	0	700	4	84
made w. *Equal*	425	24	51%	na	0	510	4	55
Coconut Cream Pie	440	33	68%	na	5	490	6	56
French Silk Pie	550	37	60%	na	53	480	4	59
Lemon Meringue Pie	395	16	36%	na	0	530	2	63
Peanut Butter Brownie	455	35	69%	na	29	435	4	44
Pecan Pie	670	26	35%	na	17	670	7	106

Pizza
Per Slice

	Cal	Fat	%FC	S.Fat	Chol	Sod	Pro	Carb
Bacon: 1/8 large	330	12	33%	na	27	440	17	39
1/8 medium	250	9	32%	na	20	330	13	29
1/4 Express Lunch	180	7	35%	na	16	240	10	21
Beef: 1/8 large	295	8	24%	na	20	480	16	39
1/8 medium	220	6	25%	na	15	360	12	29
1/4 Express Lunch	165	5	27%	na	13	260	9	21
Black Olive: 1/8 large	280	7	22%	na	18	480	14	40
1/8 medium	210	5	21%	na	13	360	11	30
1/4 Express Lunch	160	4	22%	na	12	260	8	21
Cheese: 1/8 large	270	6	20%	na	18	270	14	39
1/8 medium	200	5	22%	na	13	200	11	29
1/4 Express Lunch	150	4	24%	na	12	150	8	21
Extra Cheddar: 1/8 large	300	9	27%	na	27	330	16	39
1/8 medium	225	7	28%	na	19	235	12	29
1/4 Express Lunch	180	6	30%	na	19	195	10	21
Extra Mozzarella: 1/8 large	320	10	28%	na	31	350	18	39
1/8 medium	235	7	27%	na	22	250	13	29
1/4 Express Lunch	175	6	31%	na	18	185	10	21
Green Pepper: 1/8 large	270	6	20%	na	18	270	14	39
1/8 medium	205	5	22%	na	13	200	11	30
1/4 Express Lunch	155	4	23%	na	12	150	8	21
Ham: 1/8 large	275	6	20%	na	21	330	15	39
1/8 medium	210	5	21%	na	15	245	11	29
1/4 Express Lunch	155	4	23%	na	14	190	9	21
Jalapeno: 1/8 large	270	6	20%	na	18	335	14	39
1/8 medium	205	5	22%	na	13	245	10	30
1/4 Express Lunch	150	4	24%	na	12	200	8	21
Mushroom: 1/8 large	205	5	22%	na	13	200	11	30
1/8 medium	180	4	20%	na	12	180	9	29
1/4 Express Lunch	155	4	23%	na	12	150	8	21
Onion: 1/8 large	270	6	20%	na	18	270	14	39
1/8 medium	205	5	22%	na	13	200	10	30
1/4 Express Lunch	155	4	23%	na	12	150	8	21
Pepperoni: 1/8 large	310	9	26%	na	24	555	15	39
1/8 medium	230	7	26%	na	18	430	12	29
1/4 Express Lunch	170	6	32%	na	15	290	9	21
Pineapple; Tomato: 1/8 large	275	6	20%	na	18	270	14	40
1/8 medium	205	5	22%	na	13	200	10	30
1/4 Express Lunch	155	4	23%	na	12	150	8	22
Salami: 1/8 large	290	8	25%	na	23	340	15	39
1/8 medium	215	6	25%	na	17	255	11	29
1/4 Express Lunch	165	5	27%	na	15	200	9	21
Sausage: 1/8 large	300	8	24%	na	21	520	16	39
1/8 medium	225	6	24%	na	15	375	12	29
1/4 Express Lunch	180	6	30%	na	14	360	10	21

Pizza Hut®

	Cal	Fat	%Fc	S.Fat	Chol	Sod	Pro	Carb
Medium Size Pizza: Per Slice								
Stuffed Crust: Cheese	380	11	26%	5	25	1160	21	49
Beef Topping	410	14	30%	6	30	1270	20	49
Ham	380	14	33%	6	45	1250	22	43
Pepperoni	410	17	37%	7	40	1250	20	46
Italian Sausage	430	19	39%	8	35	1200	20	46
Pork Topping	420	16	34%	7	30	1290	22	46
Meat Lover's	500	23	41%	10	60	1510	25	47
Veggie Lover's	390	14	32%	6	25	1140	18	48
Pepperoni Lover's	480	22	41%	9	60	1440	24	47
Supreme	440	16	33%	7	40	1380	25	47
Super Supreme	470	20	38%	8	50	1440	24	51
Chicken Supreme	390	13	30%	6	40	1130	23	46
Stuffed Crust w. Pepperoni: Cheese	455	18	36%	8	56	1255	24	49
Beef Topping	475	20	38%	9	54	1520	26	49
Ham	430	17	36%	7	49	1300	23	48
Pepperoni	460	20	39%	8	53	1355	23	48
Italian Sausage	495	23	42%	9	63	1415	25	49
Pork Topping	495	22	40%	9	56	1445	25	49
Meat Lover's	540	26	43%	11	69	1655	28	49
Pepperoni Lover's	530	25	42%	11	73	1585	27	49
Supreme	505	23	41%	9	59	1580	26	50
Super Supreme	500	22	40%	9	58	1610	26	50
Thin 'n Crispy: Cheese	210	9	38%	4	20	530	12	21
Beef Topping	240	11	41%	5	20	790	13	22
Ham	190	6	28%	3	15	560	10	23
Pepperoni	220	9	37%	4	20	610	10	22
Italian Sausage	300	16	48%	6	35	740	15	24
Pork Topping	270	13	43%	6	25	780	14	22
Meat Lover's	310	16	46%	7	35	900	16	25
Veggie Lover's	170	6	32%	2	10	460	7	23
Pepperoni Lover's	270	12	40%	6	25	780	15	26
Supreme	250	11	40%	5	20	710	13	24
Super Supreme	280	13	42%	5	30	810	15	26
Chicken Supreme	220	7	28%	2	25	550	14	26
Hand Tossed: Cheese	280	10	32%	5	25	770	16	32
Beef	280	10	32%	5	20	860	15	32
Ham	230	6	23%	3	25	710	13	30
Pepperoni	260	9	31%	4	30	750	12	31
Italian Sausage	300	12	36%	5	30	780	15	32
Pork Topping	290	11	34%	5	25	850	14	33
Meat Lover's	290	11	34%	4	35	820	15	32
Veggie Lover's	240	7	26%	3	20	650	11	34
Pepperoni Lover's	320	13	37%	6	35	910	17	31
Supreme	270	9	30%	5	25	760	13	32
Super Supreme	290	10	31%	5	35	830	15	34
Chicken Supreme	240	6	23%	3	25	660	14	31

	Cal	Fat	%FC	S.Fat	Chol	Sod	Pro	Carb
Medium Size Pizza: *Per Slice*								
Pan Pizza: Cheese	300	14	42%	6	25	610	15	30
Beef	310	14	41%	5	20	720	14	31
Ham	250	9	32%	4	10	590	12	31
Pepperoni	280	12	39%	4	20	640	12	31
Italian Sausage	350	18	46%	6	40	740	16	31
Pork Topping	300	13	39%	5	30	720	14	31
Meat/Pepperoni Lover's	360	19	48%	6	40	870	17	30
Veggie Lover's	240	9	34%	3	10	480	10	30
Supreme	300	13	39%	5	25	670	13	32
Super Supreme	340	16	42%	5	30	790	15	33
Chicken Supreme	280	11	35%	3	25	570	14	32
Personal Pan Pizza: Cheese	630	24	34%	11	45	1160	28	76
Pepperoni	670	29	39%	12	60	1250	29	73
Supreme	710	31	39%	13	60	1380	32	76
Entrees/Sandwiches								
Cavatini Pasta	480	14	26%	6	25	1170	21	66
Cavatini Supreme Pasta	560	19	31%	8	30	1400	24	73
Spaghetti w.Meatless Sauce	560	6	10%	<1	5	1285	18	107
Spaghetti w.Meat Sauce	600	13	19%	5	25	910	23	98
Ham & Cheese Sandwich	550	21	34%	7	65	2150	33	57
Supreme Sandwich	640	28	39%	10	85	2150	34	62
Sides: Buffalo Wings, (12)	630	36	51%	9	390	2700	66	12
Wings Dip 'n Blue Cheese	220	24	98%	4	40	440	2	2
Wings Dip 'n Ranch	260	29	100%	4	5	380	0	1
Breadsticks (5)	650	20	28%	5	0	850	15	100
Breadsticks Dipping Sce, 3 oz	70	2	26%	<1	2	550	2	11
Garlic Bread, 1 slice	150	8	48%	2	0	240	16	3
Garlic Dipping Sauce	150	17	100%	3	0	220	0	0

Pizzeria Uno®

	Cal	Fat	%FC	S.Fat	Chol	Sod	Pro	Carb
Thin Crust Pizza: 9" Individual								
Vegetarian: w. Cheese	850	22	23%	12	55	1660	46	127
No Cheese	620	5	7%	1	0	1100	20	124
Soup: Tomato Garden Veg.	125	1	7%	0	0	900	2.5	25
Light Lunch w. Soup	745	6	7%	1	0	2000	23	150
Entrees								
Veggie Burger Meal	610	15	22%	1	0	1800	15	104
Tomato Basil Chicken	570	8	13%	1.5	55	1280	42	83
Zesty Pasta Marinara	380	3.5	8%	0.5	0	800	13	75
Salads: Special House	90	1	10%	0	0	860	4	17
Light Lunch w. Salad	710	6	7%	1	0	1960	24	141
Pasta Green Salad	410	9	13%	1	0	700	14	69
Veggie Dip Platter	460	11	22%	2	0	770	14	77

Popeye's®

	Cal	Fat	%Fc	S.Fat	Chol	Sod	Pro	Carb
Chicken Breast: Mild/Spicy, Fried	270	16	53%	4	60	660	23	9
Chicken Leg: Mild/Spicy, Fried	120	7	52%	2	40	240	10	4
Chicken Thigh: Mild/Spicy, Fried	300	23	69%	6	70	620	15	9
Chicken Wing: Mild/Spicy, Fried	160	11	62%	4	40	290	9	7
Cajun Rice, 4 oz	150	5	30%	1	25	1260	10	17
Coleslaw, 4 oz	150	11	66%	2	3	270	1	14
Corn on the Cob	130	3	21%	1	0	20	4	21
French Fries, 3 oz	240	12	45%	4	10	610	3.5	31
Nuggets, 1 serving	410	32	70%	12	55	660	17	18
Onion Rings, 3 oz	310	19	55%	6	25	210	5	31
Potatoes & Gravy	100	6	54%	2	3	460	5	11
Red Beans & Rice, 6 oz	270	17	57%	4	10	680	8	30
Shrimp	250	16	58%	5	110	650	15	13
Apple Pie	290	16	50%	8	10	820	3	37
Biscuit	250	15	54%	6	3	430	4	26

Quincy's® Family Steak House

	Cal	Fat	%Fc	S.Fat	Chol	Sod	Pro	Carb
Breakfast: Bacon	35	3	77%	1	5	100	2	0
Corned Beef Hash	210	15	64%	8	45	795	10	11
Scrambled Eggs	95	7	66%	2	215	270	7	1
Country Ham	90	6	60%	2	35	1100	9	1
Oatmeal	175	2	10%	0	0	285	4	18
Pancakes	95	3	28%	1	30	250	3	12
Syrup	75	0	0%	0	0	15	0	20
Sausage Gravy	70	6	77%	2	10	150	2	3
Sausage Links	225	22	88%	8	20	390	7	0
Sausage Patties	230	23	90%	9	45	350	7	0
Steak Fingers	360	25	62%	11	50	690	16	18
Steak								
Chopped, 8 oz	500	42	76%	20	89	350	31	0
Country Style Steak w. Gravy	530	25	42%	7	54	1160	32	44
Cowboy Steak, 14 oz	580	33	51%	15	176	1310	61	9
Filet w. Bacon	340	17	45%	7	125	310	48	2
N.Y.Strip Steak, 10 oz	450	26	52%	13	148	155	53	1
Porterhouse Steak	680	46	61%	23	154	345	67	0
Ribeye, 10 oz	450	29	58%	13	116	155	48	0
Sirloin: Large	370	20	49%	9	119	390	46	2
Regular	285	16	50%	7	71	320	34	0
Sirloin Junior	195	10	46%	5	69	200	25	0
Sirloin Tips	205	8	35%	3	63	790	27	4
Smothered Strip Steak	620	41	59%	16	148	240	55	12
T-Bone, 13 oz	520	35	60%	18	118	265	51	0

Continued Next Page

Quincy's® Family Steak House (Cont)

	Cal	Fat	%Fc	S.Fat	Chol	Sod	Pro	Carb
Soups: Chili with Beans	235	11	42%	2	15	920	13	21
Clam Chowder	180	9	45%	1	0	835	3	21
Cream of Broccoli	170	10	53%	1	0	770	2	18
Vegetable Beef	90	2	20%	1	0	325	5	14
Entrees								
Grilled Chicken, regular	125	2	14%	0.5	55	540	25	1
Homestyle Chicken Filet	220	9	37%	2	25	680	13	21
Grilled Salmon	230	4	16%	1	109	110	46	1
Sth Breaded Shrimp	545	31	51%	6	135	820	19	47
Steak & Shrimp	680	39	52%	12	170	820	48	33
Roasted Herb Chicken	875	65	67%	17	340	1240	70	4
Roasted BBQ Chicken	940	65	62%	17	340	1550	70	21
Grilled Trout	300	12	36%	3	115	520	41	2
Sandwiches: No Mayo/Extras								
Bacon Cheeseburger	665	41	55%	17	87	1000	37	33
Grilled Chicken Sandwich	325	4	11%	1	55	1185	33	39
Philly Cheese Steak	590	30	46%	11	87	1685	37	38
Smothered Steak	430	15	31%	6	69	850	34	36
Spicy BBQ Chicken	370	5	12%	1	55	1610	34	45
Breads: Banana Nut	165	7	38%	1	5	195	2	22
Biscuit	270	15	50%	4	11	610	5	29
Cornbread	140	5	32%	1	0	340	3	19
Yeast Roll	160	4	23%	<1	0	285	1	29
Sides: Baked Potatoes	370	0	0%	0	0	25	8	86
Corn on the Cob	140	1	6%	0	0	540	5	33
Rice Pilaf	105	2	17%	0	0	270	2	20
Salad Dressings: Bleu Cheese	155	16	93%	3	10	165	2	2
French: Regular	125	12	86%	1	0	500	0	4
Light	85	4	42%	1	0	285	2	13
Honey Mustard	100	6	54%	1	0	220	2	10
Italian: Regular	135	14	93%	2	0	230	0	3
Light	20	2	90%	0	0	485	2	2
Light Creamy Italian	65	4	55%	0	0	485	2	8
Light Thousand Island	65	4	55%	0	20	340	2	8
Parmesan Peppercorn	150	14	84%	0	0	280	1	4
Ranch	110	11	90%	2	10	195	1	1
Desserts: Banana Pudding	240	12	45%	9	10	240	3	30
Brownie Pudding Cake	310	5	15%	<1	0	395	4	66
Chocolate Chip Cookie	60	3	45%	1	5	35	1	8
Apple Cobbler	255	8	28%	2	5	285	1	49
Cherry Cobbler	410	8	18%	2	5	185	1	55
Peach Cobbler	305	8	24%	2	5	190	1	50
Frozen Yogurt	135	2	13%	1	5	85	5	25
Sugar Cookie	60	3	45%	1	5	30	<1	8
Toppings: Caramel	105	1	8%	<1	0	120	0	24
Fudge	105	4	34%	1	0	75	1	15
Pineapple	70	0	0%	0	0	20	0	20

Rally's Hamburgers®

	Cal	Fat	%Fc	S.Fat	Chol	Sod	Pro	Carb
Rallyburger	435	22	46%	7	63	1175	20	35
with Cheese	490	27	50%	13	78	1375	23	35
Big Buford	745	48	56%	20	151	1860	41	35
Chicken Fillet Sandwich	400	15	34%	4	42	790	21	43
Chili w. Cheese & Onion, 7 oz	360	22	55%	9	74	1145	23	20
13 oz size	670	41	55%	17	137	2125	43	37
Super Barbecue Bacon	595	31	47%	12	88	1710	29	49
Super Double Cheeseburger	760	48	57%	26	154	1735	41	37
French Fries								
Regular	210	11	47%	4	7	295	3	26
Large	320	16	45%	5	10	440	5	39
X-Large	425	21	44%	7	13	585	7	52
Shakes								
Vanilla, small	320	11	31%	6	38	200	9	49
Other flavors, small	410	12	26%	7	38	260	10	73

Rax®

	Cal	Fat	%Fc	S.Fat	Chol	Sod	Pro	Carb
Sandwiches								
Regular Rax	340	22	59%	7	54	710	16	31
Deluxe	520	35	60%	12	69	785	18	34
BBC (Beef Bacon & Cheddar)	715	51	64%	20	102	1455	28	36
Grilled Chicken	525	33	56%	8	69	995	24	32
Jr. Deluxe	370	25	61%	10	42	510	11	25
Barbeque Beef	400	20	45%	7	40	1030	13	43
Mushroom Melt	600	37	56%	13	104	1690	30	35
Turkey Bacon Club	680	46	61%	15	76	1900	29	37
Turkey	485	32	60%	8	50	1285	17	32
Cheddar Melt	345	23	60%	12	41	540	10	26
Philly Melt	540	32	54%	16	78	1295	28	35
Potatoes								
Plain	210	0	0%	0	0	10	0	50
Cheese/Broccoli	280	6	19%	3	4	620	7	50
Cheese	270	6	20%	3	4	620	7	47
Cheese/Bacon	400	19	51%	14	82	875	7	50
Butter	305	11	32%	9	0	30	0	50
Sour Cream Topping	260	4	14%	3	0	30	4	50
Soups								
Cream of Broccoli	170	10	53%	1	0	770	2	18
Chili w. Beans	235	11	42%	2	15	920	13	21
Salads								
Grilled Chicken Caesar	160	5	28%	3	50	1150	23	6
Caesar Side Salad	40	2	45%	1	5	330	2	3
Side Salad	40	4	90%	1	0	90	0	2
Gourmet Garden	220	9	37%	3	5	840	23	12

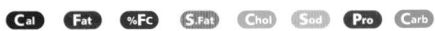

	Cal	Fat	%Fc	S.Fat	Chol	Sod	Pro	Carb

Fish: Per Lunch Portion (5 oz raw wt.)
(For **Dinner Portion** of 10 oz, double the figures.)
Prepared with No Added Fat
Add extra for butter sauce. [1 tsp = 30 cals; 3g fat (90%); 30mg sodium]

	Cal	Fat	%Fc	S.Fat	Chol	Sod	Pro	Carb
Catfish	170	10	53%	3	85	50	20	0
Cod (Atlantic)	100	1	9%	0	70	200	23	0
Flounder	100	1	9%	0	70	95	21	1
Grouper	110	1	8%	0	65	70	26	0
Haddock	110	1	8%	0	85	180	24	2
Halibut	110	1	8%	0	60	105	25	1
Lemon Sole	120	1	7%	0	65	90	27	1
Mackerel	190	12	57%	4	100	250	20	1
Monkfish	110	1	8%	0	80	95	24	0
Norwegian Salmon	230	12	47%	3	80	60	27	2
Ocean Perch (Atlantic)	130	4	28%	1	75	190	24	1
Pollock	120	1	7%	0	90	90	28	1
Rainbow Trout	170	9	48%	3	90	90	23	0
Red Rockfish	90	1	10%	0	85	95	21	0
Red Snapper	110	1	8%	0	70	140	25	0
Sockeye Salmon	160	4	22%	1	50	60	28	2
Swordfish	100	4	36%	1	100	140	17	0
Tilefish	100	2	18%	1	80	60	20	0
Yellowfin Tuna	180	6	30%	2	70	70	32	0
Shellfish								
King Crab Legs 16 oz	170	2	11%	0	100	900	32	6
Snow Crab Legs, 16 oz	150	2	12%	1	130	1630	33	1
Calamari, breaded, fried, 5 oz	360	21	52%	6	140	1150	13	30
Langostino, 5 oz	120	1	8%	0	210	410	26	2
Maine Lobster, 18 oz	240	8	30%	2	310	550	36	5
Rock Lobster, 1 tail, 13 oz	230	3	12%	1	200	1090	49	2
Calico Scallops, 5 oz	180	2	10%	0	115	260	32	8
Deep Sea Scallops, 5 oz	130	2	14%	0	50	260	26	2
Shrimp, 8-12 pces., 7 oz	120	2	15%	0	230	110	25	0
Steaks/Chicken								
Sirloin, 8 oz	350	15	39%	na	150	110	51	0
Strip Steak, 7 oz	690	64	83%	na	140	70	29	0
Hamburger, 1/3 lb	320	23	65%	na	105	70	27	0
Filet Mignon, 8 oz	350	16	41%	na	140	105	47	0
Rib Eye Steak, 12 oz	980	82	75%	na	220	150	56	0
Skinless Chicken Breast, 4 oz	140	3	19%	na	70	60	26	0

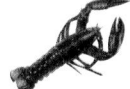

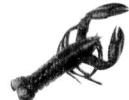

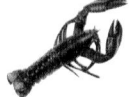

Round Table® Pizza

		Cal	Fat	%Fc	S.Fat	Chol	Sod	Pro	Carb

Large Pizza: Per Slice
(Thin = $1/16$ whole; Pan = $1/12$ whole)

		Cal	Fat	%Fc	S.Fat	Chol	Sod	Pro	Carb
Alfredo Contempo:	Thin	170	6.5	34%	4	25	210	9	17
	Pan	220	7.5	31%	4	25	240	12	27
Bacon Super Deli:	Thin	200	13	58%	5	25	360	9	16
	Pan	260	14	48%	5	25	380	12	26
Cheese:	Thin	160	6	34%	4	20	240	7	16
	Pan	210	7	30%	5	20	250	10	26
Chicken & Garlic Gourmet:									
	Thin	170	7	37%	4	25	280	9	17
	Pan	230	8	31%	4	25	310	11	27
Classic Pesto:	Thin	170	8	42%	4	15	210	7	18
	Pan	230	9	35%	4	15	240	9	27
Garden Pesto:	Thin	170	8	42%	4	15	200	7	18
	Pan	230	8.5	33%	4	15	230	9	28
Gourmet Veggie:	Thin	160	6.5	37%	3	15	200	7	18
	Pan	220	7.5	31%	4	20	230	9	28
Guinevere's Garden Delight:									
	Thin	150	5.5	33%	3	15	250	7	18
	Pan	200	6	27%	4	15	250	9	27
Italian Garlic Supreme:									
	Thin	200	10	47%	4	25	220	8	17
	Pan	250	11	40%	4	25	240	10	27
King Arthur's Supreme:									
	Thin	200	10	45%	3	25	340	9	18
	Pan	240	9	33%	4	25	320	10	27
Pepperoni:	Thin	170	8	42%	3	20	240	8	17
	Pan	220	8	33%	4	20	240	9	26
Salute Chicken & Garlic:									
	Thin	150	5.5	33%	3	20	250	8	18
	Pan	200	6	27%	3	20	270	9	28
Salute Veggie:	Thin	140	5	32%	2	10	170	6	19
	Pan	190	5	24%	3	10	190	8	28
Western BBQ Chicken Supreme:									
	Thin	170	5.5	29%	4	25	330	8	17
	Pan	220	6.5	27%	4	30	360	11	27
Zesty Santa Fe Chicken:									
	Thin	180	8	40%	4	25	310	9	17
	Pan	240	9	34%	5	30	360	11	27
Sandwiches									
Chicken Club		800	38	43%	14	115	1510	39	72
Ham & Honey Mustard		760	33	39%	13	95	1630	36	76
Garden Vegetable		670	29	39%	10	55	990	25	75
Garlic Parmesan Twists (3)		430	15	31%	6	25	690	17	55
Turkey Pesto		830	40	43%	14	85	1200	42	71
Turkey Santa Fe		840	44	47%	16	95	1360	39	72

	Cal	Fat	%Fc	S.Fat	Chol	Sod	Pro	Carb
Breakfast Items: Biscuit	390	21	48%	6	0	1000	6	44
Cinnamon 'N' Raisin Biscuit	370	18	44%	5	0	450	3	48
Sausage Biscuit	510	31	55%	10	25	1360	14	44
Sausage & Egg Biscuit	560	35	56%	11	170	1400	18	44
Bacon Biscuit	420	23	49%	7	5	1140	9	44
Bacon/Ham & Egg Biscuit	470	26	50%	8	150	1190	14	44
Ham & Cheese Biscuit	450	24	48%	8	25	1570	11	48
Ham, Egg & Cheese Biscuit	500	27	49%	10	170	1620	16	48
Sourdough Ham, Egg & Cheese	480	24	45%	9	185	1440	20	45
Big Country Breakfast: with Bacon	740	43	52%	13	305	1800	25	61
with Sausage	920	60	59%	19	340	2230	33	61
with Ham	710	39	49%	11	330	2210	24	67
3 Pancakes	280	2	6%	1	15	890	8	56
with 1 Sausage	430	16	33%	6	40	1290	16	56
with 2 Bacon	350	9	23%	3	25	1130	13	56
Bagel, all types, average	300	2	6%	0.5	0	520	10	60
Hashrowns	230	14	55%	3	0	560	3	24
Burgers								
Hamburger	260	9	31%	4	20	460	11	33
Cheeseburger	300	13	39%	7	25	690	13	34
1/4 lb Hamburger	430	18	38%	8	25	450	25	41
1/4 lb Cheeseburger	470	22	42%	10	30	680	27	42
Sourdough Bacon Cheeseburger	730	46	57%	18	65	1470	35	43
Sourdough Grilled Chicken	500	21	38%	6	45	1530	30	46
Bacon Cheeseburger	490	28	51%	13	35	800	30	29
Sandwiches: Roast Beef	260	4	14%	1	60	700	24	30
Chicken Fillet	500	24	43%	5	20	1050	19	49
Grilled Chicken	340	11	29%	2	30	910	25	32
Fisherman's Fillet (seasonal)	490	21	39%	5	15	1040	21	56
Chicken: Fried: Breast	370	15	36%	4	75	1190	29	29
Wing	200	8	36%	2	30	740	10	23
Thigh	330	15	41%	4	60	1000	19	30
Leg	170	7	37%	2	45	570	13	15
1/4 Roy's Roaster: White Meat	500	29	52%	9	240	1450	56	3
No Skin	190	6	28%	2	100	700	32	2
Dark Meat	490	34	62%	10	225	1120	43	2
No Skin	190	10	47%	3	110	400	24	1
Nuggets: 6 piece	290	18	56%	4	15	610	12	20
Salads: Grilled Chicken	120	4	30%	1	60	520	18	2
Garden	190	14	66%	9	40	280	12	3
Fries: Regular	350	15	39%	4	0	150	5	49
Large	430	18	38%	5	0	190	6	59
Baked Potato: w. Margarine	240	13	49%	2	0	220	3	27
Cornbread	310	17	49%	3	30	260	4	35
Coleslaw, 5 oz	295	25	78%	4	15	430	2	16
Desserts: Hot Fudge Sundae	320	10	28%	5	25	260	8	50
Strawberry Sundae	260	6	21%	3	15	95	6	44

Rubio's Baja Grill®

	Cal	Fat	%Fc	S.Fat	Chol	Sod	Pro	Carb
HealthMex®								
All HealthMex® items have less that 22% of calories from fat.								
Bean & Rice Burrito	340	7	20%	1	5	990	11	58
Burrito w. Chicken/Mahi Mahi	380	9	20%	2	30	960	28	48
Combo	690	13	15%	3	72	1735	51	93
Taco w. Chicken	180	3	15%	1	20	340	14	24
Taco w. Mahi Mahi	190	2	10%	0	35	260	18	25
Taco Combo: w. Chicken	480	8	15%	1	47	1195	33	68
w. Chicken & Mahi Mahi	490	7	15%	1	62	1115	37	69
w. Mahi Mahi	500	7	15%	1	77	1035	41	70
Tacos: Carne Asada	210	7	30%	1	20	520	12	25
Carnitas	290	14	45%	2	45	125	15	24
Fish Taco	280	14	45%	3	30	280	11	28
Fish Taco Especial	370	21	50%	5	45	380	15	29
Grilled Chicken	200	5	20%	1	20	260	14	24
Grilled Mahi Mahi Fish	300	14	40%	3	55	270	21	23
Shrimp	260	13	45%	2	90	430	12	23
Burritos: Bean & Cheese	490	20	35%	4	45	1000	20	57
Carne Asada	470	21	40%	4	45	1460	25	48
Carnitas	640	36	50%	10	100	540	33	47
Chicken	540	25	40%	6	70	1000	35	47
Especial: w. Carne Asada	690	39	50%	6	75	1680	29	56
w. Chicken	670	36	50%	6	75	1220	34	55
w. Carnitas	820	51	55%	8	120	990	36	55
Fish	590	30	45%	4	45	830	21	60
Mahi Mahi	640	31	45%	9	100	870	39	52
Shrimp	480	22	40%	8	130	1200	19	52
Combos: Baja Grill Combo	1100	45	35%	12	65	2440	50	129
Cabo Combo	1190	55	40%	25	160	2200	41	137
Pesky's Combo	1170	61	45%	15	90	1480	41	115
Baja Bowls: Grilled Chicken	260	6	20%	2	10	1440	19	35
Grilled Steak	380	8	20%	3	30	2640	23	55
Los Otros: Nachos Grande	1400	91	60%	18	145	1900	44	109
w. Steak	1520	97	55%	21	180	2650	58	110
w. Chicken	1500	94	55%	19	175	2200	68	110
Kid Pesky® Meals								
Beans	80	1	20%	0	5	200	5	13
Bean/Cheese Burrito	480	20	35%	8	45	810	20	55
Cheese Quesadilla	520	19	35%	9	80	820	22	41
Chips	350	18	45%	6	3	500	6	44
Fish Taco	280	14	45%	9	30	140	11	26
Rice	50	2	35%	0	7	335	1	7
Taquitos	320	17	50%	6	840	420	20	22
Churro, mini	65	4	55%	1	5	60	1	7

Note: Rubio's uses only skinless chicken breast & lean trimmed steak.
Canola oil is used – no lard or MSG. Saturated fat counts are author estimates only.

	Cal	Fat	%Fc	S.Fat	Chol	Sod	Pro	Carb
Microwave Sandwiches								
Oscar Mayer:								
Big Bite w. Bun	300	19	57%	8	30	800	10	22
1/4 Pound Big Bite	480	36	66%	15	60	1370	16	23
Mesquite Jalapeno Bite	380	26	60%	10	0	1100	15	23
Spicy Bite	380	25	60%	10	55	1140	16	22
Croissants								
Egg, Cheese & Bacon	410	28	60%	10	155	880	16	26
Egg, Ham & Cheese	350	22	57%	7	155	950	17	25
English Muffin								
w. Egg/Cheese/Canadian Bacon	270	25	85%	7	240	940	18	21
Biscuit: Sausage/Egg/Cheese	560	41	66%	14	170	1330	16	36
Burritos								
Ramona: Beef & Bean	290	9	27%	4	76	290	16	37
Potato & Beef	340	14	37%	6	33	280	13	41
Bean & Cheese	340	13	34%	6	34	300	15	41
Reynoldos Jumbo Burritos:								
Beef & Bean	630	20	28%	5	10	1470	25	88
Beef & Potato	550	16	26%	5	15	1650	19	82
Bean & Cheese	680	25	33%	10	22	1335	25	88
Red Hot	600	20	30%	5	15	1810	22	82
Green	640	22	31%	7	22	1680	23	85
Chimichanga								
Don Miguel: Chicken	270	8	27%	1.5	20	580	11	37
Shredded Beef	260	9	31%	2	20	610	11	35
Hot & Spicy Beef	280	9	29%	2	15	580	10	39
Fountain Drinks								
(Figures Assume 1/4 Ice)								
Coca-Cola/Pepsi/Dr.Pepper/7Up:								
Gulp, 16 oz	150	0	0%	0	0	15	0	38
Big Gulp, 32 oz	300	0	0%	0	0	30	0	75
Super Gulp, 44 oz	410	0	0%	0	0	40	0	102
Double Gulp, 64 oz	600	0	0%	0	0	60	0	150
Diet Coke/Diet Pepsi:								
(Negligible Calories/Fat)								
Slurpees								
Average All Flavors:								
16 oz size	200	0	0%	0	0	15	0	50
22 oz size	275	0	0%	0	0	20	0	69
32 oz size	400	0	0%	0	0	30	0	100
44 oz size	550	0	0%	0	0	40	0	138

Schlotzsky's® Deli

	Cal	Fat	%FC	S.Fat	Chol	Sod	Pro	Carb
Light/Grilled Sandwiches								
Chicken Breast: Small	350	7.5	20%	1.5	20	1425	24	50
Regular	540	11	20%	3	30	2215	35	77
Dijon Chicken Breast: Small	340	6	15%	1	20	1335	26	50
Regular	520	9	15%	2	30	1965	40	75
Grilled Chicken Breast, small	430	11	25%	3	20	1255	31	52
Santa Fe Grilled Chicken, small	490	16	30%	4	30	1930	35	53
Smoked Turkey Breast: Small	340	5	12%	1	20	1405	23	51
Regular	510	6.5	12%	1	30	2185	34	78
The Vegetarian: Small	340	10	25%	1	0	860	14	50
Regular	510	15	25%	2	0	1260	21	73
Original Sandwiches								
Per Regular Sandwich								
Deluxe	1030	53	45%	16	80	3970	57	79
Ham & Cheese	770	32	40%	12	60	3350	44	78
The Original	800	38	45%	15	60	2315	36	75
Turkey	900	42	45%	12	50	3075	50	78
Local Favorites: Per Regular Sandwich								
BLT	860	48	50%	20	60	1785	28	72
Cheese Original	830	43	45%	13	60	2005	38	75
Classic Italian	780	33	40%	10	60	3405	37	78
Corned Beef	570	16	25%	8	80	2855	37	73
Corned Beef Reuben	840	36	40%	18	90	3560	47	76
Fiesta Schlotzsky's	680	24	30%	10	50	2075	28	90
Pastrami Reuben	960	45	45%	18	90	3860	52	80
Roast Beef	650	20	30%	8	70	1795	42	72
Smoked Brisket BBQ	610	17	25%	8	60	2900	34	81
Texas Schlotzsky's	850	41	45%	14	50	3290	44	78
The Philly	820	29	35%	8	40	2525	57	80
Tuna Melt	790	38	45%	12	40	1825	34	78
Tuna Salad	700	33	45%	10	30	1670	20	78
Turkey Guacamole	760	30	35%	8	30	2870	35	85
Turkey Reuben	900	40	40%	10	50	3800	52	80
Vegetable Club	620	27	40%	7	0	1475	18	74
Western Vegetarian	630	30	40%	8	0	75	18	42
Deli Sandwiches: Per Regular Sandwich								
Grilled Chicken Club	520	20	35%	5	30	1460	35	52
Pastrami & Swiss	920	40	40%	10	50	4055	54	80
Roast Beef & Cheese	870	37	40%	10	60	2510	56	75
Turkey & Bacon Club	1000	53	45%	15	60	3080	56	73
BBQ Sandwiches: Per Regular Sandwich								
Barbeque Beef	710	15	20%	6	50	2440	46	93
Barbeque Pork	870	39	40%	10	50	2650	44	84
Bread (Regular Size)								
Dark Rye Bun	330	1.5	5%	0	0	790	11	68
Sourdough Bun	330	1.5	5%	0	0	860	10	68
Wheat Bun	330	2	5%	0	0	840	13	64

	Cal	Fat	%FC	S.Fat	Chol	Sod	Pro	Carb
Leaf Salads: (No dressing, croutons, chow mein noodles, crackers)								
Caesar Salad	65	4.5	60%	1	0	175	5	2
Chef's Salad	250	13	45%	3	10	1490	23	14
Chicken Caesar Salad	160	5	30%	1	10	445	20	4
Chinese Chicken Salad	180	3	15%	1	10	275	17	13
Greek Salad	190	12	55%	3	10	595	9	14
Smoked Turkey Chef's Salad	230	10	40%	3	10	1340	23	14
Tossed Salad	70	3	40%	0	0	115	2	10
Deli Salads: Per 1/2 Cup								
American Potato Salad	190	7	35%	1	0	1010	2	32
Pasta Salad, 3/4 cup	330	23	60%	6	20	770	5	27
Red Potato Salad w. Dill	260	13	45%	2	0	560	3	20
San Francisco Style Potato Salad	260	17	60%	3	0	600	3	25
White Cole Slaw	250	16	55%	3	10	220	1	14
Soups: Per 8 oz Cup Serving								
7-Bean Medley	200	3	15%	0	0	2000	10	34
Boston Chowder	440	10	25%	3	30	1820	10	26
Chicken Noodle (Old Fashioned)	180	4	15%	1	10	1680	10	24
Cream of Broccoli	380	7	50%	2	10	1860	6	24
Minestrone	140	2	15%	0	0	1740	6	26
Vegetable Vegetarian	100	0	0%	0	0	1420	6	20
Sourdough Crust Pizzas (8")								
Mediterranean	510	19	35%	4	30	815	20	67
Smoked Turkey & Jalapeno	580	17	25%	5	30	1465	36	71
The Original Combination	600	25	40%	12	60	845	24	70
Vegetarian Special	500	15	25%	4	20	570	25	68
Desserts: Per Serving								
Cookies: Chocolate Chip/Chunk	160	7	40%	3	20	140	2	24
Oatmeal Raisin	150	5	35%	2	10	140	1	24
Peanut Butter	170	8	40%	3	20	190	2	24
Other Cookies, average	170	8	40%	3	20	160	2	22
Fudge Brownie Cake	410	25	35%	6	40	135	5	46
New York Style Cheesecake	310	18	55%	8	50	230	7	31
Kid Schlotzsky's								
Kid's Cheese Pizza	450	13	25%	4	20	395	18	66
Peanut Butter & Jelly, small	500	15	25%	4	0	750	14	78
Cheese Sandwich, small	410	17	40%	7	20	970	18	46
Ham & Cheese, small	440	18	35%	7	30	1340	22	47

Note: Figures for saturated fat and cholesterol are author estimates only.

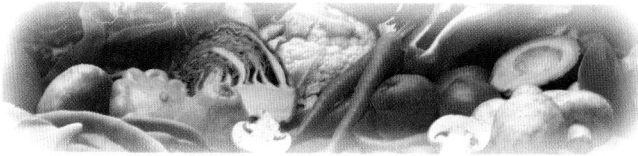

Shakey's®

	Cal	Fat	%FC	S.Fat	Chol	Sod	Pro	Carb
Pizzas (12"): Per Slice (¹/₁₀ Pizza)								
Cheese only:								
Thin Crust	135	5	33%	3	15	320	8	13
Thick Crust	170	5	26%	3	15	420	7	22
Homestyle Pan	305	14	41%	7	20	590	14	31
Onion/Olives/Mushrooms:								
Thin Crust	125	5	36%	3	10	315	7	14
Thick Crust	160	4	22%	2	15	420	9	22
Homestyle Pan	320	15	42%	7	20	650	15	32
Sausage Pepperoni:								
Thin Crust	165	8	44%	5	15	395	9	13
Thick Crust	205	8	35%	5	20	425	11	22
Homestyle Pan	375	20	48%	11	25	680	17	31
Sausage Mushroom:								
Thin Crust	140	6	39%	3	15	335	8	13
Thick Crust	180	6	30%	3	15	420	10	22
Homestyle Pan	340	17	45%	8	25	680	16	31
Pepperoni:								
Thin Crust	150	7	42%	4	15	400	8	13
Thick Crust	185	6	29%	4	15	420	10	22
Homestyle Pan	345	15	39%	9	25	740	16	31
Shakey's Special:								
Thin Crust	170	9	48%	5	15	475	13	13
Thick Crust	210	8	34%	4	20	420	13	22
Homestyle Pan	385	21	49%	11	30	880	18	32
Other Items								
Spagh. w.Meat Sce/Garlic Bread	940	33	32%	10	na	1900	26	134
Potato Wedges, 15 pieces	950	36	34%	10	na	3700	17	120
Shakey's Super Hot Hero	810	44	49%	15	na	2690	36	67
Hot Ham & Cheese Sandwich	550	21	34%	10	na	2135	36	56
5-Piece Fried Chicken & Potato	1700	90	48%	30	na	5330	97	130
3-Piece Chicken & Potato	945	56	53%	18	na	2290	57	51

Note: Saturated fat figures are author estimates only.

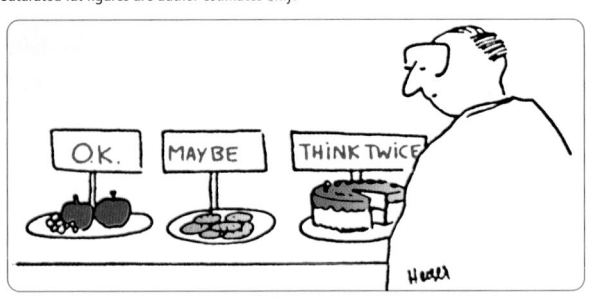

	Cal	Fat	%FC	S.Fat	Chol	Sod	Pro	Carb
Main Menu								
All-American Burger	500	33	59%	11	86	600	25	27
Bacon Burger	590	40	61%	13	86	800	28	29
Baked Fish	170	1	5%	0	83	1640	34	2
Baked Ham Sandwich	290	10	31%	4	42	1265	19	28
Baked Potato, 10 oz	265	0	0%	0	0	15	6	61
Charbroiled Chicken S'wich	450	17	34%	5	90	1000	43	28
Chicken Fillet Sandwich	465	21	41%	7	51	585	30	39
Country Fried Sandwich	590	26	40%	10	29	1500	25	67
Fish 'N Chips w. Fries	640	35	49%	11	103	875	32	50
French Fries, 4 oz	250	10	36%	3	0	365	4	39
Fried Fish, Light	300	14	42%	5	65	535	19	22
Grilled Bacon & Cheese S'wich	440	28	57%	13	36	1200	18	28
Grilled Cheese S'wich	300	17	51%	8	36	880	12	25
Half O'Pound	435	34	70%	12	123	280	32	0
Hawaiian Chicken	260	7	24%	3	85	595	43	7
Italian Feast	500	20	36%	6	74	370	38	44
Lasagna	300	10	30%	3	26	870	8	45
Mushroom Swiss Burger	615	42	61%	13	106	1135	32	29
Old-Fashioned Burger	470	28	54%	11	82	680	25	26
Patty Melt	640	42	59%	19	171	825	39	30
Philly Steak S'wich	675	44	59%	17	103	1245	32	37
Reuben Sandwich	595	35	53%	12	138	3875	33	32
Seafood Platter	566	28	45%	9	127	895	33	46
Shoney Burger	500	36	65%	12	79	785	23	22
Shrimper's Feast	385	22	51%	7	125	215	17	30
Large	575	33	52%	11	188	325	25	45
Slim Jim Sandwich	485	24	45%	8	57	1620	27	40
Spaghetti	495	16	29%	4	55	390	24	63
Steak 'N Shrimp (Charbroiled)	360	23	57%	7	141	200	37	1
Steak "N Shrimp (Fried)	510	33	58%	12	150	250	37	15
Turkey Club/Whole Wheat	635	33	47%	10	100	1290	44	44
Children's Menu								
All-American Jnr Burger	235	11	42%	4	30	545	14	20
Kid's: Chicken Dinner	245	13	48%	4	40	150	21	11
Fish 'N Chips w. Fries	335	17	46%	5	41	460	13	33
Fried Shrimp	195	12	55%	4	70	635	10	12
Spaghetti	250	8	29%	2	27	195	13	32
Desserts								
Apple Pie	490	23	42%	8	35	575	6	67
Carrot Cake	500	26	47%	6	37	475	9	56
Strawberry Pie	330	17	46%	4	0	250	2	45
Walnut Brownie	575	34	53%	15	35	435	10	61
Icecream/Sundaes								
Hot Fudge Cake	525	20	34%	9	27	485	7	82
Hot Fudge Sundae	450	22	44%	10	60	225	7	60
Strawberry Sundae	380	19	45%	8	70	145	2	48

Skipper's ®

	Cal	Fat	%FC	S.Fat	Chol	Sod	Pro	Carb
Chowder: Smoked Salmon	165	7	38%	2	20	75	13	14
Clam: 1 cup	100	3.5	32%	1	12	525	3	14
Entrees: Per Serving								
Chicken: Tenderloin Strip								
w. Fries, 5 pces	795	38	43%	13	77	800	44	69
'Lite Catch', 3 pces	305	15	44%	5	58	675	26	17
Chicken: Strips, Create A Catch	80	4	45%	2	15	150	8	4
Strips, Fish, Fries	805	40	45%	13	100	860	80	72
Strips, Shrimp, Fries	800	39	44%	13	97	1035	36	77
Clam: Strips w. Fries	1005	70	63%	14	50	570	22	90
Strips, Fish, Fries	870	54	56%	18	61	670	25	81
Cod: 3 pces. w. Fries	665	32	43%	10	38	1055	27	68
4 pces. w. Fries	760	36	43%	12	50	1390	34	74
5 pces. w. Fries	855	41	43%	14	62	1725	42	80
Fish Meal: 1 fillet w/Fries	560	28	45%	9	55	410	17	51
2 fillets w. Fries	735	38	47%	13	108	765	28	71
2 pces w. Salad, Lite Catch	410	23	51%	7	120	940	25	27
3 fillets, w. Fries	910	48	48%	16	160	1120	39	82
3 fillets + Salad, small	410	23	51%	7	119	940	25	27
'Create a Catch'	175	10	51%	3	53	360	11	11
Fish, Oysters, Fries	885	44	45%	16	80	810	25	95
Oyster w. Fries, 'Basket'	1040	51	44%	17	52	855	28	118
Salmon, baked	270	11	37%	2	70	505	39	1
Shrimp, Fish, Fries:	730	37	46%	12	105	945	24	77
Jumbo, w. Fries, Basket	710	35	45%	11	73	910	20	79
Original, Fries, Basket	725	36	45%	12	102	1120	20	82
Skipper's Platter Basket	1040	63	55%	20	111	1200	32	97
Sandwiches								
Chicken, 'Create a Catch'	605	32	48%	11	82	975	31	44
Fish: 'Create a Catch', regular	525	33	57%	9	86	1190	19	43
Double	700	73	94%	19	139	1550	30	54
French Fries	385	18	42%	4	2	50	6	50
Potato, baked	145	0	0%	0	0	5	4	32
Salads: Coleslaw	290	27	84%	4	50	330	2	10
Green, small, Lite Catch	60	3	46%	1	13	225	3	6
Shrimp & Seafood	170	3	16%	1	80	660	23	15
Side	25	0	0%	0	0	10	0	4
Salad Dressings & Sauces								
Blue Cheese	220	23	93%	10	8	240	1	4
Italian Gourmet	140	15	96%	3	0	200	0	2
Low Cal	15	1	53%	0	6	80	0	2
Ranch House	190	20	96%	4	0	300	1	2
Thousand Island	160	14	79%	3	6	415	0	8
Barbeque Sauce, 1Tbsp	25	1	36%	0	0	225	0	5
Cocktail Sauce, 1 Tbsp	20	0	0%	0	0	215	0	5
Tartar Sauce, 1Tbsp	65	7	97%	2	4	100	0	0
Root Beer Float	300	10	30%	3	10	65	3	33

Sizzler®

	Cal	Fat	%Fc	S.Fat	Chol	Sod	Pro	Carb
Hot Entrees								
Hamburger	625	33	47%	12	142	335	45	36
Dakota Ranch Steak: 6 oz	315	20	57%	8	100	255	30	0
8 oz	420	27	58%	11	135	340	37	0
9^1/2 oz	500	32	58%	13	160	400	47	0
Hibachi Chicken Breast	195	3	14%	1	65	685	28	13
w. Pineapple								
Lemon-Herb Chicken Breast	140	3	19%	1	65	380	27	0
Malibu Chick. Patty, each	310	19	55%	3	75	590	23	11
Salmon	250	12	44%	2	41	230	32	0
Santa Fe Chicken Breast	150	3	18%	1	65	350	30	0
Shrimp, Broiled	150	6	36%	0	218	375	23	0
Fried, 4 only	225	2	8%	0	118	705	18	35
Mini	150	1	6%	0	80	480	13	24
Shrimp Scampi	145	3	19%	1	150	385	27	0
Swordfish	315	14	40%	3	89	330	45	0
Accompaniments								
Cheese Toast, 1 pce	275	21	69%	5	5	495	6	16
French Fries	360	12	30%	6	0	245	5	45
Potato, Baked, Flesh Only	105	0	0%	0	0	5	2	24
Rice Pilaf	260	5	18%	1	0	865	4	47
Condiments: *Per 1^1/2 oz*								
Sauces:								
Buttery Dipping	330	37	100%	7	0	0	0	0
Cocktail	40	0	0%	0	0	395	0	8
Hibachi	60	0	0%	0	0	710	0	11
Malibu	285	31	99%	6	28	355	0	0
Marinara, 1 oz	15	0	0%	0	0	90	0	3
Nacho Cheese, 2 oz	120	10	75%	5	30	600	5	3
Sour Dressing	90	9	91%	8	0	45	0	0
Tartar	170	17	90%	3	14	455	0	6
Margarine, Whipped, 1^1/2 T.	105	12	100%	2	0	145	0	0
Hot Bar								
Broccoli Cheese Soup, 4 oz	140	9	58%	2	8	355	3	10
Chicken Noodle Soup, 4 oz	30	1	29%	0	7	495	2	4
Chicken Wings, 1 oz	75	4	49%	1	20	135	4	4
Clam Chowder, 4 oz	120	6	46%	0	6	510	3	11
Focaccia Bread, 2 pces	110	7	58%	1	0	135	2	9
Meatballs, 4 balls	155	11	63%	5	30	460	9	5
Minestrone Soup, 4 oz	35	0	0%	0	0	445	1	7
Pasta, Fettucine, 2 oz	80	1	11%	0	5	5	3	15
Pasta, Spaghetti, 2 oz	80	0	0%	0	0	0	3	16
Potato Skins, 2 oz	160	8	45%	1	0	465	2	22
Refried Beans, ^{1}/4 cup	60	1	15%	2	5	270	4	11
Saltine Crackers, 2 crackers	25	1	36%	0	2	75	1	4
Taco Filling, 2 oz	105	9	79%	4	16	230	2	3
Taco Shells, each	50	2	36%	0	0	20	1	7

	Cal	Fat	%FC	S.Fat	Chol	Sod	Pro	Carb
Salads & Toppings								
Prepared Salads: *Per 2 oz*								
Carrot & Raisin	130	10	69%	2	10	105	1	10
Chinese Chicken	55	2	33%	0	10	120	4	6
Mediterranean Minted Fruit	30	0	0%	0	0	10	1	7
Mexican Fiesta	55	1	17%	0	0	100	2	10
Old Fashioned Potato	85	5	53%	1	10	230	1	10
Red Herb Potato	120	9	67%	1	10	270	1	9
Seafood Louis Pasta	65	2	28%	0	15	140	3	9
Seafood	55	3	48%	1	7	255	3	4
Spicy Jicama	15	0	0%	0	0	30	0	4
Teriyaki Beef	50	2	37%	1	7	135	4	5
Tuna Pasta	135	10	68%	1	10	190	6	6
Sides								
Cottage Cheese, 2 oz	50	1	18%	1	5	230	8	2
Eggs, 1 oz	45	3	61%	1	120	35	4	0
Garbanzo Beans, 1/4 cup	65	1	14%	0	0	255	3	11
Turkey Ham, 1 oz	60	5	73%	2	19	375	4	0
Kidney Beans, 1/4 cup	50	0	0%	0	0	220	3	10
Olives, 1 oz	60	6	87%	1	0	180	1	1
Peas, 1/4 cup	30	0	0%	0	0	35	2	6
Peaches, 1/4 cup	35	0	0%	0	0	5	0	9
Real Bacon Bits, 1 Tbsp	30	2	67%	0	0	165	2	2
Dressings & Condiments: Per 1 oz								
Dressing: Blue Cheese	110	12	98%	4	8	170	1	1
Honey Mustard	160	16	90%	2	10	110	0	4
Italian, Lite	15	0	0%	0	0	350	0	2
Japanese Rice Vinegar, Fat Free	10	0	0%	0	0	180	0	2
Parmesan Italian	100	10	90%	2	0	450	0	2
Ranch	120	12	90%	2	10	240	0	2
Ranch, Reduced-Calorie	90	8	80%	2	10	270	0	4
Thousand Island	145	15	94%	2	10	125	0	3
Guacamole	40	4	86%	1	0	425	0	2
Salsa	10	0	0%	0	0	155	0	2
Sour Dressing, 2 Tbsp	60	6	90%	5	0	30	0	0
Dessert Bar								
Choc/Van. Soft Serve, 4 oz	135	4	26%	4	0	100	1	24
Chocolate Syrup, 1 oz	90	0	0%	0	0	15	0	21
Strawberry Topping, 1 oz	70	0	0%	0	0	5	0	18
Whipped Topping, 1 Tbsp	10	1	75%	1	0	0	0	1

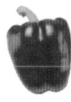

	Cal	Fat	%FC	S.Fat	Chol	Sod	Pro	Carb
Soups: Per 1 Cup								
Low Fat: Soup: Chicken Tortilla	100	3	27%	1	20	990	12	5
Chicken/Turkey Noodle	160	3	17%	2	20	480	15	17
Sweet Tomato Onion	110	3	25%	1	0	450	2	12
Vegetable Medley	90	1	10%	0	0	520	2	14
Regular Soup: Albondigas Buenas	190	9	43%	4	15	720	12	17
Chesapeake Corn Chowder	310	13	38%	5	20	720	12	43
Chicken Fajitas & Black Bean	280	7	23%	2	20	980	22	33
Chicken Jambalaya	160	7	39%	2	30	980	12	13
Chunky Potato Cheese	210	10	43%	6	30	480	10	19
Cream of Broccoli/Chicken	250	15	54%	6	40	350	11	14
Cream of Mushroom	290	21	65%	8	30	820	10	15
Irish Potato Leek	260	16	55%	8	35	680	5	23
Minestrone w.Italian Sausage	210	11	47%	4	20	890	13	14
Navy Bean w.Ham	340	10	26%	4	40	980	35	30
New England Clam Chowder	330	20	55%	10	80	630	18	21
New Orleans Style Jambalaya	160	8	45%	3	30	900	8	14
Shrimp Bisque	300	19	57%	8	70	880	11	20
Split Pea Ham; Turk. Cassoulet	350	10	26%	4	40	980	36	32
Turkey Vegetable	270	12	40%	4	40	990	22	16
Vegetarian Harvest	190	8	38%	2	0	990	5	23
Chili: Arizona /Texas Red	230	8	31%	4	20	680	14	30
Yucatan Chili	280	10	32%	4	40	890	28	31
House Chili	230	3	12%	2	15	560	15	26
Santa Fe´ Black Bean Chili	190	3	14%	0	0	580	9	26
Fresh Tossed Salads: Per 1 Cup								
Antipasto Salad; BBQ Aver.	140	10	64%	3	15	350	5	6
Caribbean Krab Salad	120	7	68%	1	110	180	5	10
Classic Caesar Salad	190	14	66%	2	10	280	5	10
Ensalada Azteca	130	9	62%	3	15	230	6	7
Greek Salad	120	9	68%	3	10	320	3	4
Mandarin Spinach w.Walnuts	170	11	58%	1	0	150	3	14
Roma Tomato, Mozzarella & Basil	120	9	68%	2	10	180	4	5
Shrimp & Krab Louis; Spinach	180	12	60%	4	190	340	10	6
Sonoma w. Artichokes	160	12	68%	2	0	640	2	8
Spinach & Pasta w.Raspb. Vin.	180	6	40%	0	0	620	6	22
Won Ton Chicken Salad	150	8	48%	1	10	220	6	12
Prepared Salads: Per 1/2 Cup								
Artichoke Rice	160	8	45%	1	3	780	3	21
Aunt Doris' Red Pepper Slaw	70	0	0%	0	0	480	18	18
Baja Bean & Cilantro	180	3	15%	0	0	190	9	29
BBQ Potato	160	8	45%	1	5	270	2	20
Carrot Raisin	90	3	30%	0	5	80	1	17
Chinese Krab	160	8	45%	1	3	260	5	19
Confetti Pasta w. Cheddar & Dill	160	9	45%	2	10	380	5	16
Cucumber Tomato w.Chile Lime	20	0	0%	0	0	20	1	4
Dijon Potato w. Garlic Dill Vin.	140	7	51%	1	0	260	3	16

	Cal	Fat	%Fc	S.Fat	Chol	Sod	Pro	Carb
Salads (Cont): *Per 1/2 Cup*								
German Potato; Gemeilli Pasta	130	3	21%	0	5	380	5	20
Greek Couscous w. Feta Cheese	170	9	42%	1	4	480	6	19
Mazatian Krab & Pasta	160	9	45%	1	2	480	4	15
Mandarin Krab Salad	150	3	18%	0	2	280	5	26
Mandarin w. Broccoli/Almonds	120	3	23%	0	0	380	3	19
Marinated Summer Vegetables	80	0	0%	0	0	210	1	19
Mediterranean Harvest	120	3	23%	1	2	180	3	17
Mediterranean Krab & Rotini	170	10	53%	1	2	380	4	15
Moroccan Marinated Vegetables	90	3	30%	0	0	230	2	9
Old Fashioned Macaroni w. Ham	180	11	55%	2	10	360	4	15
Oriental Ginger Slaw w. Krab	70	3	39%	0	2	80	2	8
Pesto Pasta; Picnic Potato	160	7	39%	1	2	320	4	18
Pineapple Coconut Slaw	150	10	60%	3	15	190	1	14
Poppyseed Coleslaw	120	9	68%	1	10	130	1	9
Rst. Potato w. Chipotle Chile	140	6	39%	1	0	250	3	18
Southern Dill Potato	120	3	23%	2	5	300	4	20
Spicy Southwestern Pasta	130	3	21%	0	0	350	5	21
Spinach Krab	230	12	47%	2	15	550	5	25
Summer Barley w. Black Beans	110	3	25%	0	0	280	4	19
Thai Noodle w. Peanut Sce	170	8	42%	1	0	310	5	17
Three Bean Marinade	170	6	32%	1	0	320	4	27
Tortellini Salad w. Basil	170	10	53%	2	2	260	4	14
Tumbleweed Tortellini	140	9	58%	1	2	330	4	11
Tuna Tarragon	240	14	53%	2	10	480	6	21
Turkey Chutney Pasta	230	9	35%	2	30	310	14	21
Zesty Tortellini	190	15	71%	2	10	460	4	18
Dressing & Croutons: *Per 2 Tbsp*								
Garlic Parmesan w. Croutons (10)	40	3	68%	1	2	160	2	2
Blue Cheese Dressing	140	14	90%	2.5	10	230	1	3
Blush Vinaigrette	120	12	90%	2	0	320	0	3
Creamy Cucumber Dressing	80	7	79%	1	0	290	0	4
Garden French Tomato	40	1.5	34%	0	0	270	0	7
Honey Mustard Dressing	150	13	78%	2	10	230	0	8
Fat Free	45	0	0%	0	10	160	0	10
Parmesan Pepper Cream	160	17	97%	2.5	5	330	1	2
Ranch House Dressing	130	13	90%	2	10	180	1	1
Fat Free	50	0	0%	0	0	180	1	2
Raspberry Vinaigrette	120	13	98%	2	0	150	0	3
Thousand Island Dressing	110	11	90%	1.5	5	250	0	3
Zesty Italian Dressing	160	18	100%	2.5	0	280	0	1
Fat Free	20	0	0%	0	0	340	0	5
Hot Tossed Pastas: *Per Cup*								
Bruschetta	260	4	(14%)	2	10	450	10	41
Creamy	360	16	(40%)	8	45	510	12	43
Chipotle Chicken w. Cilantro	390	16	(37%)	9	50	560	22	42
Creamy Pesto w. Sundried Tomatoes	430	21	(34%)	9	45	410	14	44

	Cal	Fat	%Fc	S.Fat	Chol	Sod	Pro	Carb
Tossed Pastas (continued)								
Fettucine Alfredo	390	18	42%	10	50	580	15	41
Garden Vegetable: w. Meatballs	270	7	23%	3	10	460	11	42
w. Italian Sausage	300	10	30%	3	20	540	12	42
Italian Vegetable Beef	270	6	20%	2	10	470	12	43
Jalapeno Salsa	240	4	42%	2	10	430	10	41
Nutty Mushroom	390	20	46%	9	45	410	12	41
Smoked Salmon & Dill	360	16	40%	8	45	390	13	41
Vegetarian Marinara w. Basil	260	4	14%	2	10	750	10	44
Muffins: Per Muffin								
96% Fat Free: All types	80	0.5	5%	0	0	110	2	17
Regular: Apple Raisin	150	7	42%	1	10	190	2	22
Apricot/Banana/Cherry Nut	150	7	42%	1	10	190	2	22
Carrot Pineapple w. Oat Bran	150	6	36%	1	10	230	3	23
Chili Corn	140	3	19%	1	10	320	3	22
Chocolate Varieties	170	8	42%	2	10	190	3	22
Georgia Peach Poppyseed	150	6	36%	1	10	210	2	20
Lemon	140	4	35%	1	10	190	2	19
Mandarin Almond w. Oat Bran	140	7	45%	1	10	210	3	20
Nutty Peanut Butter	170	8	42%	1	10	210	4	21
Peanut Butter Choc. Chip	190	9	43%	2	10	230	5	23
Pumpkin Raisin	150	6	36%	1	10	210	2	25
Strawberry Buttermilk	140	6	39%	1	10	210	2	21
Wild Maine Blueberry	140	5	32%	1	10	180	2	22
Large	310	12	35%	2	20	380	5	40
Zucchini Nut	150	7	42%	1	10	190	2	22
Breads: Buttermilk Corn	140	2	13%	0	10	270	3	27
Indian Grain	200	1.5	7%	0	15	260	11	35
Sourdough	150	0.5	3%	0	0	240	9	27
Focaccia: Garlic Parmesan	100	3	27%	0	0	170	2	15
Pizza /Tomarillo	140	6	39%	2	10	270	5	16
Desserts: Per 1/2 Cup								
Apple Medley	70	0	0%	0	0	5	1	18
Banana Royale	80	0	0%	0	0	5	1	20
Chocolate Chip Cookie, small	70	3	39%	1	5	90	1	10
Chocolate Pudding	140	4	26%	0	10	220	4	23
Ghirardelli Chocolate Frozen	95	0	0%	0	0	80	3	21
Jello, flavored	80	0	0%	0	0	40	1	20
Rice Pudding	110	2	16%	1	10	50	3	20
Tapioca Pudding	140	3	19%	0	10	160	4	24
Tropical Fruit Salad	75	0	0%	0	0	5	1	19
Vanilla Pudding	140	3	19%	0	10	160	4	24
Vanilla Soft Serving	140	4	26%	3	20	70	3	22
Choc. Syrup, 2 Tbsp	70	0	0%	0	10	15	0	18
Candy Sprinkles, 1 Tbsp	70	2	26%	0	0	0	0	11
Granola Topping, 2 Tbsp	110	4	33%	2	0	14	2	16

Sonic® Drive-In

	Cal	Fat	%Fc	S.Fat	Chol	Sod	Pro	Carb
Hamburgers: #1. Hamburger	410	27	59%	10	58	445	20	23
with Cheese	480	32	60%	15	76	710	24	24
#2. Hamburger	325	16	44%	5	50	550	20	23
with Cheese	395	21	48%	10	67	815	24	24
Bacon Cheeseburger	550	39	64%	18	87	840	28	23
Hickory Burger	315	16	46%	6	50	460	20	23
Jalapeno Burger	640	41	58%	12	136	1360	44	22
Super Sonic w. Mayonnaise	730	52	64%	14	144	1025	44	24
with Mustard	645	41	57%	12	136	1130	44	24
Mini Burger	245	12	44%	4	36	510	14	20
Mini Cheeseburger	280	14	45%	6	45	645	17	20
Sandwiches: Steak (breaded)	630	42	60%	14	50	1050	19	46
Chicken (breaded)	455	25	49%	9	42	755	23	36
Grilled Chicken, no dressing	215	4	17%	1	63	715	21	23
Fish	280	7	23%	2	6	655	17	38
B-L-T	325	19	52%	7	9	600	8	27
Grilled Cheese	290	17	53%	8	36	840	12	25
Coneys/Local Flavors: Chili Pie	330	23	63%	8	28	315	12	20
Regular Hot Dog	260	15	52%	6	23	240	8	21
Regular Cheese Coney	360	23	58%	10	40	340	14	23
Extra-Long Cheese Coney	635	39	55%	18	65	630	24	45
Corn Dog	280	15	48%	7	35	700	7	30
Sides: French Fries; regular	235	8	31%	3	8	50	3	37
Large	315	11	31%	4	11	70	5	50
w. Cheese, large	420	20	43%	10	38	470	11	51
Onion Rings: Regular	405	27	60%	13	na	370	5	38
Tater Tots	150	7	42%	3	10	330	2	19
Tater Tots, w. Cheese	220	13	53%	6	28	570	6	19

Spaghetti Warehouse®

	Cal	Fat	%Fc	S.Fat	Chol	Sod	Pro	Carb
Lunch: Minestrone Soup	80	1.5	17%	0.5	2	1040	4	12
Grilled Chicken Marinara	530	8	14%	1.5	96	400	46	65
Seafood Marinara	385	5	12%	1	48	400	19	65
Spaghetti: w. Tomato Sauce	425	5	10%	0.5	0	490	13	82
w. Marinara Sauce #12	440	5	10%	1	0	400	14	84
Spicy Marinara Sce Spaghetti	280	4	13%	1	2	280	9	52
Vegetable Primavera	340	4	10%	0.5	0	345	12	65
Dinner: Minestrone, 1 bowl	110	2	16%	1	3	1495	6	18
Grilled Chicken Marinara	640	10	14%	2	96	550	50	85
Grilled Halibut	880	14	14%	2	93	780	78	106
Grilled Marinated Chick. Breast	910	17	17%	3	145	825	74	116
Marinara Sauce #12	520	6	16%	1	0	390	17	99
Seafood Marinara	520	8	14%	1	77	605	27	86
Spaghetti w. Tomato Sauce	525	6	10%	1	0	650	17	101
Spicy Marinara Sce Spaghetti	330	6	16%	1.5	3	410	10	60
Vegetable Primavera	610	8	12%	1	0	660	21	116

	Cal	Fat	%FC	S.Fat	Chol	Sod	Pro	Carb
Steakburgers & Sandwiches								
Steakburger	275	7	23%)	2	60	425	18	33
with Cheese	355	13	33%	6	80	660	23	33
Super	375	12	29%	4	100	445	30	33
Super with Cheese	450	18	36%	8	120	680	35	33
Triple	475	17	32%	8	160	470	43	33
Triple with Cheese	625	30	43%	15	180	935	52	34
Ham Sandwich	450	22	44%	7	na	1860	29	37
Grilled Cheese Sandwich	250	13	47%	6	20	610	9	24
Grilled Chicken Sandwich	510	22	39%	5	85	1150	26	53
Other Items: French Fries	210	10	43%	3	10	300	3	28
Chili & Oyster Crackers	335	14	38%	4	na	1160	16	37
Chili Mac & 4 Saltines	310	12	35%	3	na	1300	15	34
Chili 3 Ways & 4 Saltines	410	16	35%	4	na	1730	19	45
Baked Beans	175	4	21%	1	0	655	9	27
Lett./Tom/ Salad/1oz 1000 Island	170	15	79%	3	15	225	1	7
Chef Salad	315	18	51%	5	120	1580	41	6
Cottage Cheese, $^1/_2$ cup	95	4	38%	1	20	200	12	3
Desserts: Apple Danish	390	24	55%	6	30	350	6	35
Brownie	260	12	42%	4	10	165	3	39
Cheesecake	370	11	27%	5	60	295	7	61
with Strawberries	385	11	26%	5	60	295	7	65
Pies: Apple	405	18	40%	5	40	480	4	61
Cherry	335	14	38%	4	30	270	6	48
Apple, A La Mode	550	25	41%	9	80	525	4	76
Cherry, A La Mode	475	22	42%	7	70	315	6	63
Sundaes: Brownie Fudge	645	35	49%	15	30	260	7	81
Hot Fudge Nut	530	34	58%	14	60	120	5	51
Strawberry	330	22	60%	8	50	80	2	29
Vanilla Ice Cream	215	12	50%	6	40	70	1	23
Shakes & Drinks: Hot Chocolate	685	19	25%	6	50	670	17	129
Floats: Coca-Cola	515	17	30%	8	0	230	16	76
Orange	500	17	31%	8	0	225	16	74
Lemon	555	19	31%	9	0	250	18	82
Root Beer	530	17	29%	8	0	240	17	78
Freezes: Lemon	550	25	41%	10	0	215	15	69
Orange	515	24	42%	10	0	200	14	63
Shakes: Chocolate/Vanilla	610	38	56%	10	100	180	13	57
Strawberry	650	40	55%	11	100	190	16	62

(Cholesterol & Saturated Fat Figures - Estimates only)

Sub Station®

	Cal	Fat	%FC	S.Fat	Chol	Sod	Pro	Carb
Sandwiches: Ham/Turkey & Cheese	510	30	53%	na	na	1160	18	40
Roast Beef/Turkey & Cheese	525	31	54%	na	na	1045	24	39
Salami, Pepperoni, Turkey								
Bologna, Ham, Cheese	635	42	60%	na	na	1590	23	40

Subway®

	Cal	Fat	%Fc	S.Fat	Chol	Sod	Pro	Carb
6" Cold Subs: Cheese & Condiments Not Included								
Classic Italian BMT	450	21	44%	8	52	1580	21	45
Cold Cut Trio	375	14	33%	5	47	1435	19	45
Ham	295	5	15%	2	25	1340	18	45
Roast Beef	295	5	15%	2	20	930	19	45
Subway Club	305	5	16%	2	26	1240	21	46
Subway Seafood & Crab w. Light Mayo.	340	9	24%	2	14	1355	14	51
Tuna w. Light Mayonnaise	380	14	33%	3	32	940	18	45
Turkey Breast	280	4	13%	1	20	1170	17	45
& Ham	290	4	14%	2	23	1255	18	45
Veggie Delite	230	3	11%	1	0	580	9	43
6" Hot Subs: Cheese & Condiments Not Included Unless Indicated								
Meatball	415	15	33%	6	35	1025	19	50
Roasted Chicken Breast	340	6	16%	2	48	965	26	46
Steak & Cheese	365	10	24%	4	37	1160	24	47
Subway Melt (w. cheese)	370	11	27%	5	35	1025	20	23
Super Subs: Cheese & Condiments Not Included								
Classic Italian BMT	670	39	52%	14	104	2575	33	47
Cold Cut Trio	520	7	12%	2	52	1895	29	47
Subway Club	380	7	16%	2	52	1895	32	48
Wraps: Condiments Not Included								
Chicken Parmesan Ranch	335	5	96%	2	45	1395	17	56
Steak & Cheese	355	9	0%	4	37	1450	16	53
Turkey Breast & Bacon	355	10	0%	4	39	1825	14	52
Deli Style Sandwiches: Cheese & Condiments Not Included Unless Indicated								
Bologna	290	12	37%	4	20	745	10	38
Ham	225	3	12%	0	12	830	12	37
Roast Beef	235	4	15%	0	13	680	14	37
Tuna w. Light Mayonnaise	270	8	26%	1	16	630	12	37
Turkey Breast	230	3	12%	0	13	840	13	37
Salads: Cheese & Condiments Not Included Unless Indicated								
Classic Italian BMT	270	20	66%	7	52	1305	14	11
Cold Cut Trio	195	12	55%	4	47	1160	12	12
Ham	110	3	24%	1	25	1070	12	11
Meatball	230	13	51%	5	35	750	13	17
Pizza (w. cheese)	320	20	56%	10	50	1335	12	13
Roast Beef	115	3	23%	1	20	655	12	11
Roasted Chicken Breast	160	4	23%	1	48	695	20	13
Steak and Cheese	180	8	40%	4	37	900	17	13
Subway Club	125	3	22%	1	26	965	14	12
Subway Melt (w. cheese)	190	9	42%	4	41	1345	16	12
Subway Seafood & Crab w. Light Mayo	160	7	39%	1	14	760	7	17
Tuna Salad w. Light Mayonnaise	200	12	54%	2	32	670	11	11
Turkey Breast and Ham	105	2	17%	1	23	980	11	11
Turkey Breast Salad	100	2	18%	0	20	895	11	12
Veggie Delite Salad	50	1	18%	0	0	310	2	10

	Cal	Fat	%FC	S.Fat	Chol	Sod	Pro	Carb
Breads/Wraps								
6" White Bread	190	1	5%	1	0	420	7	38
6" Wheat Bread	210	3	13%	1	0	430	8	39
Deli Style Roll	170	2	10%	1	0	350	6	31
10 oz Tortilla	200	2	10%	1	0	720	0	45
Condiments & Extras								
Bacon, 2 strips	40	3	64%	1	9	160	3	0
Cheese, 2 triangles	40	3	67%	2	10	205	2	0
Mayonnaise, 1 Tbsp	40	4	90%	1	3	30	0	0
Light Mayonnaise, 1 Tbsp	15	2	100%	0	2	35	0	0
Mustard, 2 tsp	10	1	90%	0	0	115	0	0
Olive Oil Blend, 1 Tbsp	45	5	100%	1	0	0	0	0
Vinegar, 1 Tbsp	1	0	0%	0	0	0	0	0
Salad Dressings: Per 2 oz Packet								
Creamy Italian, 1 pkt	260	28	97%	4	16	530	0	12
Fat-Free Italian, 1 pkt	20	0	0%	0	0	610	0	4
French, 1 pkt	280	24	85%	4	0	400	0	20
Fat-Free, 1 pkt	70	0	0%	0	0	390	0	16
Thousand Island, 1 pkt	260	28	97%	4	32	620	0	12
Ranch, 1 pkt	350	40	73%	8	24	470	0	8
Fat-Free, 1 pkt	60	0	0%	0	0	710	0	16
Cookies: Per Cookie								
Brazil Nut	215	10	42%	3	14	155	2	29
Chocolate Chip/Chunk; M & M	215	10	42%	3	15	145	2	29
Macadamia Nut	220	11	45%	2	12	145	2	28
Oatmeal Raisin	200	8	36%	2	14	160	3	29
Low Fat Oatmeal Raisin	170	3	16%	1	15	170	3	33
Peanut Butter	225	12	48%	2	0	215	3	27
Sugar Cookie	225	12	48%	3	18	180	2	28

Sweet Tomatoes®

~ Same Menu & Data as Souplantation (Page 233) ~

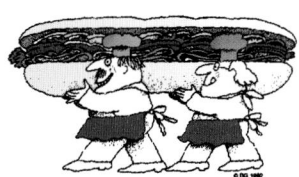

Taco Bell®

	Cal	Fat	%FC	S.Fat	Chol	Sod	Pro	Carb
Tacos								
Taco, regular	170	10	53%	4	30	340	9	12
Taco Supreme®	210	14	60%	6	40	350	9	14
Soft Taco	210	10	43%	4	30	570	11	20
Soft Taco Supreme®	260	13	45%	6	40	590	11	22
Double Decker® Taco	330	15	40%	5	30	740	14	37
Double Decker® Taco Supreme	380	18	42%	7	40	760	15	39
Grilled Steak Soft Taco	200	7	31%	2.5	25	570	14	19
Grilled Steak Soft Taco Supreme®	240	11	41%	5	35	580	15	21
Grilled Chicken Soft Taco	200	7	31%	2.5	35	530	14	20
Gorditas								
Gordita Supreme™ Beef	300	16	48%	5	35	550	17	27
Gordita Supreme™ Chicken; Steak	300	13	40%	5	45	530	16	28
Grodita Santa Fe™ Beef	380	23	54%	5	35	700	14	31
Grodita Santa Fe™ Chicken; Steak	370	20	48%	4	40	610	17	30
Gordita Baja™ Beef	380	21	50%	5	35	920	13	29
Gordita Baja™ Chicken; Steak	340	18	47%	4	40	930	17	28
Chalupas								
Chalupa Supreme™ Beef	380	23	55%	8	40	580	14	29
Chalupa Supreme™ Chicken	360	20	50%	7	45	490	17	28
Chalupa Supreme™ Steak	380	23	55%	7	35	500	17	27
Chalupa Santa Fe™ Beef	440	29	60%	7	35	650	14	31
Chalupa Santa Fe™ Chicken; Steak	420	26	56%	5	40	580	17	30
Chalupa Baja™ Beef	420	27	58%	7	35	760	14	30
Chalupa Baja™ Chicken; Steak	400	24	54%	6	35	660	17	28
Burritos								
Bean Burrito	370	12	30%	3.5	10	1080	13	54
Burrito Supreme®	430	17	36%	6	40	1210	17	50
Big Beef Burrito	400	23	52%	9	50	1320	19	43
Big Beef Burrito Supreme®	510	23	40%	10	60	1500	23	52
Chili Cheese Burrito	330	13	35%	5	25	900	13	40
7-Layer Burrito	520	22	38%	7	25	1210	18	65
Grilled Chicken Burrito	380	16	38%	4	40	1240	19	45
Big Chicken Burrito Supreme®	460	11	21%	6	70	1200	27	50
Speciality Items								
Big Beef Meximelt®	290	16	49%	7	45	830	15	22
Cheese Quesadilla	350	18	46%	9	50	880	16	31
Chicken Quesadilla	400	19	43%	9	75	1050	25	33
Mexican Pizza	540	35	58%	10	45	1030	20	42
Chicken	520	32	55%	8	50	940	23	41
Steak	530	33	56%	9	45	950	24	39
Tostada	250	12	43%	5	15	640	10	27
Taco Salad w. Salsa & Shell	850	52	55%	14	70	2250	30	69
Taco Salad w. Salsa, w/out Shell	430	22	46%	10	70	1990	25	36
Nachos and Sides: Nachos	320	18	50%	4	5	560	5	34
Big Beef Nachos Supreme	440	24	50%	7	35	820	14	44
Nachos BellGrande®	760	39	46%	11	35	1300	20	83

	Cal	Fat	%FC	S.Fat	Chol	Sod	Pro	Carb
Nachos and Sides (Cont):								
Nachos BellGrande® Chicken; Steak	740	36	44%	9	40	1200	23	82
Pintos 'N Cheese	180	8	40%	4	15	640	9	18
Mexican Rice	190	10	47%	3.5	15	750	5	23
Cinnamon Twists	180	8	40%	2	3	190	1	25
Side Items/Condiments								
Border/Picante Sauce, 1/3 oz	0	0	0%	0	0	90	0	0
Fiesta Salsa, 3/4 oz	5	0	0%	0	0	55	0	1
Green Sauce, 1 oz	5	0	0%	0	0	150	0	1
Guacamole, 3/4 oz	35	3	77%	0.5	0	80	0	2
Nacho Cheese Sauce, 2 oz	120	10	75%	3	5	470	2	5
Pepper Jack Cheese Sauce, 1/2 oz	30	2	1%	1.5	5	45	2	0
Red Sauce, 1 oz	10	0	0%	0	0	220	0	2
Santa Fe Sauce, 1/2 oz	100	10	90%	1.5	10	75	0	1
Sour Cream, 3/4 oz	40	4	90%	3	10	10	1	1
Southwest Salsa, 4/5 oz	15	0	0%	0	0	15	1	3
Three Cheese Blend, 1/4 oz	25	2	1%	1	5	60	2	0

	Cal	Fat	%FC	S.Fat	Chol	Sod	Pro	Carb
Burritos								
Bean Burrito Soft	550	21	35%	7	20	1030	22	68
w/o Cheese	460	14	27%	4	0	895	17	65
Casita, no Sour Cream/Chse	430	17	36%	6	25	1245	23	46
Combo, Soft	550	24	39%	10	48	1230	30	55
w/o Cheese	460	14	27%	5	0	1095	17	65
Meat Soft, w/o Cheese	470	19	37%	6	53	1295	32	40
Veggie	535	20	34%	8	20	890	21	71
w/o Sour Cream	500	17	30%	6	14	885	21	71
w/o Sour Cream/Cheese	480	13	25%	4	0	800	18	69
Cheeseburger, Taco: no Dressing/Chse	400	13	29%	4	17	1070	20	49
Refried Beans, no Cheese	295	11	34%	3	0	835	11	38
Rice, Brown, Mexican	160	2	11%	0	0	540	2	28
Taco: Chicken, Soft	390	12	28%	5	70	320	31	34
Chicken, Soft, no cheese	335	8	21%	2	56	240	29	32
Flour, Soft, no cheese	330	12	33%	3	26	600	19	34
Tostada: no Sour Cream/Chse	410	17	37%	5	25	915	22	42
Salads: Taco, no dressing	350	16	41%	5	35	720	23	22
Chicken Taco, no dressing	435	19	39%	7	70	520	31	35
Chicken Taco, no dress./chse	380	15	35%	5	56	435	29	33
Side Order, no dress./cheese	300	13	39%	4	0	715	12	36
Veggie, no dressing/cheese	300	13	39%	4	0	715	12	36
Sauce: Casa	40	0	0%	0	0	180	0	10
Enchilada	15	0	0%	0	0	115	0	3
Hot	10	0	0%	0	0	120	0	2
Ranchero	20	1	50%	0	0	115	1	3

Taco John's®

	Cal	Fat	%FC	S.Fat	Chol	Sod	Pro	Carb
Burritos/Fajitas								
Bean Burrito	390	11	25%	4	18	870	15	57
Beef Burrito	330	18	49%	8	52	645	20	23
Chicken Fajita Burrito	370	12	29%	5	49	1540	21	45
Chicken Fajita Softshell	200	7	31%	3	33	905	13	20
Combination Burrito	420	15	32%	7	35	865	19	50
Meat and Potato Burrito	500	25	45%	7	25	1340	17	53
Mucho Grande Burrito	802	37	42%	13	77	1605	31	78
Ranch Burrito	450	23	46%	8	74	805	18	44
Super Burrito	465	19	37%	9	41	920	20	53
Tacos								
Crispy	180	11	59%	4	26	270	9	12
Softshell	230	10	39%	4	26	520	13	23
Bravo	345	14	37%	5	28	680	15	39
Burger	280	12	39%	5	32	580	15	28
Machaco	340	12	32%	4	34	645	21	37
Mucho Grande	580	34	53%	11	66	835	28	41
Platters: *Per Meal*								
Chimichanga	980	38	35%	15	59	2340	33	127
Double Enchilada	970	43	39%	15	89	1920	42	106
Sampler	1410	61	39%	24	126	2875	61	156
Smothered Burrito	1030	40	35%	16	70	2350	39	132
Sandwiches								
Sierra Chicken Fillet	535	29	49%	8	68	1410	30	40
Kid's Meals: Crispy Taco	580	34	53%	10	35	790	13	54
Softshell Taco	620	33	48%	10	35	1040	15	64
Specialities								
Super Nachos	920	57	56%	13	48	1485	26	72
Mexi Rolls w. Nacho Cheese	865	48	50%	11	54	1390	30	72
Taco Salad (no dressing)	585	38	58%	11	46	770	20	43
Sides								
Beans, Refried	360	9	23%	2	17	1030	18	53
Chili	350	21	54%	10	56	865	20	19
Mexican Rice	350	18	28%	5	0	1295	8	40
Nachos	335	21	56%	2	0	600	7	27
Nacho Cheese	300	10	30%	0	na	600	5	0
Potato Oles: Regular	365	23	57%	6	na	965	3	38
Bravo	580	38	59%	7	7	1550	11	47
w. Nacho Cheese	570	38	60%	7	0	985	8	46
Sour Cream, 1 oz	60	5	75%	na	na	15	1	1
Desserts								
Apple Flauta	85	1	10%	0.2	0	75	1	19
Cherry Flauta	145	4	25%	0.5	0	110	2	27
Cream Cheese Flauta	180	8	40%	3	10	135	2.5	27
Choco Taco	320	17	48%	11	20	100	3	38
Churro	150	8	48%	2	4	160	2	18
Italian Ice	80	0	0%	0	0	5	0	19

TCBY® Frozen Yogurt

	Cal	Fat	%Fc	S.Fat	Chol	Sod	Pro	Carb
Frozen Yogurt								
Regular, all flavors: Medium	285	6.5	21%	4.5	33	135	9	51
Large	365	8.5	21%	5.5	42	170	11	64
Hand-Dipped: Medium	310	6.5	20%	4.5	11	175	6.5	57
Large	390	8.5	20%	5.5	14	225	9	73
Nonfat: Medium	240	0	0%	0	99	130	9	51
Large	310	0	0%	0	126	170	11	64
No Sugar Added Nonfat: Medium	175	0	0%	0	6	77	9	44
Large	225	0	0%	0	8	98	11	56
Hand-Dipped Ice Cream: Small	320	19	53%	11	56	115	6	37
Medium	440	26	53%	15	77	160	9	50
Large	560	34	53%	20	98	200	11	64
Sorbet: Medium	220	0	0%	0	0	65	0	53
Large	280	0	0%	0	0	85	0	67
Paradise Ice: Medium	430	0	0%	0	0	0	0	110
Large	550	0	0%	0	0	0	0	140

TOGO's® Eatery

	Cal	Fat	%Fc	S.Fat	Chol	Sod	Pro	Carb
Sandwiches: Per Sandwich								
Chunky Chicken Salad	680	26	34%	5	60	1000	40	72
Hot Pastrami	710	26	33%	8	100	1100	34	85
Turkey & Cheese (6") w. dressing	640	23	32%	8	60	1300	34	75
Salads: Per Serving								
Garden Salad	260	10	35%	1	0	400	12	31
Oriental Salad	490	21	38%	3	0	700	25	49
Taco Salad	950	59	56%	19	90	1300	29	76

Note: Figures for saturated fat, cholesterol and sodium are author estimates only.

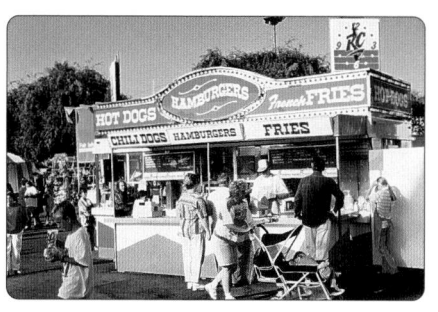

Wendy's®

	Cal	Fat	%Fc	S.Fat	Chol	Sod	Pro	Carb
Sandwiches								
Plain Single	360	16	40%	6	65	580	25	31
Single with Everything	420	20	43%	7	70	920	26	37
Big Bacon Classic	580	30	46%	12	100	1460	34	46
Jr. Hamburger	270	10	33%	3	30	610	15	34
Jr. Cheeseburger	320	13	37%	6	45	830	17	34
Deluxe	360	17	42%	6	50	840	18	36
Jr. Bacon Cheeseburger	380	19	45%	7	60	850	20	34
Kids' Meal: Hamburger	270	10	33%	3	30	610	15	33
Cheeseburger	320	13	37%	6	45	830	17	33
Grilled Chicken	310	8	23%	2	65	780	27	33
Breaded Chicken	440	18	37%	3	60	840	28	44
Chicken Club	470	20	38%	4	70	980	31	44
Spicy Chicken	410	15	33%	3	65	1280	28	43
Fresh Stuffed Pitas: Greek	440	20	41%	8	35	1050	15	50
Caesar/ Garden Chicken	490	18	33%	5	65	1320	34	48
Garden Veggie	400	17	38%	4	20	760	11	52
Garden Spot Salad Bar								
Applesauce, 2 Tbsp	30	0	0%	0	0	0	0	7
Bacon Bits, 2 Tbsp	45	2.5	50%	1	10	550	6	0
B'nas & Strawb. Glaze, $^{1}/4$ cup	30	0	0%	0	0	0	0	8
Broccoli/Carrot/Cauliflower, $^{1}/4$ c.	5	0	0%	0	0	0	0	1
Cantaloupe, 1 slice	15	0	0%	0	0	0	0	4
Chse, shred. (imitation), 2 T.	50	4	72%	1	0	260	3	1
Chicken Salad. 2 Tbsp	70	5	64%	1	0	135	4	2
Chow Mein Noodles, $^{1}/4$ cup	35	2	51%	0	0	30	1	4
Cole Slaw, 2 Tbsp	45	3	60%	0	5	65	0	5
Cottage Chse, 2 Tbsp	30	1.5	45%	1	5	125	4	1
Croutons, 2 Tbsp	25	1	36%	0	0	65	0	4
Parmesan Blend, grated, 2 T.	70	4	51%	2	10	290	4	5
Pasta Salad, 2 Tbsp	35	2	51%	0	0	180	1	4
Peaches, 1 slice	15	0	0%	0	0	0	0	4
Pepperoni, 6 slices	30	3	90%	1	5	70	1	0
Potato Salad, 2 Tbsp	80	7	79%	3	5	180	0	5
Pudding, $^{1}/4$ cup: Choc./Vanilla	70	3	39%	0.5	0	60	0	10
Red Onions, 3 rings	5	0	0%	0	0	0	0	1
Seafood Salad, $^{1}/4$ cup	70	4	51%	0.5	0	300	3	5
Sesame Breadstick, 1 each	15	0	0%	0	0	20	0	2
Strawberries, 1 each	10	0	0%	0	0	0	0	2
Sunflower Seeds & Raisins, 2 T.	80	5	56%	0.5	0	0	3	5
Tomato, wedged, 1 piece	5	0	0%	0	0	0	0	1
Turkey Ham, diced, 2 Tbsp	50	4	72%	1	25	280	3	0
Salads-To-Go: No Dressing								
Caesar Side	100	4	36%	2	10	620	8	8
Deluxe Garden	110	6	49%	1	0	350	7	10
Grilled Chicken:	200	8	36%	2	50	720	25	10
Caesar	260	10	35%	3	60	1170	26	17

	Cal	Fat	%Fc	S.Fat	Chol	Sod	Pro	Carb
Salads (Cont)								
Side Salad	60	3	45%	0.5	0	180	4	5
Taco Salad	380	19	45%	10	65	1040	26	28
Soft Breadsticks	130	3	21%	0.5	5	250	4	24
Dressings & Sauce								
Barbeque Sauce, 1 pkt	50	0	0%	0	0	100	1	11
Blue Cheese, 2 Tbsp	180	19	100%	3	15	180	1	0
French, 2 Tbsp	120	10	75%	2	0	330	0	6
French Fat Free, 2 Tbsp	35	0	0%	0	0	150	0	8
French Sweet Red, 2 Tbsp	130	10	69%	2	0	230	0	9
Hidden Valley Ranch, 2 Tbsp	100	10	100%	2	10	220	0	1
Reduced Fat	60	5	75%	1	10	240	0	2
Honey Mustard, 1 pkt	130	12	83%	2	10	220	0	6
Italian Caesar, 2 Tbsp	150	16	96%	3	20	240	1	1
Italian Red. Fat; 2 Tbsp	40	3	67%	0	0	340	0	2
Salad Oil, 1 Tbsp	120	14	97%	2	0	0	0	0
Sweet & Sour Sce, 1 pkt	50	0	0%	0	0	120	0	12
Thousand Island, 2 Tbsp	90	8	80%	2	10	125	0	2
Wine Vinegar, 1 Tbsp	0	0	0%	0	0	0	0	0
French Fries: Small	260	13	45%	3	0	85	3	33
Medium	380	19	45%	4	0	120	5	47
Biggie	460	23	45%	5	0	150	6	58
Great Biggie	570	27	43%	4	0	180	8	73
Baked Potato: Plain	310	0	0%	0	0	25	7	71
Bacon & Cheese	530	18	30%	4	20	1390	17	78
Broccoli & Cheese	470	14	27%	3	5	470	9	80
Cheese	570	23	36%	8	30	640	14	78
Chili & Cheese	630	24	35%	9	40	770	20	83
Sour Cream & Chives	380	6	14%	4	15	40	8	74
Sour Cream, 1 pkt	60	6	90%	4	10	15	1	1
Whipped Marg., 1 pkt	60	7	100%	1	0	110	0	0
Chili: Small	210	7	30%	3	30	800	15	21
Large	310	10	29%	4	45	1190	23	32
Cheddar Chse, shred. 2 Tbsp	70	6	77%	3	15	110	4	1
Saltine Crackers, 2	25	0.5	18%	0	0	80	0	4
Chicken Nuggets & Wings								
Chicken Nuggets, 5 Piece	230	16	63%	3	30	470	11	11
Spicy Buffalo Wing Sauce	25	1	36%	0	0	210	0	4
Desserts & Drinks								
Choc. Chip Cookie, 1 Tbsp	270	13	43%	6	30	120	3	36
Frosty Dairy Dessert: Small	330	8	22%	5	35	200	8	56
Medium	440	11	22%	7	50	260	11	73
Large	540	14	23%	9	60	330	14	91
Cola, small	130	0	0%	0	0	36	0	36
Lemon-Lime, small	130	0	0%	0	0	30	0	36
Lemonade, small	130	0	0%	0	0	0	0	37
Milk (2%), 8 oz	110	4	33%	2.5	15	115	8	11
Hot Chocolate, 6 oz	80	3	34%	0	0	135	1	15

Weinerschnitzel®

na - figures not available

	Cal	Fat	%FC	S.Fat	Chol	Sod	Pro	Carb
Breakfast Burrito	570	37	58%	13	530	1105	na	na
Breakfast Sando	445	27	55%	10	285	1040	na	na
Chicken Sandwich	540	32	53%	9	48	960	na	na
Chili Burger	625	40	58%	12	96	1350	na	na
Deluxe: Hamburger	580	37	57%	12	90	1145	na	na
Cheeseburger	635	42	59%	14	103	1350	na	na
Bacon Cheeseburger	690	46	60%	16	110	1520	na	na
Hickory Burger	605	37	55%	12	90	1215	na	na
Patty Melt	580	35	54%	16	108	1330	na	na
Dogs: Chili Dog	295	16	50%	5	28	935	na	na
Chili Cheese Dog	350	21	54%	8	41	1140	na	na
Corn Dog	290	23	70%	8	26	460	na	na
Deluxe Dog	275	14	45%	5	21	1620	na	na
Kraut Dog	265	14	46%	5	21	1150	na	na
Mustard Dog	260	14	48%	5	21	795	na	na
Relish Dog	280	14	45%	5	21	900	na	na
Western Dog	380	23	55%	9	43	985	na	na
Fries: Small	175	13	67%	8	19	345	na	na
Medium	270	21	70%	13	30	460	na	na
Large	380	29	69%	17	42	690	na	na
Chili Fries	470	36	69%	19	64	1000	na	na

Whataburger®

	Cal	Fat	%FC	S.Fat	Chol	Sod	Pro	Carb
Justaburger	275	11	36%	4	34	580	13	30
Whataburger:	600	26	39%	9	84	1095	30	61
Small bun, no oil	410	19	42%	7	84	840	25	34
Whataburger Jnr.	300	12	36%	4	34	580	14	35
Fajitas: Chicken	270	7	23%	0.5	33	690	18	35
Beef	325	12	33%	3	28	670	22	34
Sandwiches: Grilled Chicken	440	14	29%	3	66	1100	34	48
No Dressing	385	9	21%	2	66	990	34	46
w.Mustard, small bun	300	3	9%	1	66	990	33	35
Whatachick'n	500	23	41%	4	40	1120	27	51
Whatacatch	470	25	48%	4	33	630	18	43
Sides: No Dressing								
Baked Potato: Plain	310	0	0%	0	0	25	7	72
w. Cheese	510	16	28%	8	22	865	15	80
w. Broccoli & Cheese	450	10	20%	0	17	635	13	79
Garden Salad	55	0	0%	0	0	30	3	11
Grilled Chicken Salad	150	1	6%	0.5	49	435	23	14
French Fries: Regular	330	18	49%	3	0	210	5	37
Onion Rings: Regular	330	19	52%	3	0	595	5	34
Shakes: Vanilla, 12 oz	325	10	28%	5	37	170	9	51
Strawberry; Chocolate, 12 oz	350	9	23%	5	35	170	9	60

White Castle®

Hamburgers	Cal	Fat	%Fc	S.Fat	Chol	Sod	Pro	Carb
Hamburger	135	7	7%	3	10	135	6	11
Cheeseburger	160	9	1%	4	15	250	7	11
Sandwiches: Chicken	190	8	8%	2	20	360	8	20
Fish (w/out Tartar), 1 serving	160	6	34%	2	15	210	8	18
Breakfast Sandwich	340	25	66%	10	130	900	14	17
Bacon Cheeseburger	200	13	58%	6	25	400	10	12
French Fries: Small	115	6	47%	1	15	195	2	37
Onion Chips, small	180	9	45%	2	0	580	3	25
Onion Rings, 8 piece	540	26	43%	na	0	1300	8	69

Yoshinoya Beef Bowl®

	Cal	Fat	%Fc	S.Fat	Chol	Sod	Pro	Carb
Bowls								
Beef Bowl, 13 oz	720	29	36%	12	80	1130	31	87
Combo Bowl, 25 oz	1005	32	28%	13	110	2250	52	147
Teriyaki Chicken, 17 oz	640	11	15%	4	60	1440	31	105
Teriyaki Steak, 17 oz	720	20	25%	11	60	1400	31	105
Vegetable Bowl, 16 1/2 oz	410	1	2%	0	0	880	8	93
Vegetable Beef Bowl, 16 oz	470	21	29%	6	80	1250	25	91
Extras								
Beef, 5 1/2 oz	370	26	67%	12	60	1200	25	6
Chicken & Vegetables, 10 oz	290	10	31%	4	50	140	25	24
Rice, 7 1/2 oz	350	1	1%	0	0	40	6	81
Steak & Vegetables, 10 oz	370	19	45%	11	60	1380	25	24
Vegetable, 9 oz	60	0	0%	0	0	840	2	12

Note: Yoshinoya Beef Bowl Restaurants are based in California.

Zantiago®

Burrito	Cal	Fat	%Fc	S.Fat	Chol	Sod	Pro	Carb
Hot Cheese, Chilito	330	15	41%	7	35	466	14	35
Mild Cheese, Chilito	335	15	41%	7	35	505	14	36
Enchilada: Beef	315	15	43%	5	30	904	18	26
Cheese	390	23	53%	11	40	759	20	26
Taco: Burrito	415	19	41%	8	40	815	21	41
Regular	200	12	55%	4	20	318	10	13

Feedback *welcome*

Comments and suggestions are most welcome. Please write, fax or email the author

(Contact Details ~ Page 287)

Fats & Cholesterol Guide

Notes on Cholesterol

- **Cholesterol** is a white waxy substance produced mainly by our liver. It is also found in animal food products. Plant foods have no cholesterol.

- **Cholesterol is essential to life.** It is a structural part of every body cell wall and is the building block for vitamin D, sex hormones, and bile acids which help in the digestion of dietary fats.

- **The body makes sufficient cholesterol** for its needs and does not rely on cholesterol in the diet. Dietary fats have a major influence on blood cholesterol levels - more so than dietary cholesterol.

- **A high blood cholesterol increases** the risk of atherosclerosis - the thickening of arteries that can reduce or block blood flow to the heart muscle, brain, eyes, kidneys, sex organs and other body parts.

  This in turn increases the risk of heart attack, stroke, blindness, kidney failure, impotence and other blood circulatory problems.

  Other risk factors which increase the risk of atherosclerosis include high blood pressure, tobacco smoking, obesity and diabetes (uncontrolled).

HEART ATTACK WARNING SIGNALS

Many victims die before reaching hospital by ignoring warning signals and delaying medical help.

Symptoms vary and commonly include:

- **Chest pain,** vice-like squeezing or burning sensation in centre of chest or between shoulder blades, or feeling of severe indigestion.

- **Pain** may spread to shoulders, neck, jaw or arms.

- **Sweating,** nausea, dizziness, shortness of breath, irregular pulse.

If you experience any of the above symptoms seek IMMEDIATE medical attention!

Every minute counts.

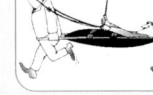

BLOOD CHOLESTEROL
Check Your Risk

Cholesterol Level (mg per deciliter)	Risk of Heart Attack
240 and above	High Risk
200 - 239	Borderline/High
Below 200	Desirable

♥ Know your cholesterol level, particularly if there is a family history of heart disease or stroke. If high, see your doctor.

♥ All adults should have their cholesterol, HDL and triglycerides tested at least every 5 years.

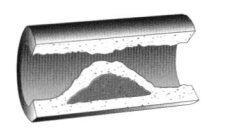

▲ Atherosclerosis can clog arteries and impede blood flow to the heart muscle or other body organs.

▼ A thrombus (blood clot) can form on unstable, festering atherosclerotic plaque and rapidly block blood flow.
A heart attack or stroke can result.

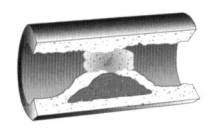

The amount and type of dietary fat has the greatest influence on blood cholesterol levels.

Fats in food are a mixture of 3 basic types: saturated, monounsaturated, and polyunsaturated. Animal fats are mainly saturated while plant oils and fish oils are mainly mono- and polyunsaturated.

Saturated fats have subgroups known as long chain, medium chain, and short chain fats. Most of the long chain fats raise blood cholesterol; and increase the risk of blood clots and thrombosis leading to artery blockage.

Long chain saturated fats are found mainly in full cream milk, cheese, butter, cream, fatty meats and sausages, and processed foods.

Monounsaturated fats tend to more selectively lower 'bad' LDL-cholesterol and maintain the protective 'good' HDL-cholesterol in the bloodstream - but only if they replace saturated fats in the diet.

Foods rich in monounsaturates include canola and olive oils, canola margarine, peanuts, and avocados.

Polyunsaturated fats consist of two main classes. **Omega-6** polyunsaturates tend to lower blood cholesterol. Rich sources include safflower, sunflower and corn oils.

Omega-3 polyunsaturated fats can lower blood cholesterol, and also confer extra benefits by lowering blood triglycerides, and reducing the risk of thrombosis, heart arrhythmias, and artery spasm.

Best practical omega-3 sources include canola oil and margarine, soybean oil and fish. (See adjoining chart)

A **balanced intake** of the two omega classes is important for optimal health. Increasing slightly omega-3 intake by Americans would help to attain a more ideal balance. Adequate vitamin E intake is also important.

All fats are high in calories and need to be limited for weight control.

DIETARY FATS COMPARISON

■ Saturated Fat   ■ Monounsaturated Fat
■ Linoleic (Omega-6)   ■ Alpha-Linolenic (Omega-3)

OILS   **PERCENTAGE CONTENT**

OILS	Saturated Fat	Monounsaturated Fat	Linoleic (Omega-6)	Alpha-Linolenic (Omega-3)
CANOLA OIL	7	63	20	10
LINSEED/FLAX OIL	9	19	17	55
SAFFLOWER OIL	9	14	77	
GRAPESEED OIL	10	22	68	
SUNFLOWER OIL	11	23	66	
CORN OIL	14	32	52	2
OLIVE OIL	14	76		10
SOYBEAN OIL	15	23	54	8
PEANUT OIL	19	45	34	2
COTTONSEED OIL	26	16	58	
PALM OIL	51	39	10	

SPREADS & FATS

Saturated Fat includes 'Trans Fats'   ☐ WATER CONTENT

SPREADS & FATS	Saturated Fat	Monounsaturated	Linoleic	Alpha-Linolenic	Water Content
LIGHT MARGARINE	14	14	21	51	
CANOLA MARGARINE	18	45	12	6	19
POLYUNSATURATED MARG.	24	20	36		20
BUTTER	57		18	2	24
LARD	41	47			12
BEEF FAT	44	37	4		15

GOOD SOURCES OF OMEGA-3 FATS

Plant Sources	Omega-3 Fats (Grams)
Canola Oil, 1 Tbsp, 1/2 fl.oz	1.5g
Flaxseed Oil, 1 Tbsp	8g
Soybean Oil, 1 Tbsp	1.2g
Canola Margarine, 1 Tbsp, 1/2 oz	1g
Soybeans, cooked, 1/2 cup, 4 oz	0.5g
Walnuts, 1/2 oz	0.5g

FISH - *Per 4 oz Serving*

High Content: Salmon (Chinook), Tuna,	3g
Trout (Lake), Sardines, Herring, Mackerel	3g
Medium Content:	
Salmon (Pink/Red/Coho), 4 oz	2g

Fair Content: Per 4 oz Serving

Bass, Catfish, Cod, Grouper, Hake, Halibut, Kingfish, Perch, Pollock, Shark, Trout (rainbow), Tuna (Skipjack), Crab, Oysters, Blue Mussel, Shrimp, Squid } 0.5-1g

How Much is Needed?

As little as 1-2 grams daily of omega-3 fats may benefit general health. High doses of fish oil supplements should only be taken as directed by your doctor.

Cholesterol in Food

Dietary Cholesterol

Cholesterol in food varies in its effect on blood cholesterol level (BCL) from person to person. Much depends on the amount and type of fat, and fiber eaten at the same meal.

Any elevating effect of dietary cholesterol on BCL is more likely to occur when the diet is high in saturated fat. Little elevation, if any, generally occurs when dietary fats are balanced in favour of mono- and polyunsaturated fats (including omega-3 fats). For example, while fish does contain cholesterol, the omega-3 fats can prevent any increase in BCL. Conversely, a meal containing no cholesterol but rich in saturated fat, may see a significant increase in BCL.

Consequently, the need to be overly concerned about dietary cholesterol is being de-emphasised in favour of a stricter approach to limiting total fats, and saturated fat in particular.

The liver usually cuts back its own cholesterol production in response to cholesterol in the diet. Many people can consume normal amounts of high cholesterol foods without concern.

However, it is difficult to identify just who is at risk - the so-called 'hyper-responders' - and because over 50% of Americans have a BCL above ideal levels, the **American Heart Association** advises all Americans to be prudent and limit their cholesterol intake to less than 300mg daily.

This limitation still allows the inclusion of most foods regularly eaten - even the overly maligned egg.

Note: Eggs contain a modest 5 grams of fat per large egg of which barely 2 grams are saturated, the rest being mono- and polyunsaturated.

By comparison, a cup of whole milk has almost 10g fat of which 6g are saturated.

CHOLESTEROL COUNTER

Cholesterol is found only in foods of animal origin. Plant foods contain no cholesterol. AHA recommends limiting dietary cholesterol to less than 300mg/day.

	Chol mg
Meat - Average all types:	
Lean Meat, cooked, 4 oz	70
Fatty Meat, cooked, 4 oz	105
Fat, thick strip, 2 oz	35
(Note: While lean meat and fat have similar amounts of cholesterol, choose lean meat to limit fat intake.)	
Chicken/Turkey, average, 4 oz	90
Organ Meats: Liver, fried, 4 oz	500
Brains, beef, pan fried, 3 oz	1700
Sausages: Frankfurter, 1.5 oz	25
Salami, 2 slices, 2 oz	40
Bacon: 3 slices, cooked, 1 oz	20
Fish: Fish fillets, average, ckd, 4 oz	70
Tuna/Salmon, canned, 3 oz	30
Scallops, 9 medium, 3 oz	30
Shrimp, 12 large, raw, 3 oz	130
Oysters, raw, 6 medium, 3 oz	45
Lobster, Crab, raw, 3 oz	80
Eggs (Chicken), 1 large	210
1 medium	180
Egg White, *Egg Beaters*	0
Milk/Yogurt: Whole, 1 cup, 8 fl.oz	35
1% Milk, 1 cup	10
Skim/Non-fat, 1 cup	5
Soy Milk	0
Cheese: Natural/Hard/Cream 1 oz	30
Cottage, lowfat, 4 oz	5
Ricotta, part skim, 4 oz	25
Fats: Butter, 2 Tbsp, 1 oz	60
Margarine, Oils (vegetable)	0
Mayonnaise, 1 Tbsp	10
Cream: Heavy, whipping, 2 T, 1 oz	40
Half & Half/Sour, 2 Tbsp, 1 oz	10
Icecream: Regular, $1/3$ cup, 4 fl.oz	30
Fruit, Vegetables, Avocados	0
Nuts, Seeds, Grains	0
Coffee, Tea, Soda, Beer, Wine	0

Fast-Foods ~ See Pages 160 - 247

Blood Cholesterol ~ Diet Hints

Dietary Hints to Lower Blood Cholesterol

1. Maintain a healthy weight.
If overweight, lose weight with lowfat eating and daily exercise.

2. Reduce saturated fat intake by:
(a) eating less dairy fat. Choose lowfat or fat-reduced varieties of milk, yogurt, cheese, and icecream. Enjoy soy drinks.

(b) replacing saturated fats with fats and oils rich in mono- and polyunsaturated fats; and carbohydrate-rich foods. Choose vegetable oils such as canola, olive, sunflower and soybean. Avoid solid frying fats.

Note: *Benecol* food products (spreads and dressings) contain plant stanol ester which can lower total and LDL cholesterol.

(c) eating less fat from meat and poultry. Choose lean cuts of meat and skinless chicken. Go easy on luncheon meats, salamis and fatty sausages. Enjoy fish.

(d) eating less saturated fats from baked and fried fast-foods. Avoid deep-fried foods. Avoid donuts, cakes, pastries and cookies unless made with healthier fats and oils.

3. Increase your 'soluble' fiber intake.
Foods rich in 'soluble' fiber include dried beans, baked beans, lentils, chick peas, hummus, nuts, seeds, psyllium seed husks and psyllium fiber supplements.
Oat bran, rice bran and barley are also useful, as are fruit, veges and avocados.

4. Eat more soya bean products such as: soy drinks, tofu, tempeh (cultured soya beans), soy flour and soy vegetarian foods.
Soy protein in place of animal protein can significantly decrease high blood cholesterol levels - as well as 'bad' LDL-cholesterol and blood triglycerides. Good' HDL-cholesterol is maintained. For best results, eat at least 25g of soy protein per day (from 3-4 servings)

5. Eat more fruit and vegetables in place of high-fat foods.
Aim for 2 fruits and 5 servings of vegetables per day. They also contain valuable antioxidants.
The fat of avocados is mainly unsaturated and lowers blood cholesterol levels.

6. Limit cholesterol to 300mg per day.
(Extra Notes ~ See Previous Page)

7. Avoid brewed unfiltered coffee
(espresso; plunger-style). It contains oil compounds (diterpenes) which can raise blood cholesterol. American style filtered coffee is fine.

8. Spread your food intake over the day.
Have 5-6 small meals per day rather than just 2-3 large meals. Nibbling, versus gorging, favors lower blood cholesterol.

ALCOHOL - WINE

Alcohol is a mixed bag. Moderate amounts of 1-2 drinks daily appear to reduce the risk of heart attack and ischaemic stroke in older persons.

However, larger amounts increase the risk of high blood pressure, obesity, heart failure and hemorrhagic stroke; and can aggravate hypertriglyceridemia - in addition to many other health hazards.
(See Alcohol Guide - p.149)

The over-riding harmful effects of excess alcohol do not allow its recommendation for any aspects of health promotion.

Note:
Red wine (more so than white) contains antioxidants which may help protect cholesterol in the blood from becoming oxidized.

Many fruits, vegetables and tea also contain protective antioxidants.

How Fats Affect Blood Flow

Fats in the diet not only affect blood cholesterol levels. They can also strongly influence blood clot formation and thrombosis, as well as blood flow and ultimate oxygen delivery to body parts and organs.

While advanced atherosclerosis can impede blood flow to the heart and other organs, it is thrombosis (complete blockage by blood clots) or arterial spasm which commonly result in a heart attack or stroke.

Plant and fish oils rich in omega-3 fats lessen the risk of blood clots, thrombus formation and artery spasm by reducing platelet stickiness and adhesion to artery walls. This reduces the risk of atherosclerotic plaque becoming unstable and reactive.

Omega-3 fats also improve blood flow by reducing blood viscosity; and increasing the flexibility of red blood cells (**RBC**) that need to flex and twist on themselves in order to squeeze through tiny narrow capillaries often half their diameter.

A diet high in saturated fats has the opposite effect by stiffening RBC membranes and increasing blood viscosity thereby hindering blood flow. The stiffening of the RBC membrane also reduces its ability to release vital oxygen to body cells and take up carbon dioxide.

Stiff red blood cells may also form aggregates like coin stacks. In narrow blood vessels, this further impedes blood flow and impairs oxygen release through the much lessened surface area of red blood cell membranes exposed to blood. (Smoking, lack of exercise, and stress can have similar adverse effects on thrombosis, red blood cell flexibility and blood flow.)

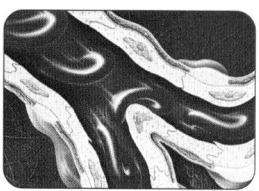

▲ Picture of Healthy Blood Flow

Flexible red blood cells twist and slide through tiny capillaries - often half the diameter of red blood cells.

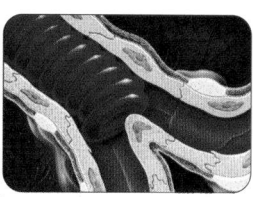

▲ A Not-So-Healthy Picture!

Red blood cells have lost their flexibility and ability to twist and slip through capillaries. They are stacked up thereby impeding blood flow.

A diet high in saturated fats can contribute to this picture - as can smoking, lack of exercise and stress.

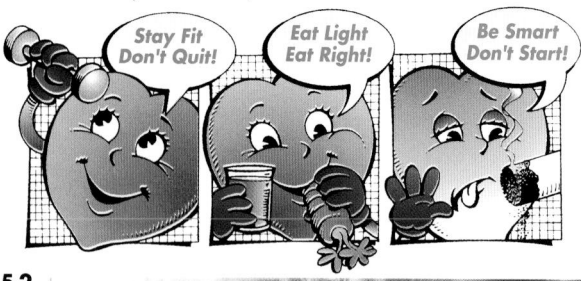

Ongoing research suggests that it may be the **oxidation of cholesterol** in the blood that promotes atherosclerosis in artery walls; and that taking steps to prevent this oxidation may well complement the benefits of controlling blood cholesterol levels.

Vitamin E appears to be the major antioxidant that defends cholesterol against oxidation. Low blood levels of vitamin E are associated with a greater incidence of heart disease deaths. Vitamin C and beta-carotene also appear to play important support roles (as may other food substances).

This research strengthens the current dietary advice to moderate fat intake, and to eat plenty of antioxidant-rich plant foods such as whole-grain cereals, fresh fruit and vegetables (5 serves daily), legumes, soybeans, nuts, seeds, and garlic.

While future research may prove the value of supplemental antioxidants in persons at high risk of heart attack, such supplements will not replace the current preventive advice to lower the risk of heart disease and stroke by: lowering saturated fat intake, not smoking, losing weight if overweight, exercising regularly, and controlling hypertension.

Extra Notes for High-Risk Persons:

- **Vitamin E supplements** are required to attain the pharmacological doses (400 - 800 IU daily) suggested in some research reports to provide maximum oxidative protection in persons at high coronary risk. Check with your doctor before taking large doses of vitamin E or other supplements.

- **Daily supplemental intake** of beta-carotene and vitamin C may also complement vitamin E.

- **Eat at least 3 different colors of fruit** and vegetables from at least 5 servings daily. There are many non-vitamin antioxidants that cannot be put in vitamin supplements.

LDL PARTICLE - CHOLESTEROL CARRIER

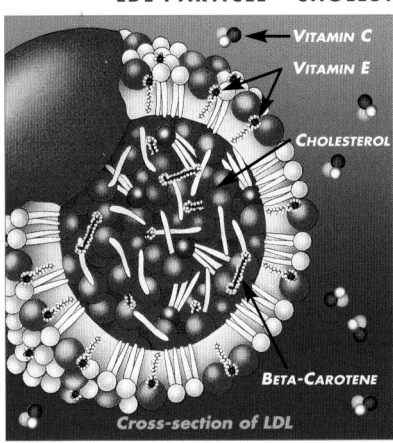

VITAMIN C
VITAMIN E
CHOLESTEROL
BETA-CAROTENE
Cross-section of LDL

- Low density protein particle (LDL) transports cholesterol in the blood since cholesterol is not soluble in blood (largely water).

- 'Free radical' attack on the LDL particle can oxidise it into a toxic form that may injure artery walls and promote atherosclerosis.

- Vitamin E molecules embedded in LDL shell provides the first line of defence against 'free radical' attack and oxidation.

- Vitamin C may help to directly neutralise 'free radicals' and to also regenerate vitamin E. Beta-carotene in the LDL core provides a second oxidation barrier.

- An antioxidant-rich diet will boost antioxidant blood levels and provide better resistance to LDL oxidation.

- **Moderate caffeine intake** is probably not harmful to healthy adults. However, regular large amounts (over 350mg/day) may cause dependency ('caffeinism') and adversely affect health.

- **Symptoms of excessive caffeine** intake include chronic insomnia, persistent anxiety and depression, restlessness, heart palpitations, stomach upset and increased need to urinate. (It can take 4-6 hours for caffeine's effects to wear off.)

- **Caffeine-withdrawal** headaches, fatigue and irritability are more commonly experienced on weekends when any heavy coffee drinking at work is suddenly reduced. Such headaches are relieved by drinking coffee. As little as 100-200 mg caffeine daily can produce withdrawal effects. (Withdrawal symptoms only last one week or less.) Reduce gradually by mixing with decaffeinated.

- **Sensitivity to caffeine** may increase during pregnancy and with age. To be safe, limit caffeine to 200mg/day.

- **Persons wise to avoid caffeine** entirely include those who get irritable and jittery from just one cup of coffee, pregnant and nursing women, children under eight, people with stomach ulcers or heart arrhythmia.

- **Large amounts of cola drinks** (4-6 cans per day) as well as coffee may also lead to excessive caffeine intake, particularly in children. Caffeine-free colas are available.

- **Coffee alternatives** such as *Postum, Kaffree Roma, Teeccino Caffre* are caffeine-free. Decaffeinated coffee is also suitable.

> - **Blood cholesterol can be raised** by several drinks daily of boiled unfiltered coffee (such as espresso and cafetiere/plunger pot style). American-style filtered coffee does not contain the oil compounds (diterpenes) which appear to raise blood cholesterol.
>
> - **Coffee does not sober up** an inebriated person. It simply turns him or her into a wide-awake drunk!

Coffee   Caffeine (mg)

Instant Coffee:	
Weak, 1 level tsp	45
Medium, 1 rounded tsp	60
Strong, 1 heaping tsp	90
Decaffeinated, 1 rnd tsp	2
Bags(*Folgers*), 1 bag (6-8 fl.oz)	115
Decaffeinated, 1 bag	3
Brewed: Percolator, 8 oz cup	120
Drip Method, 8 oz cup	160
Ground, 1 Tbsp, 6g	60
Decaffeinated, 1 Tbsp	2
Bottled (Ready-To-Drink), 9.5 fl.oz	75

Flavoured Coffee Mixes

Coffee with Chicory, 1 rnd tsp	40
General Foods: Irish Mocha Mint	25
Orange Cappuccino	70
Other flavors, average	50

Coffee Shop Style

Coffee: Drip-brew, average, 8 fl.oz	160
Percolated, 8 fl.oz	120
Cappuccino, 8 fl.oz	80
Decappuccino (decaffeinated)	5
Espresso: Regular/Solo	80
Double (Doppio) Espresso	160
Latte/Macchiato	80
Iced Coffee, 8 fl.oz	80
Mocha, 8 fl.oz	90
Vienna Coffee, 8 fl.oz	80
Cocoa, 8 fl.oz	10

Starbucks (Franchise Chain)

Drip Coffee: Short, 8 fl.oz	140
Tall, 12 fl.oz	210
Grande, 16 fl.oz	280
Cappuccino: Short or Tall	70
Grande	100
Caffe Americano: Tall, 14 fl.oz	150
Grande, 16 fl.oz	220
Venti, 20 fl.oz	250
Caffe Latte, Short or Tall	75
Grande	150
Cafe Mocha, Short or Tall	85
Grande	170
Espresso (Reg./Macchiato): Solo	75
Doppio	150
Frappuccino, Reg./Mocha, Tall	75
Grande	100

Coffee Alternatives
(Roasted Cereals - Caffeine-Free)

	Caffeine (mg)
Kaffree Roma/Postum/Teeccino Caffe	0

Bottled Milk Coffee (Ready-To-Drink):
Starbucks/ Nestle: Average, 9.5 fl.oz	75

Tea
Brewed or Tea Bags: Weak, 1 cup	20
Medium Strength	40
Strong	70
Instant Tea Powder: 1 tsp	30
w. lemon flavor, 1 tsp	25
+ sugar, 3 rnd tsp	30
Decaffeinated Tea (*Kaffree*)	1
Herbal Tea	0
Iced Tea, regular: 8 oz Glass	20
12 oz Glass	30
16 oz Glass	40
Flavored Teas, Ready to drink, Average, 12 fl.oz	25

Cola Soft Drinks: Per 12 fl.oz
Coca Cola: Can/Bottle	30
Fountain/Restaurant	38
Diet Coke: Can/Bottle	40
Fountain/Restaurant	45
Pepsi: Can/Bottle	32
Fountain/Restaurant	37
Diet Pepsi: Can/Bottle	30
Fountain/Restaurant	37
Caffeine Free Coke/Pepsi	0

Other Colas: Per 12 fl.oz
Cherry Coke	35
Cherry Cola (Shasta)	40
Diet Rite Cola	48
Jolt Cola	55
K-Mart Amer. 1 Can Fare Cola/Diet	12
Kroger Big K Cola	5
Diet Cola	30
Pepsi Kona	55
RC Cola	43
Diet RC Cola	50
Shasta Cola	42
Diet Shasta Cola	37
Slice Cola	10
Slice: Dr. Slice, Cherry Spice, Red	35
Surge	53
TAB	50
Wal-Mart Sam's Choice/Diet	12
Wild Cherry Pepsi	38
Winn-Dixie Chek Cola	8

Non-Cola Soft Drinks
Per 12 fl.oz Can/Bottle

	Caffeine (mg)
National: Cherry Spice; Dr Slice	35
Dr Pepper, Reg./Diet	42
Java Juice, all flavors, 20 fl.oz	140
Josta (Pepsi)	60
Kick	55
Mello Yellow	50
Mountain Dew, Reg./Diet	55
Mr PiBB, Reg./Diet	43
Red	35
Sunkist Orange	43

Store Brands - Non- Cola Drinks
Kroger Big K Citrus Drop, Reg./Diet	26
Kroger Dr K, Reg/Diet	17
Wal-Mart Sam's Choice: Green Lightning	50
Southern Lightning	30
Winn-Dixie: Dr Chek	18
Chek Kountry Mist	53

Caffeinated Waters
Aqua Java; Water Joe 17 fl.oz	60
Java Johnny, 20 fl.oz	70
Krank20, 17 fl.oz	100
Java Juice all flavors, 20 fl.oz	140

Chocolate/Cocoa
Chocolate: Milk Choc., 2 oz	20
Dark Chocolate/Bakers, 2 oz	35
Choc Chips, 1/4 cup., 1.5 oz	15
Candy Bars, average, 1.5 oz	10
Cocoa, dry, unsw. 1 Tbsp, 5g	12
Cocoa/Hot Choc. Mix, 1 oz pkt	5
Chocolate Milk, 8 fl.oz	8
Chocolate. Cake, 1 pce	10
Choc Chip Cookie, 1 oz	4
Chocolate Icing, 1 serving	5
Chocolate Icecream, 1/2 cup	2
Chocolate Pudding, 1/2 cup	5
Chocolate Syrup, 2 Tbsp	6

Pharmaceuticals & Guarana
Anacin/Empirin/Midol, 2 tabs	65
Aqua-Ban (diuretic), 2 tabs	200
Dexatrim (weight control), 1 tab	200
Excedrin, 2 tablets	130
NoDoz: Regular Strength, 1 tab	100
Maximum Strength, 1 tab	200
Tylenol, 1 tablet	0
Vivarin, 1 tablet	200
Guarana: Powder, 1 tsp, 3 g	120
Tablet/Capsules (800mg), 1	30
Drinks/Soda, average, 1 fl.oz	50

Calcium's Role in the Body

Calcium plays a vital role in nerve and muscle function, clotting of blood, enzyme regulation, insulin secretion and overall bone strength. Bones and teeth store 99% of the body's calcium.

The calcium level in blood is kept at a steady level by the continual exchange of calcium between blood and bone. When insufficient calcium is obtained from food the body draws calcium out of the bones.

This bone loss over a period of years may lead to **osteoporosis** - thinning of the bones (*porous bones*).

The bones become weak, brittle and easy to fracture, particularly the bones of the wrist, hips and spine. Loss of height and curvature of the spine may also result, as may periodontal disease - the deterioration of the jaw bones that support the teeth.

Osteoporosis - Common in Women

While osteoporosis also occurs in men, women are particularly vulnerable (1 in 4 by age 60). They have about 30% less bone than men, and a greater bone loss at menopause when estrogen levels drop. Slender framed women are at greater risk. (A woman in her eighties can have lost up to two thirds of her skeleton.)

Insufficient dietary calcium during pregnancy and breastfeeding will see bone reserves drawn upon, increasing the risk of osteoporosis.

Causes of Osteoporosis

The major factors associated with the bone loss of osteoporosis appear to be:

- **Hormone changes of menopause.**
- **Insufficient calcium in the diet.** (Absorption decreases with age.)
- **Insufficient exercise (weight bearing - such as walking, cycling.)**
- **Family history of osteoporosis.**
- **Other contributing factors may include:** excess amounts of alcohol, protein and phosphorus (from meats and soft drinks); insufficient vitamin D and magnesium; and cigarette smoking.

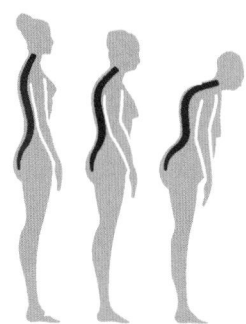

As osteoporosis progresses after menopause, vertebrae may collapse causing the spine to curve and shoulders to hunch.

RECOMMENDED DAILY INTAKE OF CALCIUM

		Calcium
Infants:		
	0-6 mths ~	360mg
	6-12 mths ~	540mg
Children:		
	1-10 yrs ~	800mg
	10-12 yrs ~	1200mg
Teenagers:		
	13-18 yrs ~	1200mg
	16-18 yrs ~	800mg
Adults: 19+ yrs	~	800mg
Women:		
Pre-menopausal	~	1000mg
Menopausal(beginning)	~	1200mg
Post-menopausal	~	1500mg
Pregnancy/breastfeeding:		
10-18 yrs	~	1600mg
19+ yrs	~	1200mg

Early Prevention Important

Gradual loss of bone begins in the thirties after maximum bone mass is reached. The stronger the bones at that time, the less trouble is likely to occur later. The earlier that prevention or treatment begins the greater the benefit. **The key to prevention** is to build strong, dense bones early in life. **By age 16,** some 80% of peak bone mass is reached.

Young women may lessen the risk by eating high-calcium foods, not engaging in excessive dieting that results in period cessation (less estrogen), taking regular exercise and not smoking.

In menopausal women, hormone therapy as well as calcium supplements and exercise, can help retard osteoporosis. Your doctor can advise you.

Dietary Sources of Calcium

Milk, yogurt, calcium-enriched soy drinks and cheese are the richest sources of calcium. (Lowfat and nonfat varieties contain similar calcium.)

Canned fish with edible bones (salmon/sardines) are high in calcium. Tofu (soybean curd), tempeh, broccoli and dried beans are also good sources.

- Soy drinks (calcium-enriched) may be preferable to cow's milk. Body calcium losses are much greater with animal protein. Soy protein is relatively 'bone-sparing'.
- Phytoestrogens in soy foods may also lessen calcium losses at menopause. Soy drinks are suitable for persons with lactose intolerance.

Extra Notes on Calcium

Persons who have difficulty eating sufficient calcium-rich foods should consider a **calcium supplement.** Prescribed high doses of calcium (1.5-2g/day) may benefit persons with osteoporosis - as well as vitamin D (up to 400 IU), and magnesium (100mg).

Calcium in food reduces iron absorption by up to 60% when eaten with iron-containing foods. Consume calcium-rich foods/supplements at smaller meals and mid-meal snacks.

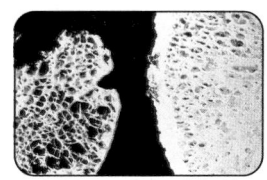

▲ Osteoporotic Fragile Bone   ▲ Healthy Dense Bone

GOOD SOURCES OF CALCIUM (MILLIGRAMS)

MILK
8 fl.oz
300

YOGURT
8 oz
300

CHEESE
1 oz
200

RICOTTA CHEESE
Part Skim, 1/2 Cup
330

SOY DRINK
Calcium Enriched
8 fl.oz
300

SALMON
w. Bones
3 oz
300

ALMONDS
1 oz
70

BROCCOLI
1 Cup
100

BAKED BEANS
1/2 Cup
50

Milk & Milk Drinks

	Calcium (mg)
Milk Fluid:	
Whole: 1 cup, 8 fl.oz	300
1 small glass, 6 fl.oz	220
1% or 2%: 1 cup, 8 fl.oz	300
Lowfat/Skim: 1 cup, 8 fl.oz	300
Hi-Calcium *(Borden)*, 1 cup	1000
Viva, w. extra Calcium, 1 cup	500
Condensed Milk, sweet, 1 Tbsp	110
Evaporated Milk: Skim, 1 fl.oz	90
Whole/Lowfat	80
Dry/Powder: Whole, 1/4 cup	290
Skim/Nonfat, 1/4 cup	380

Other Milks & Drinks

Buttermilk, average, 1 cup	300
Chocolate Milk, average, 1 cup	300
Cocoa/Chocolate w. Milk, 1 cup	300
Goats Milk, 1 cup	320
Malted Milk, 1 cup	350
Milkshakes: Small, 10 fl.oz	280
Medium, 15 fl.oz	450

Milk Drink Powders:

Malted Milk, dry powder, 1 oz	80
Chocolate, Instant, 3 Tbsp	10
Cocoa Powder: Regular, 1 Tbsp	10
Cocoa Mix: *Hershey*, 1/3 cup	40
Alba High Calcium, 1 envelope	320

Soy & Grain Drinks: *Per 8 fl.oz Cup*

Soy: Regular, non-fortified	60
Calcium-fortified *(e.g. Edensoy Extra)*	300
Dry Powder, 1 oz	80
Rice/Oat Drinks: Average, 1 cup	10

Yogurt

Average All Brands	350
Fruit-flavored, 1 cup, 8 oz	250
Small cup, 6 oz	230
4 1/2 oz cup	350
Plain: Average, 1 cup, 8 oz	430
Dannon, Nonfat/Lowfat, 8 oz	200
Custard-style, 6 oz	100
Frozen Yogurt, average, 1/2 cup	100

Fats/Oils

Butter, Lard, fats	0
Margarine, Regular/Imitation	0
Oils, Salad Dressings	0

Cream

	Calcium (mg)
Average: Unwhipped, 1 Tbsp	15
Whipped, 1 heaping Tbsp	15
Half & Half, 1 Tbsp	15
Non-dairy Creamers, 1 tsp	0

Ice Cream & Ices

Ice Cream: Regular, 1 scoop	65
1/2 cup	90
Premium, 1 serve, 4 oz	150
Soft Serve, 1/2 cup	120
Ice Milk, average, 1/2 cup	100
Sherbet, average, 1/2 cup	50
Fruit Sorbet	0
Sundae, regular, 6 fl.oz	200
Tofu Ices, average, 1/2 cup	10

Cheese: *Per 1 oz (1 1/2" cube)*

Natural, Hard: Average, 1 oz	200
Processed Cheese: Average, 1 oz	150
Single-wrapped, 3/4 oz	120
Cheese Substitutes: Average, 1 oz	200
Specific Cheeses:	
Blue, 1 oz	150
Brie	50
Camembert	110
Cheddar	200
Cottage Cheese: 1 round Tbsp, 1 oz	20
1/2 cup, 4 oz	80
Cream Cheese	20
Dorman's Light, average 1 oz	200
Edam, Gouda	200
Feta	140
Goat, semi-soft	85
Gruyere	290
Kraft Light Naturals, average	250
Light-Line *(Borden)*, singles	200
Monterey Jack	210
Mozzarella, average	170
Parmesan, grated, 1 Tbsp	70
Processed, average	160
Provolone	210
Ricotta, part skim, 1/2 cup, 4 1/2 oz	330
Swiss	270
Cheese Dishes:	
Souffle, 4 oz	240
Macaroni & Cheese, 1 cup, 8 oz	150
Ham & Cheese Crepes, 8 oz	350
Quiche, 1 serve, 6 oz	200

Eggs	Calcium (mg)
1 large Egg	30
Scrambled, with Milk	50
Omelet w. Cheese (1/2 oz)	260

Fish & Seafood

Canned Fish:

Salmon: with bones, 3 oz	190
without bones, 3 oz	10
Sardines, with bones, 3 oz	90
Tuna, canned, 3 oz	10
Fresh Fish: cooked, average, 4 oz	35
Seafood: Lobster, cooked, 4 oz	60
Mussels/Oysters, (10), 4 oz	95
Crabmeat, cooked, 4 oz	50

Meats & Poultry

Average all types, cooked, 4 oz	20

Soups

Average all types:

No Milk or Cheese added, 1 serve	30
with Milk, 1/2 cup, 1 serve	180

Sauces

Average all kinds, 1 Tbsp	10
Cheese/White Sauce, 2 Tbsp	40

Spices

Average all types, 1 tsp	5-20

Bread, Bagels

Bread: White, 1 slice	30
Wholewheat, Rye, 1 slice	30
Bagels, average	30
Buns/Rolls: Small	40
Large	90
English Muffins, 2 oz	90
Pita, 6 1/2 " diameter, 2 oz	50
Tortillas, Corn, 1 oz	40

Breakfast Cereals

Ready To Eat:

Average all types, 1 oz	20
with 3/4 cup Milk/Soy (enriched)	250
Total (General Mills), 1 oz	200

Hot Type, cooked

Corn (Hominy) Grits, 1 cup	5
Cream of Wheat, 1 cup	50
Oatmeal/Rolled Oats:	
Regular, non-fortified, 1 cup	20
Instant, fortified, 1 pkt	100

Note: Breakfast cereals are a good medium for calcium-rich milk or soy drinks (150mg per 1/2 cup).

Flours, Grains	Calcium (mg)
Wheat Flour: All-purpose, 1 cup	20
Self-rising, 1 cup	330
Whole-wheat, 1 cup	50
Carob Flour, 1 cup, 3 1/2 oz	360
Corn meal, 1 cup, 4 oz	20
Soybean Flour, 1 cup, 3 oz	170
Grains, Barley, Rice, average:	
Cooked, 1 cup	15

Pasta, Spaghetti

Average all types, cooked, 1 cup	15
Lasagne, average, 1 serve	300
Macaroni & Cheese, aver., 1 cup	150
Spaghetti w. Meat Sce, 1 serve	20
with 1 Tbsp Parmesan	90

Sugar & Syrups

Sugar: White	0
Brown, 1 Tbsp	10
Syrups: *Per 2 Tbsp, 1 oz*	
Choc., Thin type, 2 Tbsp	5
Fudge type, 2 Tbsp	40
Molasses: Light, 2 Tbsp	70
Blackstrap, average, 1 Tbsp, 3/4 oz	270
Table Syrup, 2 Tbsp	0

Honey, Jam, Jelly

Contain negligible calcium.

Cookies & Cakes

Cookies: Average all types, 1 only	5
Crackers, average, 1 only	5
Cake: Plain, average, 2 oz	40
Carrot Cake with Icing	45
Cheesecake, 1 piece	80
Fruitcake, 1 piece	40
Croissants, average, 2 oz	20
Danish pastry, average, 2 oz	60
Donuts, average, 2 oz	20
Muffins:	
Regular, average, 1 1/2 oz	40
English Muffins, 2 oz	90
Pancakes, 4" diameter, average, 1 oz	40
Pies:	
Apple/Fruit, average, 5 oz	20
Custard Pie, average, 5 oz	140
Pecan Pie, 1 piece, 5 oz	70
Pumpkin Pie, 1 piece, 5 oz	80
Waffles, 7" diameter average	160

Desserts

	Calcium (mg)
Custard, average, $^1/_2$ cup	150
Gelatin, plain w. water, $^1/_2$ cup	2
Puddings: Canned, aver., 5 oz	80
Dry Mix, made w. milk, $^1/_2$ cup	150
Rice Pudding, $^1/_2$ cup	120
Snack Can, 5 oz	60
Pancakes, 4" diam., 2	120

Candy, Chocolate

Chocolate: Milk	50
Plain/Fruit, 1 oz	65
with Almonds, 1 oz	80
Kit Kat Wafer, $1^1/_2$ oz	80
Mars Bar	80
Milky Way Bar, 2 oz	60
Carob Bar, average, 2 oz	220
Plain candy, uncoated, 1 oz	0
Jelly Beans, Marshmallow, 1 oz	0

Snacks & Bars

Breakfast Bars (*Carnation*)	20
Corn Chips; Tortilla Chips, 1 oz	40
Granola Bars, average	30
Popcorn, 1 cup	5
Potato Chips, 1 oz	10
Power Bar	300
Tiger's Milk/Sport	350

Nuts & Seeds (Shelled)

Almonds, 12-15 nuts, $^1/_2$ oz	40
Brazil Nuts, 4 medium, $^1/_2$ oz	30
Cashews, 6-8 nuts, $^1/_2$ oz	5
Coconut, fresh, $^1/_2$ oz	5
Filberts (Hazelnuts), $^1/_2$ oz	40
Macadamias, 6 medium, $^1/_2$ oz	10
Peanuts, raw, 1 oz	25
Walnuts, 1 oz	20
Seeds: Pumpkin, 1 oz	15
Sesame, 1 Tbsp	10
Sunflower, 1 oz	30
Tahini, 1 Tbsp, $^1/_2$ oz	20

Beverages – Alcohol, Soda

Beer, Cider, Wine, 1 glass	5
Spirits, 1 fl.oz	0
Coffee, Tea, Soda, Fruit Drinks	5
Water: Tap, average, 1 cup	5
Perrier, 1 glass, 6 oz	20

Fruit & Fruit Juice

	Calcium (mg)
Fresh Fruit: Average all types, 1 serve	20
Apple, 1 medium	10
Avocado, 1 medium	20
Banana, 1 medium	10
Orange, 1 medium	50
Pear, 1 medium	20
Rhubarb, cooked, $^1/_2$ cup	170
(calcium largely not available to body)	
Dried Fruit: Average, 1 oz	20
Figs, 3 medium, $1^1/_2$ oz	55
Fruit Juice: Average, 1 cup, 8 fl.oz	25
Orange Juice, calcium fortified:	
Citrus Hill Plus Calcium, Hi-C	300
Minute Maid (Premium Calcium)	300
Jui2ce, 8 fl.oz	200
Tropicana Grapefruit & Calcium	300

Vegetables

Average all types, $^1/_2$ cup	20
1 cup	40
Higher Calcium Content:	
Beans, dried: cooked, $^1/_2$ cup	50
Baked/Refried Beans, $^1/_2$ cup	60
Broccoli, chopped, 1 cup	100
Chickpeas, boiled, $^1/_2$ cup	40
Collards, cooked, 1 cup	150
Dandelion Greens, cooked, 1 cup	150
Kale, 1 cup	130
Mustard Greens, 1 cup	100
Potato: Plain, 1 large	20
Au Gratin, 1 cup	200
Mashed w. Milk, 1 cup	60
Spinach, cooked, $^1/_2$ cup	120
Soybeans, cooked, $^1/_2$ cup, 3 oz	90

Tofu:

Tofu: *Mori Nu:* Silken, 4 oz	90
Azumaya: Silken, 3 oz	20
Firm/Extra Firm, 3 oz	150
Hinoichi: Regular, 1" slice, 3 oz	100
Firm/Extra Firm, 3 oz	150
Soft, 1" slice, 3 oz	60
Nasoya: Firm, 3 oz	120
Extra Firm, 3 oz	150
Soft, 3 oz	120
Silken, 3 oz	60
Miso: $^1/_2$ cup, 5 oz	100
Tempeh: 4 oz serving	100

Frozen Entrees/Meals	Calcium (mg)
Budget Gourmet Light	
Chicken Parmigiana; Ziti Parmesano	160
Three Cheese Lasagne	360
Lean Cuisine: Cheese Ravioli	160
Cheese Lasagna w. Chicken	360
Chicken Fettucine	160
French Bread Pizza, Deluxe	360
Stouffer's: Cheese Manicotti	320
Chicken Enchilada; Fettucini Alfredo	200
Extra Cheese Pizza	280
Five Cheese Lasagna	400
Turkey Pie/Tetrazzini	80
Weight Watchers	
Bowtie Pasta & Mushroom Marsala	160
Lasagna w. Meat Sauce	320
Tuna Noodle Casserole	160

Frozen Pizzas	
Average All Brands: Cheese, 1/4 pizza	350
Meats (Sausage/Pepperoni), 1/4 pizza	250

Calcium Supplements	
Caltrate 600, 1 tablet	600
Citracal, 1 tablet	200
Ethical Nutrients 'Bone Builder', 1	200
IDN LifePak: Reg./Prime, 2 pkts	500
Women, 2 pkts	1000
Nature's Life 'Super Cal-Mag', 1	500
Os-cal; 1 tablet	500
Posture Calcium, 1 tablet	600
Tums: Regular, 1 tablet	200
Extra Strength, 1 tablet	300

Exercise enhances bone growth, bone density and strength.

Fast-Foods, Restaurants	Calcium (mg)
Chicken:	
Grilled/BBQ, 1/4 chicken	20
Battered & Fried, 2 pieces	80
Nuggets, 6 pack	20
Crispy Chicken Deluxe Sandwich	50
Croissant Sandwich: Plain	40
with Cheese, 1 oz	240
Fish Sandwich: no Cheese	60
with Cheese	140
Fish Filet Deluxe	70
Fish, fried, 2 pieces	20
French Fries: Small Serving	10
Hamburgers: Average all outlets,	
Regular, no Cheese	120
Cheeseburger, regular	120
McDonald's: Big Mac	160
Arch Deluxe w. Bacon	70
Quarter Pounder w. Cheese	120
Egg McMuffin	120
Hot Dog: Plain	60
with Cheese	150
Mexican: Burrito	120
Enchilada	300
Nachos, regular	200
Taco, regular	140
Taco Bell Salad	400
Pizza: Average all types,	
Medium (12"), 2 slices	250
Double Cheese, 2 slices	350
Large (16"), 2 slices	350
Double Cheese, 2 slices	500
Pizza Hut, Medium:	
Cheese, 2 slices	290
Pepperoni, 2 slices	300
Potato: Plain, baked, 8 oz	20
Stuffed w. Cheese Topping	100
with Cheese Filling	300
Sandwiches: Average	
no Cheese	60
with 1 oz Cheese	200
with 2 oz Cheese	460
Subway: 6" Sandwich average	100
Tuna, 6"; Tuna Salad (small)	100
Salads, small, average	100
Salads: Chef, regular	300
Coleslaw, small	20
Shakes, average	330

Introduction

Fiber is the general term for those parts of **plant** food that we cannot digest (although bacteria in the large bowel partly digests fiber through fermentation). It is not found in foods of animal origin (meats, dairy products).

Fiber promotes intestinal health, bowel regularity, can benefit diabetes and blood cholesterol levels, and may help prevent colon cancer. High fiber foods also assist weight control.

Most Americans don't eat enough fiber - less than 20 grams/day - instead of a **healthier 25 to 35 grams/day.**

Types of Fiber

Plant foods contain a mixture of different fibers in varying proportions. Insoluble and soluble fiber categories are based on their solubility in water. All types of fiber are beneficial to the body.

◆ Insoluble fibers (cellulose, hemi-celluloses, lignin) make up the structural parts of plant cell walls. The **best sources** are wheat bran, corn bran, rice bran, wholegrain cereals and breads, dried beans and peas, nuts, seeds and the skins of fruits and vegetables.

These fibers absorb many times their own weight in water. They create a soft bulk and hasten the passage of waste products through the intestines.

They promote bowel regularity, and aid in the prevention and treatment of uncomplicated forms of **constipation, diverticulosis and haemorrhoids.**

The risk of colon cancer may also be reduced by fiber's diluting effect of potentially harmful substances.

◆ Soluble fibers (pectin, gums, mucilages) are found mainly within plant cells, soy milk (whole bean) and products.

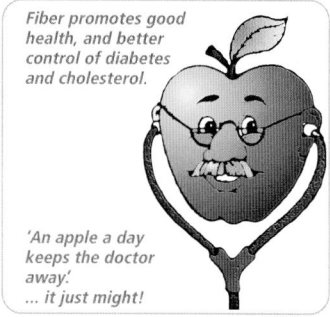

Fiber promotes good health, and better control of diabetes and cholesterol.

'An apple a day keeps the doctor away'.
... it just might!

Types of Fiber (Cont)

Best Sources of Soluble Fiber:
Fruits and vegetables, oat bran, barley, dried beans and peas, psyllium and flax seed.

These fibers form a gel which slows both stomach emptying and the absorption of sugars from the intestines. This helps to control **blood sugar** levels.

Weight control is also aided by the slower emptying of the stomach and the feeling of **fullness provided by soluble fiber.**

Some soluble fibers can lower **blood cholesterol** by binding bile acids and excreting them. More body cholesterol must then be broken down to supply bile acids for emulsification of dietary fats. **Rice bran, while not high in soluble fiber can also lower blood cholesterol.**

◆ Resistant starch is that part of starchy foods (approx. 10%) which is tightly bound by fiber and resists normal digestion. Friendly bacteria in the large bowel ferment and change the resistant starch into short-chain fatty acids which are important to bowel health and may protect against colon cancer.

Starchy foods include bread, cereals, rice, pasta, potatoes and legumes.

Fiber & Weight Control

Fiber can assist weight control in several ways. Fiber-rich foods such as fresh fruit and vegetables, potatoes and whole-grain bread contain few calories for their large volume (due to their lowfat, high water content).

Their bulk fills the stomach and satisfies appetite much earlier than fiber-depleted foods. The extra chewing time also contributes to satiety, and gives the stomach time to register a feeling of fullness. Excessive calories are less likely to be consumed.

Fiber-depleted foods and drinks are more concentrated in calories; e.g. fats, sugar, candy, soft drinks, fruit juices, alcohol. They require little or no chewing. Large amounts with excessive calories can be consumed before appetite is satisfied.

Example: Whereas one fresh apple might satisfy our appetite, an apple juice drink with the equivalent sugars and calories of 2-3 apples does little to satisfy appetite. (See illustration below.)

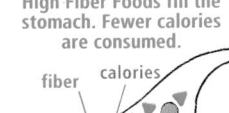

High Fiber Foods fill the stomach. Fewer calories are consumed.

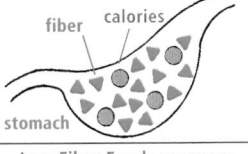

Low Fiber Foods are more concentrated in calories. More food must be eaten to fill the stomach.

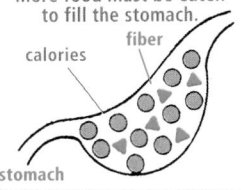

EFFECTS OF REMOVING FIBER FROM FOOD

2-3 pieces of fresh fruit produces 1 glass of fruit juice. The removal of fiber concentrates the sugar and calories.

FIBER REMOVED

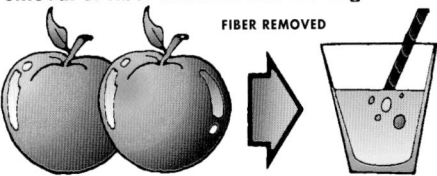

Fresh Fruit		Fruit Juice
High Fiber	←	Negligible Fiber
Low Calorie Density	←	High Calorie Density
Long Eating Time	←	No Eating Time (Drink)
Satisfies Hunger	←	Does Not Satisfy Hunger
Sugar Slowly Absorbed	←	Sugar More Quickly Absorbed
Less Insulin Required	←	More Insulin Required

Fiber Guide – Constipation

Constipation

Constipation can reasonably be defined as a failure to have a bowel movement at least every second day - and just as importantly, without straining or pain.

Typically, stools are too hard, too narrow, and too small . . . *sinkers* rather than *floaters*.

The **main cause** is simply a lack of dietary fiber. Other contributing factors include insufficient fluids, too little exercise, emotional stress, gastro-intestinal disease, lack of proper dentition to chew high-fiber foods, and some medications (e.g. some antacids, antidepressants, tranquilizers).

Note: Check with your doctor to rule out any underlying medical problem – especially if you have a change in bowel habits in middle-age or later years.

DESIRABLE FIBER INTAKE

Adults: 25-35gm per day
Children (under 18): Age + 5gm
Example: 6-year old (6 + 5)= 11gm

SAMPLE FOOD QUANTITIES

For 35 Grams of Fiber/Day **Fiber**

Breakfast Cereal (higher-fiber)	5g
plus 4 slices whole wheat Bread	6g
plus 3 servings fresh Fruit	9g
plus 1 medium Potato (w. skin) **or** 1 cup Brown Rice **or** 1/2 cup whole-wheat Pasta	4g
plus 3-4 servings Veges/Salad	6g
plus 1 cup Bean Soup **or** 1/4 cup Baked/Soy Beans **or** 1/2 cup Corn/Peas/Lentils **or** 1 1/4 oz Almonds (natural) **or** 3 medium Figs	5g

Hints to Increase Fiber and Avoid Constipation

1. Breakfast is an important contributor to daily fiber intake. Eat high-fiber breakfast cereals (bran-based cereals, oatmeal etc.). Add 1-2 tablespoons of unprocessed bran (wheat/ barley/ rice) and wheat germ if required.

Dried fruits, chopped nuts, soy grits, and seeds are also excellent additions to cereals.

Note: A gradual increase in fiber will prevent bloating, gas or pain. Persons intolerant to bran may benefit from psyllium-based fiber supplements and cereals.

2. Drink 6-8 glasses of water daily. Fiber works by absorbing many times its own weight of water.

3. Eat wholegrain breads, or fiber-enriched breads. One slice of whole-wheat bread has over double the fiber of regular white bread.

4. Enjoy fruit as fresh fruit with skins rather than as fruit juice. Enjoy whole-wheat pasta, barley, brown rice, nuts and seeds.

5. Eat more vegetables, salads and legumes - especially dried beans, baked beans, lentils, potatoes with skins, avocado, broccoli, brussel sprouts, cabbage, carrots, celery, and peas.

6. Add bran (barley/rice/wheat) or soy grits to soups, casseroles, yogurt, desserts, biscuits, cakes. Also use wholemeal flour or soy flour in place of white flour. Use nuts and seeds.

7. Snack on fresh or dried fruits, carrot or celery sticks, popcorn, nuts or seeds, wholegrain crackers, high-fiber bars (low-fat). Limit amounts if overweight.

8. Exercise regularly to strengthen abdominal muscles and stimulate the gut. Keep up fluids, especially in warm weather.

9. Avoid indiscriminate and regular use of harsh laxatives. They can overstimulate the intestinal muscles and may make normal bowel activity impossible. It may take several weeks to restore normal bowel function.

FOODS WITH ZERO FIBER

- **Dairy Products (Milk, Cheese, etc)**
- **Meats, Poultry, Fish, Eggs**
- **Fats/Oils, Sugar/Syrups**

(Only foods of plant origin contain fiber.)

Breakfast Cereals	Fiber
General Mills: Cheerios, 1 cup, 1 oz	3
Basic 4, 1 cup, 2 oz	3
Crispy Wheaties, 1 cup, 1 oz	3
Fiber One, 1/2 cup, 1 oz	13
Raisin Nut Bran, 3/4 cup, 2 oz	5
Oatmeal Crisp, 1 cup, 2 oz	4
Wheat Chex, 1 cup, 1 3/4 oz	5
Health Valley: Amaranth Flakes, 3/4 cup	4
Banana Gone Nuts! 3/4 c., 2 oz	4
Bran w. Apple & Cinnamon, 3/4 cup	7
Bran w. Raisins, 1 1/4 cup	6
Blue Corn/Bran Flakes, 3/4 cup	4
Fiber 7 Flakes, 3/4 cup	4
Golden Flax, 1/2 cup	6
Granola (Fat Free), 2/3 cup	6
Healthy/Honey Crunches & Flakes, 3/4 cup	4
Healthy Fiber Flakes, 3/4 cup	4
Honey Crunch O's, 3/4 c., 1 oz	3
Oat Bran Flakes, all types, 3/4 cup	4
Real Oat Bran, 1/2 cup	5
Rice Crunch-Ems, 1 1/4 cup, 1 oz	4
10 Bran O's, 3/4 cup	4
Kellogg's:	
All-Bran, 1/2 cup, 1 oz	10
All-Bran w. Extra Fiber, 1/2 cup	13
Bran Buds, 3/4 cup, 2 oz	12
Bran Flakes, 3/4 cup	5
Corn Flakes, Fruit Loops, Smacks, 3/4 cup	1
Cracklin' Oat Bran, 3/4 cup, 2 oz	6
Cocoa/Rice Krispies, 3/4 cup	0
Complete Wheat, 3/4 cup, 1 oz	5
Frosted Mini Wheats, 1 cup, 2 oz	6
Healthy Choice, all types, 1 cup	5
Nutri-Grain (Almond Raisin), 1 1/4 cup	4
Mueslix (Almond. Raisin, Date), 2/3 cup	4
Raisin Bran, 1 cup, 2.2 oz	8
Smart Start, 1 cup	2
Special K; Product 19, 1 cup	1
Nabisco: 100% Bran, 1/2 cup, 1 oz	8
Shredded Wheat, 2 biscuits	5
Shredded Wheat & Bran, 1 1/4 cup, 2 oz	8

Fiber ~ Fiber (grams)

Breakfast Cereals (Cont)	Fiber
Nature Valley: Average, 1/3 cup, 1 oz	1
Quaker:·Per 1 oz	
Cap'n Crunch; Cr. Nut Oh's, 3/4 cup	1
Crunchy Bran, 3/4 cup, 1 oz	5
Life Cereal (3/4 cup), Oat Squares (1/2 c.)	2
Oat Bran, 1/3 cup	6
Oatmeal, average, 1 packet	3
100% natural cereals, average, 1/2 cup	3
Puffed Rice, 1 cup	1
Puffed Wheat, 1 cup	2
Toasted Oatmeal; Honey Nut, 1 cup	3
Post: Banana Nut Crunch, 1 cup, 2 oz	4
Blueberry Morning, 1 1/4 cup, 2 oz	2
Bran Flakes (Natural), 3/4 cup, 1 oz	5
Cocoa/Fruity Pebbles, 3/4 cup	0
Cranberry Almond Crunch, 1 cup, 2 oz	3
Frosted Alpha Bits, 1 cup	1
Fruit & Fiber, 1 cup, 1 3/4 oz	5
Grape-Nuts, 1/2 cup, 2 oz	5
Grape-Nuts Flakes, 3/4 cup, 1 oz	3
Great Grains, 2/3 cup, 2 oz	4
Honey Bunches of Oats, 3/4 cup, 1 oz	1
Oat Flakes, 1 cup, 1 oz	2

Brans & Supplements	
Oat Bran: 1 Tbsp (level)	0.8
1/3 cup, (5 1/3 Tbsp), 1 oz	4.2
Rice Bran: 1/3 cup, 1 oz	6
Wheat Bran: unprocessed: 1 Tbsp	1.6
2 Tbsp (level), 1/4 oz	3.2
1/4 cup, (4 Tbsp), 1/2 oz	6.4
1/2 cup, 1 oz	13
Corn Germ: 1/4 cup, 1 oz	5
Wheat Germ: 1/4 cup, 1 oz	3
Psyllium Seed Husks, 2 Tbsp	8
Bios Life 2(Rexall), 1 pkt	5
Metamucil, 1 dose	3.4

Hot Cereals, Oatmeal	
Bulgur (cracked Wheat), ckd, 1 cup	8
Cream of Wheat, ckd, 2/3 cup	1
Hominy Grits, dry, 3 Tbsp, 1 oz	1.2
Kashi (Breakfast Pilaf), 1/2 cup, cooked	6
Kashi 'Go', all varieties, 1/2 cup	6
'From Kashi to Good Friends', 3/4 cup	8
Puffed Kashi, 1 cup, 0.8 oz	2
Oatmeal, uncooked, 1/3 cup, 1 oz	2.7
cooked, 2/3 cup	2.7

Breads & Crackers — Fiber

	Fiber
Bread: White, 1 slice, 1 oz	0.7
Whole-wheat, 1 slice, 1 oz	1.5
Whole-grain, 1 slice, 1 oz	2
Rye, Pumpernickel, 1 oz	1.5
Bagel/Roll/Bun, 1 medium, 2 oz	1.5
Pita, whole wheat, 5" pocket	4.5
Crackers: Graham, average, 2	1.4
Saltine, 4 crackers	0.3
Crispbreads (Rye), average, 2	4
Matzo 1 board, 1 oz	1
Rice Cakes: Average, 1 cake	0.3
Tortilla: Regular, 6"	0.5
Whole-wheat, 6"	1.3

Barley, Pasta, Rice & Flours

Barley, pearled, raw, 1/4 cup, 1.7 oz	5
Rice: White, cooked, 1 cup, 7 oz	1.6
Brown, cooked, 1 cup	3.2
Rice-A-Roni, average, 1 cup	1.5
Spaghetti/Noodles: cooked, 1 cup	2
Whole-wheat, cooked, 1 cup	7
Amaranth (Health Valley), 1 cup	9
Flour: Wheat, All-purpose, 1 cup, 41/2 oz	3.5
Whole-wheat, 1 cup, 41/2 oz	15
Cornmeal, stone ground, 1 cup, 41/2 oz	13
Carob Flour, 1 cup, 31/2 oz	13
Rye Flour, 1 cup, 31/2 oz	15
Soy Flour: Defatted, 1 cup, 31/2 oz	17
Full-fat, raw, 1 cup, 3 oz	8
Soy Meal, defatted, 1 cup, 41/2 oz	14

Frozen Entrees & Dinners

Average All Brands: Per Serving

Potato/Pasta base, average	4-6
Vegetable base, average	3
Meat/Chicken base, average	2-3
Pizzas, 1/4 large, average	3

Soups

Chicken Noodle, 1 cup	<0.5
Tomato Soup, average, 1 cup	<1
Vegetable Soup, average, 1 cup	3
Health Valley: Per 1 Cup Serving	
Black Bean; Minestrone	10
Tomato	4
Organic Split Pea Soup	8
5-Bean Vegetable; Lentil & Carrots	13
Mushroom & Barley; Vegetable	7
Chili:	
w. Beans, average, 1 cup, 8.8 oz	7
without Beans, average, 1 cup, 8.3 oz	3

Fast Foods & Restaurants — Fiber

	Fiber
Hamburgers: Small, average	1.5
Large/Whopper, average	2.5
Hot Dog, Regular	1.5
French Fries: Small serving, 21/2 oz	2.5
Regular/Medium, 31/2 oz	3.5
Chicken Nuggets, 6 pack	<0.5
Chicken Sandwich, average	2
Taco, average	4
Sundaes, Shakes, Soft Drinks	0
Arby's: Baked Potato w. Broccoli	9
Roast Beef Sandwich, regular	3
Denny's: Oriental Chicken Salad	7
Dennyburger w. fries	3
Club Sandwich	3
Grilled Chicken Sandwich	1
Domino's (Pizza): Veggie, 2 sl. (12")	4
Pepperoni, 2 slices (12")	2.5
Cheese., Saus/Mushr., 2 slices, (12")	3
McDonald's: Arch Deluxe; Crispy Chicken	3
Big Mac	4
Egg McMuffin	1
Salads: Garden; Grilled Chicken	2
Pizza Hut: Per 2 slices, Medium	
Pan Pizza: Cheese, Pepperoni	2
Supreme	4
Thin 'n Crispy: Supreme	4
Hand-Tossed, average	3
Personal Pan Pizza, 1 whole	5
Subway: Sandwich, white roll	2.5
w. honey Wheat Roll	3.2
Footlong, w.Wheat Roll	6.4
Salads, average	2

Cakes, Cookies, Snack Bars

Apple/Fruit Pie, 1 serving	2
Cake, w. plain flour, 1 serving	1
w. whole-wheat flour, 1 serving	3
Carrot Cake, 1 serving	2
Cookies, oatmeal, (3 small/1 large)	3
Donuts	0
Fruit Cake, 1 serving	3
Fi-Bar (Natural Nectar), 1 bar	4
Fig Bars, 2	1.3
Granola Bars, average	1
Health Valley: Fat-Free Fruit Bars	3.7
Oat Bran Jumbo Fruit Bars	7
Fat-Free Cookies, 2	2
Fat-Free Fruit Muffins, 1	5
IDN Fiberry Snack Bar	3
Muffins, Oat Bran (2 small, 1 large)	5

Chocolate, Chips, Popcorn Fiber

Cheese Balls/Curls/Twists	0
Chocolate, Hard Candy, Cheese Balls	0
Chocolate with nuts/fruit, 2 oz bar	1
Mars Bar	1
Potato Chips, corn chips, 1 oz	1
Popcorn, 3 cups	2
Pretzels, Twists, 6	1

Nuts, Seeds

Almonds: Natural, 25 kernels, 1 oz	4
Blanched (skins removed), 1 oz	3
Cashews, Filberts, Pecans, 1 oz	1.7
Peanuts, Mixed Nuts, Coconut, 1 oz	2.5
Peanut Butter, 2 Tbsp, 1 oz	1.8
Pistachio Nuts, dried, shelled, 1 oz	3
Walnuts, Black/English, dried, 1 oz	1.5
Seeds: Amaranth, $2^1/2$ Tbsp, 1 oz	3.5
Flax Seeds, 3 Tbsp, 1 oz	7
Psyllium Seed Husks, 5 Tbsp, 1 oz	20
Quinoa Seeds, 3 Tbsp, 1 oz	2.7
Sesame Seeds, whole, 1 oz	3
Sesame Butter/Tahini, 2 Tbsp, 1.1 oz	3
Sunflower kernels, $1/4$ cup, 1 oz	4.4
Teff Seeds, 1 oz	3.8

Fruit – Fresh

Apples: 1 medium, 6 oz (whole)	
with skin + core	5.5
with skin, no core	4.5
without skin, no core	3.7
Apricots, 2 medium, 4 oz	2
Avocado, average, $1/2$ medium	3
Banana, 1 medium, 6 oz (w. skin)	2
Blueberries, raw, $1/2$ cup, 5 oz	4.4
Cherries, sweet, raw, 10 fruits, $2^1/2$ oz	1.5
Grapefruit, average, $1/2$ fruit, $8^1/2$ oz	1
Grapes, 1 medium bunch, seedless, 7 oz	3
Kiwifruit, 1 medium, 3 oz	3
Mango, 1 medium, 11 oz (whole)	1.6
Melons, cantaloup, 4 oz (edible)	1
Nectarine, 1 medium, 4 oz	1.8
Olives, average all types, 7 jumbo, 2 oz	1.5
Oranges, 1 medium (7-8 oz w. skin)	
$5^1/2$ oz (peeled)	3.8
Passionfruit, 2 medium, $2^1/2$ oz	5
Peaches, 1 large, 6 oz	2
Pears, raw, 1 medium, 6 oz	4.5
Pineapple, 1 slice, 3 oz	1.8
Plums, 2 medium, 6 oz	2.8
Strawberries, 6 medium/3 large, 2 oz	1.5
Watermelon, 4 oz (edible)	0.5

Fruit – Dried, Juice Fiber

Dried Fruit: Apricots, 8 halves, 1 oz	2.2
Dates (3 med); Raisins (2 Tbsp), 1 oz	1.5
Figs, 3 medium,$1^1/2$ oz	5
Prunes, 4 medium, 1 oz	2
Fruit Juice: Orange/Apple etc, 1 glass	<0.5
Prune Juice, 5 oz	1.4
Carrot Juice, 8 oz	1.8

Vegetables

Asparagus, 4 spears	2
Bean Sprouts, $1/2$ cup, $2^1/4$ oz	1.5
Beans: Snap/Green, $1/2$ cup, $2^1/2$ oz	2
Baked Beans in Tom Sce, $1/2$ c, $4^1/2$ oz	10
Dried Beans, ckd, average, $1/2$ cup	7
Beets, ckd, slices, $1/2$ cup, 3 oz	1.5
Broccoli, ckd, $1/2$ cup, 3 oz	2.2
Brussels Sprouts, ckd, $1/2$ cup, 3 oz	3.5
Cabbage: White, ckd, $1/2$ cup, $2^1/2$ oz	1
Red, ckd, $1/2$ cup, $2^1/2$ oz	2
Carrots, 1 medium ($7^1/2$"), $1/2$ cup, 3 oz	2.7
Cauliflower, cooked, $1/2$ cup, 3 oz	2.8
Celery, raw, diced, $1/2$ cup, $2^1/2$ oz	1
Chick Peas (Garbanzos), ckd, $1/2$ c., $3^1/2$ oz	6
Corn, kernels, ckd, $1/2$ cup, $2^1/2$ oz	2.5
Cream-style, $1/2$ cup, $4^1/2$ oz	1.5
Cucumber/Lettuce/Mushrooms, 2 oz	0.5
Eggplant, raw, sliced, $1/2$ cup	2.5
Lentils, cooked, $1/2$ cup, $3^1/2$ oz	4
Onions, 1 medium, 4 oz	2
Spring Onions, chop., $1/4$ cup, 1 oz	1.5
Peas: Green, $1/2$ cup, 3 oz	3
Cowpeas (Black-eyed), ckd, $1/2$ cup	10
Split Peas, ckd, $1/2$ cup, $4^1/2$ oz	6.5
Peppers, sweet, raw, 1 large, $3^1/2$ oz	1.5
Potatoes: 1 medium, with skin, 5 oz	4
without skin	2
$1/2$ cup mashed, $3^1/2$ oz	1.5
French Fries, 3 oz serving	3
Spinach, cooked, $1/2$ cup, 3 oz	2
Squash: Summer, cook'd, 3 oz	1.2
Winter, cooked, 3 oz	2.4
Tomatoes: 1 medium, 5 oz	2
Tomato Sauce, 1 cup	0.3
Frozen: Mixed Vegetables, ckd, $1/2$ cup	3
Soybean Products: Miso, $1/2$ c., 5 oz	7.7
Tempeh, 1 piece, 3 oz	
Tofu, 4 oz	1.4
Salads: Side Salad, average	1
Bean Salad, $1/2$ cup	5
Coleslaw, $1/2$ cup	1
Potato Salad, $1/2$ cup	2

Protein Guide

General Notes

- **Protein has many important body functions.** It builds and repairs muscle, and is the basis of our body's organs, hormones, enzymes, and antibodies to fight infection.

- **Protein is also an emergency fuel** in the absence of sufficient carbohydrate and fats. For this reason, weight loss should be gradual so as to preserve protein levels in muscle, the heart and other body organs.

- **It is easy to obtain sufficient protein**, even if vegetarian. **Plant proteins are not inferior to animal proteins.** In fact, eating more soy and other plant proteins, and less animal protein, may help to build stronger bones and prevent osteoporosis; and may help to control blood cholesterol levels.

- **When changing to a vegetarian diet**, include soybeans, and other dried beans, soy milk drinks (calcium-enriched), lentils, tofu, tempeh, nuts, and wholegrain breads and cereals. Milk, yogurt, cheese and eggs may enhance nutrient intake.

Protein & Muscle

- Although muscles are built of protein, protein is not a special fuel for working muscle cells - carbohydrates and fats are.

- In fact, a diet high in protein (and fat) and low in carbohydrate, can significantly reduce the performance of endurance sports athletes. **Carbohydrate** is the best fuel for muscles exercised for long periods.

- Any **extra protein** required by athletes and body-builders, can easily be obtained from the extra food eaten to satisfy hunger and energy needs - even allowing an excessive 120g protein daily for a 170 lb athlete (0.7g/lb body wt; twice the RDI).

- Remember, **excess protein** in food will not build bigger muscles. Any excess is converted and stored as fat. Excess protein can also strain the kidneys which excrete the waste products of protein metabolism.

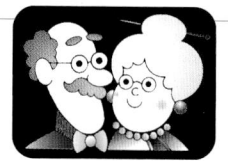

Elderly people (and dieters) must eat sufficient food to ensure adequate protein intake.

Inadequate protein leads to a drop in immune response with greater susceptibility to illness and infections. Muscle strength and muscle mass also drop.

Protein needs are easily met with sensible eating. Athletes who eat enough food for their energy needs, can obtain sufficient protein.

RECOMMENDED DAILY PROTEIN INTAKE (Grams)

(Figure in brackets - Recommended amount of protein per lb of ideal body weight.)

Infants:	0-6 mths	**13g**	(1g/lb)
	6-12 mths	**14g**	(0.7g/lb)
Children:	1-3 yrs	**16g**	(0.6g/lb)
	4-6 yrs	**24g**	(0.5g/lb)
	7-10	**28g**	(0.5g/lb)
Males:	11-14 yrs	**45g**	(0.45g/lb)
	15-18	**59g**	(0.4g/lb)
	19-24	**58g**	(0.36g/lb)
	25+	**50g**	(0.4g/lb)
Females:	11-14 yrs	**46g**	(0.45g/lb)
	15-18	**44g**	(0.37g/lb)
	19-24	**46g**	(0.36g/lb
	25+	**50g**	(0.36g/lb)
Pregnancy:		**60g**	
Breastfeeding:		**65g**	

Note: Above figures allow for a large safety margin for most persons.

Iron & Anemia Guide

- **Iron deficiency** is one of the most common nutritional deficiencies in women. The risk is increased in dieters who do not eat well-balanced meals. Chronic shortage of iron leads to **anemia**.

- **Women** between 11 and 50 years of age are at greater risk because of the monthly loss of menstrual blood. Pregnancy, growth, and endurance sports also demand extra iron.

- **In red blood cells**, iron combines with protein to form **hemoglobin** - the red pigment which carries oxygen in the blood. A lack of iron limits the production of hemoglobin and hence the amount of vital oxygen delivered to body cells.

Note: A blood test will tell you if your Hb and Iron stores (ferritin) are adequate. (Iron stores can be low even when Hb is normal.)

- **Vitamin C** (in fruits/veges/salads) enhances absorption of 'non-heme' iron in bread, cereals, milk, vegetables, nuts, eggs and iron supplements. Small amounts of meat, fish or poultry also help. (They contain 'heme' iron).

- **Iron absorption is lessened** by up to 60% when high calcium foods are consumed with iron-rich main meals. Tea, coffee, phytates (in bran) and oxalates lessen absorption of non-heme iron.

- **For infants to 1 year**, use iron-fortified milk/soy formula if not breast-feeding. Introduce iron-fortified baby cereals at 4-6 mths.

Note: Iron deficiency in children (even without anemia), can result in lethargy, irritability, repeated infections, and developmental problems.

Iron Supplements

- **Most people** can obtain adequate iron from their diet. A **wide variety** of animal and plant foods contain iron. (See Iron Counter)

- **Iron supplements** are only recommended for women with heavy menstrual blood losses, during pregnancy (if tests show a low-iron status), endurance athletes with low blood ferritin (iron stores) and for persons with diagnosed anemia. Check with your doctor.

- While the 5 mg of iron in multi-vitamin/mineral supplements is safe for most people, large amounts can be toxic, (especially in persons with hemochromatosis iron overload condition).

ANEMIA SYMPTOMS

Anemia reduces the amount of oxygen carried in the blood. The body tissues become starved of oxygen. Symptoms include:

- **Pale skin; brittle finger nails (may turn up into spoon shape).**

- **Excessive tiredness or fatigue**

- **Breathlessness**

- **Feeling of malaise and irritability.**

- **Always feel cold.**

- **Decrease in attention span.**

Note: Other medical conditions may also cause similar symptoms. Check with your doctor.

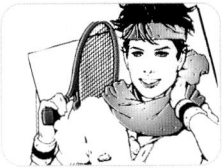

A nutritious diet with adequate iron is important - particularly for women and athletes.

RECOMMENDED DAILY IRON INTAKE (mg)

Infants (0-6 mths):			
	Breastfed	~	0.5mg
	Bottlefed	~	3mg
	6-12 mths	~	9mg
Children:	1-11 yrs	~	6-8mg
Males:	12-18 yrs	~	10-13mg
	19+ yrs	~	7mg
Females:	12-50yrs	~	12-16mg
	51+ yrs	~	5-7mg
	Pregnancy	~	22-36mg
	Breastfeeding	~	12-16mg

Pro ~ Protein (grams)   **Iron** ~ Iron (mg)

Meat

	Pro	Iron
Steak: Average all cuts, lean (no fat)		
Small (4 oz raw/3 oz ckd)	23	2.3
Medium (6 oz raw/4¹/₄ oz ckd)	34	3.4
Large (10 oz raw/7¹/₄ oz ckd)	57	5.7
Roast Beef: lean, 2 slices, 3 oz	24	2.5
Ground Beef patty, lean, ckd, 3 oz	21	2
Lamb chop, broiled, 3 oz	22	1.5
Liver, cooked, 3 oz	23	5.5
Veal cutlet, 1 medium	23	1
Pork, cooked, lean, 3 oz	24	1
Bacon, 3 medium slices	6	0.3
Ham, roasted, 2 pieces, 3 oz	18	1
Ham, luncheon, 2 slices, 1¹/₂ oz	7	1
Pastrami (*Oscar Mayer*), 3 sl., 1³/₄ oz	10	1.3
Sausages: Bologna, 2 sl., 2 oz	7	1
Braunschweiger, 2 sl., 2 oz	8	5.3
Pork link, thick, 2 oz	6	0.4
Frankfurter, 1¹/₃ oz	5	0.5
Salami, hard, 3 slices, 1 oz	7	0.5

Chicken/Turkey

	Pro	Iron
Chicken, ckd; Breast portion, 3 oz	27	1
Leg/Thigh, lean, 3 oz	24	1
¹/₂ Whole Chicken	60	2.5
Drumstick, 1 medium, 3 oz	12	0.6
Turkey, cooked: Light meat, 3 oz	24	2
Dark meat, lean, 3 oz	24	2

Fish

	Pro	Iron
Finfish: Per 4 oz, cooked		
Cod, Flounder/Sole, Pollock	28	0.5
Catfish, Haddock, Halibut, M/Mahi	28	1.3
Ocean Perch, Swordf., Orange Roughy	28	1.3
Canned Fish: Tuna, Light, 3 oz	25	1.5
White, 3 oz	23	0.5
Salmon, pink, 3 oz	17	1
Salmon, red, 3 oz	17	1
Sardines, 3 whole (3"), 1¹/₄ oz	9	1
Anchovies, 1 can, 1¹/₂ oz	13	2
Shellfish: Crabmeat, 3 oz	17.5	0.7
Clams, raw, 4 large/9 sml, 3 oz	11	12
Crayfish, cooked, 3 oz	20	1
Lobster, cooked, 3 oz	17	0.5
Oysters, raw, 6 medium, 3 oz	7	5
Scallops, 2 lge/5 small, 1 oz	5	0.1
Shrimp, raw, 6 large, 1¹/₂ oz	8.5	1
Fish Products: Fish Sticks, 4 sticks	10	0.5
Fish Portions, in batter, 4 oz	13	0.6
Gefilte Fish, 1 medium ball, 2 oz	8	1

Eggs

	Pro	Iron
1 Large Egg, whole	6	0.7
Egg Yolk	3	0.7
Egg White	3	0
Omelet: Plain, 2 eggs	13	1.7
Ham & Cheese	17	3
Egg Substitutes (liquid):		
Eggbeaters, 1 egg equiv.	4.5	1
Scramblers, ¹/₄ cup, 2 oz	6	0.7

Milk, Yogurt, Ice-Cream

	Pro	Iron
Milk: Whole/Lowfat/Skim, 8 fl.oz cup	8	0.1
Protein Enriched, 1 cup	10	0.1
Chocolate Milk, 1 cup	8	0.6
Thick Shake, Chocolate, 10 oz	9	1
Vanilla, 10 oz	11	0.3
Soymilk (fortified), average, 1 cup	7	1
Yogurt: Plain, 6 oz	10	0.1
Fruit flavors, 6 oz	8	0.3
8 oz	11	0.5
Ice-Cream: Rich, ¹/₂ cup	2	0
Regular, Vanilla, ¹/₂ cup	2.5	0
Sherbet, ¹/₂ cup	1	0
Custard, baked, ¹/₂ cup	7	0.5

Cheese

	Pro	Iron
Hard Cheeses, average, 1 oz	7	0.2
4 oz piece	28	0.8
Cottage Cheese, ¹/₂ cup	13	0.3
Ricotta, part skim, ¹/₂ cup	14	1

Bread, Bagels, Biscuits

	Pro	Iron
Bread (w. enriched flour): 1 slice, 1 oz	2	1
4 slices, 4 oz	8	4
4 thick slices, 6 oz	1.2	6
Bagel, plain 2 oz	6	1.5
Biscuits, 1 oz	2	0.7
Pita Bread, 1 pita, 1¹/₂ oz	4	1
Pumpernickel, 1 slice, 1 oz	3	1

Infant/Baby Foods

	Pro	Iron
Infant Formula Milk:		
Enfamil/Gerber/Similac, 5 fl.oz		
Regular/Low Iron	2.2	0.2
With Iron	2.2	1.8
Isomil/Nursoy/ProSobee	3	1.8
Baby Cereals: *Average All Brands*		
Dry, 4 Tbsp, ¹/₂ oz	1	7
Jars (w. fruit), 4¹/₂ oz	1	7

Breakfast Cereals

	Pro	Iron
Hot Type, cooked:		
Bulgur, cooked, 1 cup, 5 oz	9	2
Oatmeal: Reg., non-fortified., 1 cup	6	1.5
Instant, fortified, average, 1 pkt	4	8
Quaker Extra, all flavors	4	18
Total, all types, 1 pkt	4	18
Corn/Hominy Grits: Reg., 1 cup	3	1.5
Quaker: Reg., 3 Tbsp, 1 oz	2	0.8
Instant White, 1 packet	2	8
Cream of Wheat, 1 cup	4	10
Ready-To-Eat: *Per 1 oz serving*		
Arrowhead, Average, all varieties	3	1
General Mills:		
Basic 4, 1 cup, 2 oz	4	3.8
Cheerios, regular, 1 cup, 1 oz	3	6.8
Cocoa Puffs, 1 cup, 1 oz	1	3.8
Corn Flakes, 1 cup	2	6.8
Fiber One, 1 cup	2	3.8
Kix, 1 1/3 cups; Kaboom, 1 1/4 cup	2	6.8
Total, Raisin Bran, 1 cup, 2 oz	4	15
Wheaties, 1 cup	3	6.8
Health Valley:		
10 Bran O's, 3/4 cup	3	0.9
Amaranth Flakes, 3/4 cup	3	0.6
Bran Cereal w. Raisins, 3/4 cup	5	1.5
98% Fat Free Granola, 2/3 cup	5	1.2
Real Oat Bran, 1/2 cup	6	0.6
Golden Flax, 1/4 cup	6	1.2
Kellogg's: All Bran, 1/2 cup	4	4.5
Bran Flakes, 3/4 cup	3	8.5
Cocoa Krispies, 3/4 cup	2	1.8
Corn Flakes, 1 cup	2	8.4
Just Right, 1 cup	4	16
Nutrigrain Almond Raisin, 1 1/4 cup	4	1.4
Product 19, 1 cup, 2 oz	2	18
Raisin Bran, 1 cup, 2 oz	6	4.5
Raisin Squares, 3/4 cup,	4	16
Rice Krispies, 1 1/4 cup	2	1.8
Special K, 1 cup	6	8.7
Nature Valley: All varieties, 1/3 cup	2	0.7
Post: Raisin Bran, 1 oz	3	4.5
Grape Nuts, 1 oz	3	1
Quaker: Crunchy Bran, 2/3 cup	2	8
Oat Squares, 1/2 cup, 1 oz	4	6
100% natural cereal, 1/4 cup	3	1
Puffed Rice/Wheat, 1 cup, 1/2 oz	1	0.5
Shreaded Wheat, 2 biscuits	4	1

Brans & Wheatgerm

	Pro	Iron
Oat Bran, raw, 1 Tbsp	2	0.5
Rice Bran, raw, 2 Tbsp	1	1
Wheat Bran, unprocessed, 2 Tbsp	1	1
Wheat Germ, 2 Tbsp, 1/2 oz	4	1.3

Grains & Flours

	Pro	Iron
Amaranth, 1 cup, 1/2 oz	10	3
Barley, 1/2 cup, 3 1/2 oz	8	2
Buckwheat Flour, dark, 1 cup	11.5	2.7
light, 1 cup	6	1
Carob Flour, 1 cup	5	3
Corn Flour, 1 cup, 4 oz	9	2
Corn Meal, enriched, 1 cup	11	3.5
Flour: White, enriched, 1 cup, 4 1/2 oz	13	6
Wholegrain, 1 cup, 4 1/4 oz	16	5
Millet, wholegrain, 1 cup, 3 1/2 oz	10	7
Rye Flour, dark, 1 cup, 4 1/2 oz	21	6
light, 1 cup, 3 1/2 oz	10	1
Soy Flour, full fat, 1 cup, 3 oz	32	5.5
Yeast: Brewer's, dry, 1 Tbsp	3	1.5

Rice, Spaghetti

	Pro	Iron
Rice: brown/white, average		
1 cup cooked, 6 1/2 oz	5	1
Spaghetti/Macaroni/Noodles (enriched):		
Cooked, 1 cup, 4 1/2 oz	7	2
Canned: in Tomato Sauce, 1/2 cup	2	0.5
w. Meatballs, 1 cup, 8 oz	9	2

Soups

	Pro	Iron
With Noodles/Vegetables, 1 cup	3	0.5
With Meat/Beans/Peas, 1 cup	8	1.5

Fruit

	Pro	Iron
Fresh/Canned: Average, all types, 1 serving		
1 medium/2 small fruit	1	0.5
Avocado, 1/2 medium	2	1
Dried Fruit: Apricots, 8 halves, 1 oz	1	1.3
Dates, 6 dates, 2 oz	1.5	0.7
Figs, 4 medium figs, 2 oz	2	1.7
Prunes, 5 medium, 1 1/2 oz	1	1
Raisins, 1 oz	1	0.7
Fruit Juice: Average, 1 cup	0.5	0.5
Prune Juice, 6 fl.oz	1	2.5
Tomato Juice, 6 fl.oz	0.5	1

King Kong was a vegetarian

Vegetables

	Pro	Iron
Beans: Snap/green, 1/2 cup	1	0.8
Dried: Average all types, cooked, 1/2 cup	7	2.5
Baked Beans, 1/2 cup 41/2 oz	5	2
Bean Sprouts, mung, 1 cup	3	1
Broccoli, 3/4 cup pieces, 4 oz	4	1.4
Cabbage; Cauliflower, 1 cup	1	0.6
Corn, 1/2 cup kernels, 3 oz	2.5	0.3
1 ear trimmed to 31/2"	2	0.4
Lentils, cooked, 1/2 cup, 31/2 oz	9	3.3
Mushrooms, raw, 1/2 cup, sliced	0.5	0.5
Peas: green, 1/2 cup, 3 oz	4	1.2
Split Peas, cooked, 1 cup	16	2.5
Potatoes, cooked:		
1 medium, with skin, 5 oz	3.3	2
without skin, 4 oz	2.3	1
French Fries, 3 oz	2	1
Potato Salad, 1/2 cup	3.5	2.5
Pumpkin, 1/2 cup mashed	1	2.5
Seaweed, kelp, 1 oz	1	2.5
Spinach, cooked, 1/2 cup, 3 oz	2.7	2.5
Squash, ckd, all types, 1/2 cup	1	1
Tomatoes, 1 medium, 41/2 oz	1	0.6
Vegetables, mixed, ckd, 1 cup	2.5	0.7
Soybeans, cooked, 1/2 cup, 3 oz	14	4.4

Tofu, Tempeh, Miso

	Pro	Iron
Tofu, raw, firm, 1/2 cup, 41/2 oz	10	1.5
Tempeh, 1/2 cup, 3 oz	16	2
Miso, 1/2 cup, 5 oz	16	4
Soybean Protein (TVP), 1 oz	18	3

Cakes, Pastries, Pies

(Made with enriched flour)	Pro	Iron
Carrot w. cream cheese frosting, 4 oz	4	1.3
Cheesecake, 1 piece, 31/2 oz	5	0.5
Chocolate, 1 piece, 2 oz	2	2
Fruitcake, 1 piece, 11/2 oz	2	1.2
Plain, 1 piece, 3 oz	4	1.2
Croissant, plain, 2 oz	5	2
Danish Pastry, 1 pastry, 21/4 oz	4	1.3
Donuts, average, 2 oz	4	1.2
Muffins, average, 1 medium, 11/2 oz	3	1
Pancakes, 4" diam., two, 2 oz	4	1
Pies: Fruit, 1 piece, 51/2 oz	4	1.5
Pecan, 1 piece, 5 oz	7	4.5
Puddings, average, 1/2 cup, 41/2 oz	4	0.3
Waffles, 1 large, 21/2 oz	7	1.5

Sugar, Honey, Jam

	Pro	Iron
Sugar: White	0	0
Brown, 1 Tbsp	0	0.3
Molasses: Light/Medium, 1 Tbsp	0	1
Blackstrap, 1 Tbsp, 3/4 oz	0	3
Corn Syrup, 1 Tbsp, 3/4 oz	0	1
Honey, Jams, Jelly	0	0.2

Candy, Chocolate, Carob

	Pro	Iron
Candy, sugar-based	0	0
Chocolate: Plain, 2 oz bar	4	0.8
with nuts, 2 oz bar	6	0.8
Carob, plain, 2 oz	6	0.7

Cookies, Crackers, Chips

	Pro	Iron
Cookies, average, 4 cookies	2	1
Crackers: Graham, 21/2" sq., 2	1	0
Rice Cakes, average, one	1	0
Corn/Potato Chips, 1 oz	2	0.3

Nuts: Almonds, shelled, 20-25 nuts

	Pro	Iron
Almonds, shelled, 20-25 nuts	6	1
Brazil Nuts, 7-8 medium nuts, 1 oz	4	1
Cashews, 12-16 nuts, 1 oz	5	1.5
Coconut, raw, 11/2 oz pce (2"x 21/2")	1	1
Macadamias, 1 oz	2	0.5
Mixed Nuts, 1 oz	5	1
Peanuts, dry roasted, 40 nuts, 1 oz	6	0.6
Pecans, 24 halves, 1 oz	2	0.5
Walnuts, 15 halves, 1 oz	4	0.7
Peanut Butter, 1 Tbsp	1	0.5

Seeds: Per 1 oz

	Pro	Iron
Pumpkin Kernels, dry, hulled, 1 oz	7	4.2
Sesame Seeds, dry, 1 Tbsp	2	0.6
Sunflower Seeds, dried, hulled, 1 oz	6	2
Tahini, 1 Tbsp, 1/2 oz	2.5	1.4

Granola & Food/Protein Bars

	Pro	Iron
Granola Bar, average	2	0.5
Peanut Bar (*Planters*), 11/2 oz	7	0.7
Bariatrix: Nutra Bars, 1	11	3.6
Proti Bars, 1	15	1.5
Choice dm Bar, 35g	6	3.6
Diet Center Meal Repl. Bar, 65g	14	2
Fi-Protein Nutritional Bar, 1	9.5	0
Genisoy Protein Bar, 2.2 oz	14	4.5
IDN: proGram-16, 65g	16	3.6
MetaForm Bar	30	7.2
Met-Rx Bar, 100g	27	7.2
MightyBite Nutritional Bar, 25g	6	1
Power Bar, 1	10	6.3
Slim-Fast Bar, 34g	6	4.5
Source One Bar, 2.2 oz	15	4.5
Sweet Success Bar, 33g	2	2.7
Tiger Sport, 65g	11	4.5

Nutritional & High Protein Drinks

	Pro	Iron
Bariatrix Shakes, dry, 1 oz	15	3.6
Fruit Drinks, mix, 20g	15	0
Proti-Max Meal Replacement, 67g	35	6.3
Boost Nutrition Energy Drink, 8 oz	10	3.6
Ensure, all flavors, 8 oz	9	2.3
Ensure Plus, 8 oz	13	3
Carnation Instant Breakfast, 10 oz	12	4.5
Diet Center Meal Repl. Powder, 1 pkt	12	6.3
GatorPro, 11 oz can	17	5.5
GemSoy Shake: Pro-Cal 100, 1 pkt	14	3.6
IDN Appeal, 1 pkg, 1 cup	16	2.7
Kindercal, 8 fl.oz	8	2.5
Met-Rx, Drink Mix, 72g	38	9
Nature's Best, Protein Shake, 11 oz	20	3.6
Nutra Start, 11 oz	10	3.6
Resource (Novartis) Standard, 8 fl.oz	9	4.5
Slim Fast, 325 ml can	10	2.7
Sweet Success (Nestle), 10 fl.oz can	10	4.5
Sustacal/Plus, 8 oz	15	4
Ultra Slim Fast, powder, 3 Tbsp, 33g	5	6.3
Walgreens Nutritional Suppl.: Plus, 8 oz	9	4.5
Advanced, 8 oz can	13	2.7
Lite, 8 oz can	10	4.5
Weider: Muscle Builder, 2 scoops	18	9
90% Plus Protein, 3 Tbsp	24	2.7

Coffee, Tea, Soda

	Pro	Iron
Coffee, Coffee Substitutes, 1 cup	0	0.1
Tea (all types); Soft Drinks/Soda	0	0
Hot Chocolate, 6 fl.oz	2	2.2

Beer, Wine, Spirits

	Pro	Iron
Beer, 12 fl.oz	1	0
Wines, red/white, 1 glass	0	0.4
Spirits/Liquor	0	0

Fast-Foods/Burgers

Note: See Fast-Foods Section for comprehensive protein counts.

	Pro	Iron
Arby's: Roast Beef Sandwich, reg.	23	4
Giant Roast Beef S/wich	35	6
Italian Sub	30	2
Roast Turkey Deluxe	20	3
Burger King: Whopper S/wich	27	2.5
Hamburger	20	1.5
Double Bacon Cheeseburger	44	2.5
Chicken Sandwich; Big Fish Sandwich	26	2
Carl's Jr: Famous Star Hamburger	26	2
Super Star Hamburger	43	3
Chicken Club Sandwich	35	2
Hot & Crispy Sandwich	14	1

Fast Foods/Burgers (Cont)

	Pro	Iron
Domino's Pizza: Deep Dish (12"), 2 sl.		
Cheese, 2 slices	18	4
Pepperoni, Sausage/Pepperoni	21	4
X-tra Cheese & Pepperoni	24	4.5
French Fries: Medium, 3$\frac{1}{2}$ oz	4.5	0.7
KFC		
Original, Wing & Breast	38	0.4
3-Pce. Dinner, Original	51	0.4
Kentucky Nuggets, 6	16	0.4
Colonel's Chicken Sandwich	29	1.5
McDonald's: Arch Deluxe	29	2.5
Big Mac	25	2.5
Cheeseburger	15	1.5
Chicken McNuggets (6)	18	0.6
Fish Filet Deluxe	24	1.5
Grilled Crispy Chicken Deluxe	27	1.5
Hamburger	12	1.5
Quarter Pounder	23	2.5
French Fries: Small, 2$\frac{1}{2}$ oz	3	0.2
Large, 5 oz	6	0.6
Breakfast: Egg McMuffin	17	1.5
Hotcakes w. Marg/Syrup	9	1.5
Sausage McMuffin w. Egg	19	1.5
Grilled Chicken Salad Deluxe	21	1
Muffin, Lowfat, Apple Bran	6	1
Pancakes: 3 Pancakes	8	2
Pizza Hut: Per Medium, 2 slices		
Pan Pizzas, average	26	4
Thin 'n Crispy: Supreme	28	2
Hand Tossed: Pepperoni	24	3
Supreme; Personal Pan Pizza	32	4.5
Shakes, Chocolate	12	0.4
Subway: 6" Subs, average	22	2
Del Style Sandwiches, average	12	1
Subway Club Salad, reg.	16	2
Sundaes: Average all outlets	7	0.3
Taco Bell: Bean Burrito	13	3.5
Beef Burrito	22	3.7
Tostado	10	1.5
Enchirito; Nachos Bellgrande	20	3
Taco Bellgrande	18	2
Taco Light	19	2.5
Taco Salad w. Shell	35	7
Wendy's: Single w. Everything	26	3
Big Bacon Classic	34	3
Hamburger Kid's Meal	15	2
Grilled Chicken Sandwich	27	1.5
Stuffed Potatoes: Broc. & Cheese	9	2.5
Bacon & Cheese	17	2.5
Taco Salad	29	2.5

High Blood Pressure

Many American adults have hypertension (high blood pressure), and are unaware of it. It is generally symptomless, so **have your blood pressure checked annually** - particularly if there is a family history of hypertension.

Untreated hypertension overworks the heart, damages arteries and promotes atherosclerosis. This in turn greatly increases the risk of heart disease, stroke, blindness, kidney disease and impotence. The earlier hypertension is detected, the sooner it can be brought under control.

Treating Hypertension

If your blood pressure is high, consult your doctor about diet and medication. You may be referred to a dietitian for more detailed dietary advice and meal planning.

High-Normal and Stage 1 hypertension can often be treated by reducing sodium intake, losing weight if overweight, limiting alcohol to 2 drinks or less daily, exercising regularly, and dealing with stress.

Stages 2, 3 and 4 hypertension usually require drug therapy. However, salt restriction, abstaining from alcohol and the above lifestyle changes will improve the success of drug therapy, and enable smaller drug doses to be prescribed.

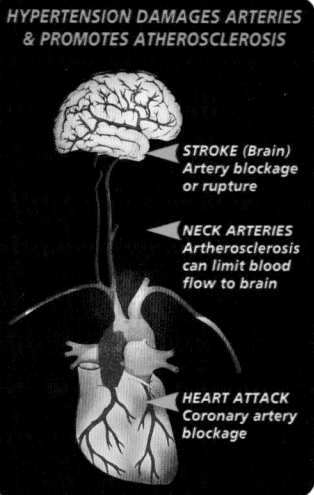

HYPERTENSION DAMAGES ARTERIES & PROMOTES ATHEROSCLEROSIS

STROKE (Brain)
Artery blockage or rupture

NECK ARTERIES
Artherosclerosis can limit blood flow to brain

HEART ATTACK
Coronary artery blockage

BLOOD PRESSURE CLASSIFICATIONS

National High Blood Pressure Educ. Prog. (1993)

	DIASTOLIC	SYSTOLIC
Normal ►	80-84	120-129
High-Normal ►	85-89	130-139
Stage 1 ►	90-99	140-159
Stage 2 ►	100-109	160-179
Stage 3 ►	110-119	180-209
Stage 4 ►	120 or over	210 or over

STROKE
KNOW THE WARNING SIGNS!

If you notice one or more of these signs, **call your doctor immediately.** They may be signalling a possible stroke or transient ischemic attack:

- **Sudden weakness** or numbness in your face, arm or leg on one side of your body.
- **Sudden dimness,** blurring or loss of vision, particularly in one eye.
- **Loss of speech,** or trouble talking or understanding speech.
- **Sudden severe headache** - 'a bolt out of the blue' - with no apparent cause.
- **Unexplained dizziness,** unsteadiness or a sudden fall, especially if accompanied by any of the other symptoms.

Salt & Sodium

- **Sodium is a mineral element** most commonly found in salt (sodium chloride). It also occurs naturally in much smaller amounts in animal and plant foods, and water - normally sufficient for our needs without having to add salt.

- **Sodium is required** for nerve and muscle function as well as to balance the amount of fluid in our tissues and blood.
  Sodium acts like a sponge to attract and hold fluids in body tissues.

- **Excess sodium** can cause water retention, and increase the risk of developing hypertension. Very high salt intake may also increase the risk of stomach cancer.

- **Too little sodium** may cause low blood pressure (hypotension), and decrease blood flow to the heart, brain and kidneys - especially during exercise. (A certain blood volume is required to sustain the blood pressure needed for adequate blood flow in the capillaries).

Salt - Sensitive Persons

- **Normally, our kidneys** excrete excess dietary sodium. The thirst we feel after a salty meal is the body calling for water to dilute the sodium, and enable the kidneys to flush out excess sodium.

- **However, 'salt sensitive'** persons (perhaps 1 in 2-3 adults) tend to retain excess sodium (above approximately 3000mg daily) instead of excreting it. Such persons are more likely to develop hypertension and would most benefit from sodium restriction. Assume you are susceptible if there is a family history of hypertension.

- **Although not everyone will benefit**, all Americans are being asked to **moderate their salt and sodium intake** as a public health measure - particularly that so many do not know whether or not they have hypertension; and also because we do not know just who is salt-sensitive.

Safe Sodium Levels

The American Heart Association recommends a maximum sodium intake of 2400mg per day for adults with normal blood pressure. Many Americans have double this amount.

Persons with hypertension and kidney ailments are usually restricted to as little as **1000mg sodium per day**. Your doctor will discuss the correct sodium level for you.

Persons engaged in prolonged strenuous work or exercise may lose sodium through heavy sweating - especially in hot, humid weather. Adequate salt (and fluids) is necessary to avoid dehydration. A little extra salt at mealtimes is usually sufficient to satisfy any extra need. Do not take salt tablets.

Finding Hidden Sodium

On average, only one third of our sodium intake comes from the salt shaker. The rest is hidden in processed foods that have salt added during manufacture.

Sodium compounds added to food or medicinals can also contribute significant sodium.

Sodium bicarbonate in particular is widely used in antacid tablets and powders, and saline drink powders (such as *Alka Seltzer*). Sodium bicarbonate contains 27% sodium by weight. Each gram contributes 270mg sodium. Large amounts of sodium can be unwittingly consumed.

Other sodium compounds include monosodium glutamate (MSG), sodium ascorbate, sodium nitrite, and sodium citrate.

ALCOHOL

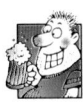

Excess alcohol causes up to 20% of hypertension in America.

Susceptible persons should abstain to normalize their blood pressure.

Salt-Sodium Guide

Sodium accounts for only 40% of the weight of salt (sodium chloride). Examples:
1 gram (1000mg) Salt has 400mg Sodium

1 teasp. (5g) Salt has 2000mg Sodium

Hints to Reduce Sodium

● **Watch the salt shaker.** Start with an easy 50% cut in sodium by using Lite Salt (*Morton*). Then gradually cut back until you can leave the salt shaker off the table.

● **Taste your food before salting.** Use the pepper shaker (small holes) for more controlled sprinkling of salt.

● **Choose low sodium,** sodium free, and reduced sodium products in place of regular salted products.

● **Check labels for sodium levels.** The following sodium descriptors may appear on labels:

Reduced Sodium: At least 75% less sodium than the original product.
Low Sodium: 140 mg or less/serving.
Very Low Sodium: 35mg or less/serving.
Sodium Free: Less than 5mg per serving.

● **Use reduced-sodium breads,** butter and margarine. Regular varieties contain up to 2% salt. This is considered high in view of their significant contribution to our diet.

● **Go easy on condiments and sauces** such as tomato ketchup, mustard, soy sauce and spaghetti sauces, plus salad dressings. Use low sodium varieties.

● **Limit pizzas and salty fast-foods.** Check the *Fast-Food Restaurant* Section.

● **Avoid salty snack foods** such as potato chips, corn chips, salted nuts, pretzels and cheesy-flavoured snacks. **Choose unsalted** popcorn, nuts or seeds. Eat more fruit.

● **Don't salt children's food** to your taste.

● **Limit or avoid antacids and saline powders** with sodium bicarbonate (such as *Alka-Seltzer*). They are high in sodium.

FOODS HIGH IN SODIUM

- Cheese, Butter, Margarine
- Pickles, Sauerkraut, Olives
- Condiments, Sauces
- Salad Dressings
- Canned vegetables/salads/beans
- Deli Salads (with dressing)
- Frozen/Packaged Meals/Entrees
- Soups: Canned/dry; bouillon cubes
- Meats: Ham, bacon, sausage, luncheon meats, smoked meats
- Canned Fish (in brine)
- Seasoning Salts (e.g. garlic, celery)
- Snack Foods (potato chips, pretzels)
- Tomato Jce (Canned), V8 Vegetable Juice
- Fast Foods: Pizza, Burgers, Chicken
- *Alka-Seltzer* Antacid

MODERATE SODIUM

- Bread (Reduced Salt)
- Meat, Fish, Poultry - Unprocessed
- Milk, Yogurt, Soy Drinks, Eggs
- Peanut Butter
- Breakfast Cereals (<200mg/serving,
- Chocolate Candy, Fruit/Nut Bars
- *Reduced & Low-Sodium Products*

FOODS LOW IN SODIUM

- Products labelled *Very Low Sodium, or Sodium Free*
- Fresh fruits and vegetables
- Canned and Dried Fruits
- Potatoes, Rice, Pasta
- Dried Beans & Lentils, Tofu
- Nuts & Seeds (unsalted)
- Corn & Popcorn (unsalted)
- Pepper, Spices, Herbs
- Jam, Honey, Syrup
- Candy, Gum
- Hard & Jelly Candy
- Coffee, Tea, Alcohol
- Fresh Fruit Juices, Water

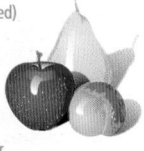

The American Heart Association recommends a sodium intake of **less than 2400mg/day**

Sod ~ Sodium (mg)

Milk & Dairy Products

	Sod
Milk: Whole/lowfat/skim, average	
1 cup, 8 fl.oz	120
Whole, low sodium, 1 cup	5
Choc Milk (*Hershey's*), 1 cup	130
Human Milk, 8 fl.oz	40
Soy Milk, 8 fl.oz	30
Buttermilk, cultured, 8 fl.oz	250
Dry/Powder, skim, $1/4$ cup, 1 oz	110
Yogurt: with fruit aver., 8 oz	130
Cheese:	
Blue, 1 oz	330
Parmesan, 1 oz	450
Kraft: Cheddar, 1 oz	180
Philadelphia Brand Cream Cheese	85
Process Cheese., average,1 oz	430
Swiss, 1 oz	40
Cottage Cheese, $1/2$ cup, 4 oz	450
Ricotta Cheese, $1/2$ cup, 4 oz	150

Icecream, Frozen Yogurt

	Sod
Icecream, average, $1/2$ cup	50
Frozen Yogurt, $1/2$ cup	50

Fats/Oils

	Sod
Butter/Margarine:	
Regular, 2 Tbsp, 1 oz	230
Unsalted, reg., 2 Tbsp, 1 oz	5
Mayonnaise, aver., 2 Tbsp, 1 oz	160
Molly McButter, 1 tsp	120
Oils/Lard/Dripping	0
Cream, average, 1 Tbsp	6
Coffee-Mate: Powdered, 1 tsp	2
Liquid, 1 Tbsp	5

Eggs

	Sod
Whole, 1 large	70
Omelet, 2 egg, plain	220
w. cheese	400
Egg Beaters (*Fleischmann's*), $1/4$ cup	80

Meats

	Sod
Meat, average all types, cooked	
(Beef/Lamb/Veal/Pork), 4 oz	80
Corned Beef, cooked, 3 oz	800
Bacon, cooked, 2 slices, $1/2$ cup	270
Ham, 3 oz	1100

Chicken & Turkey

	Sod
Chicken/Turkey, cooked, unsalted, 4 oz	80
Stuffing Mixes, average., $1/2$ cup	500

Sausages & Meats

	Sod
Bologna, 1 oz	280
Frankfurter, 2 oz	640
Ham, chopped, $3/4$ oz slice	290
Liverwurst (Braunschweiger), 1 oz	320
Pepperoni, 5 slices, 1 oz	570
Salami, cooked, 1 oz	350
dry/hard, 1 oz	600
Sausage, 1 oz link	220
Pork, 2 oz patty	260
Turkey Roll, 1 oz	160

Fish:

	Sod
Fish: Fresh Fish, average, plain	
Cooked, 4 oz (no bone)	60
Broiled w. butter, 4 oz	150
Breaded & fried, 4 oz	320
Fish fillets, bat.-dipped 3 oz	350
Fish sticks, 1 oz stick	160
Gefilte Fish (w. broth), 1 pce, $1^1/2$ oz	220
Herring, pickled, 2 pces, 1 oz	260
Lobster, meat only, 4 oz	180
Oysters, fresh, 6 med., 3 oz	95
Salmon, canned, 3 oz	460
No Salt Added, 3 oz	65
Smoked fish, average, 3 oz	650
Tuna, canned, 3 oz	330
No Added Salt, 3 oz	40

Entrees & Meals

	Sod
Frozen Meals, average	600-900
Lean Cuisine, average	900
Stouffer's, average	580
Dinners, average	900-1200
Side Dishes, average	400-600
Pizza, frozen, $1/4$ large, 6 oz	800-1200
Microwave Cup Meals	900-1200
Cup O'Noodles, average	1500

Fast-Foods & Restaurants

	Sod
(Comprehensive listings in **Fast-Foods Section**)	
Cheeseburger	750
Chicken Dinner (3 piece)	2200
Chicken Nuggets w. Sauce	800
Fish/Chicken Sandwich	1000
French Fries, small, $2^1/2$ oz	150
Hamburger: Regular	500
Large with cheese	1100
Hot Dog (Frankfurter)	800
Pizza, 2 medium slices	1200
Shake, chocolate	250
Taco	400

Sodium Counter

Sod ~ Sodium (mg)

Soups:
Condensed, 1 c., 8 oz	800-1000
Low Sodium	70
Chicken Noodle, 1 cup	900
Bouillon Cube, average	950
Cup-A-Soup, average	850
Lite, average	450
Soup Mixes, average, 1 cup	900

Condiments, Sauces, Dressings
A-1 Sauce, 1 Tbsp	270
Barbecue Sauce, 1 Tbsp	130
Bragg Liquid Aminos, 1 tsp	220
Chili Sauce, 1 Tbsp	230
Ketchup: tomato, 1 Tbsp	180
Low Sodium, 1 Tbsp	20
Mayonnaise, 1 Tbsp	80
Mustard, 1 tsp	70
Pizza Sauce, 1/2 cup	700
Salad Dressings, 2 Tbsp, 1 oz	160-400
Spaghetti Sauce, 1/2 cup	500
Soy Sauce, 1 Tbsp	900
Lite *(Kikkoman)*, 1 Tbsp	600
Sweet & Sour, 1/2 cup	250
Tabasco, 1 tsp	25
Vinegar, Lemon Juice	0
Worcestershire, 1 Tbsp	200
Tomato: Sauce, 1 cup	1200
Paste/Puree (salted), 1/2 cup	1000
No Salt Added, 1/2 cup	25

Salt & Salt Substitutes
Table Salt: 1 tsp, 6g	2400
Single Serve packet, 1 g	400
Lite Salt *(Morton)*, 1 tsp, 6g	1200
No Salt Alternative, 1 tsp	5
Garlic/Seasoned Salt 1 tsp, 4g	1300
Sea Salt, 1 tsp, 5g	2250

Seasonings, Herbs & Spices
Baking Powder, 1 tsp, 3g	340
Baking Soda (Sodium bicarb), 1 tsp, 3g	810
Accent (Flavor Enhancer), 1 tsp	600
Chili Powder, 1 tsp, 3g	25
Herbs/Spices: Curry Powder	0
Lemon Pepper *(Lawry's)*, 1 tsp	340
Meat Tenderizer, 1 tsp, 5g	1750
MSG (Monosodium glutamate), 5g	500
Mrs Dash (Herb/Spice Blend), 1 tsp	0
Pepper, Mustard (dry), 1 tsp	1
Yeast, Nutritional, 1 Tbsp	10

Breakfast Cereals
Kellogg's: All-Bran, 1/3 cup, 1 oz	260
Bran Flakes, 2/3 cup, 1 oz	220
Corn Flakes, 1 cup, 1 oz	290
Just Right, 2/3 cup, 1 oz	200
Shredded Wheat Squares, 1/2 cup, 1 oz	5
Health Valley Cereals, 1 serving	5
Quaker: Crunchy Bran, 1 oz	320
100% Natural, 1 oz	15
Puffed Rice/Wheat, 1 oz	1
Total, 1 cup, 1 oz	140
Nature Valley: Average, 1 oz	90
Oatmeal: Regular, 3/4 cup	1
Instant *(Quaker)*, 2/3 cup (1 pkt)	270

Breads, Bagels, Crackers
Bread: Average all types, 1 oz	140
Low Sodium, 1 oz	10
Bagels, plain, 2 oz	200
Sara Lee, 3 oz	500
Biscuits, average, 1 oz	180
Bun/Roll, 1 medium, 1 1/2 oz	200
Crackers: Saltine, 2 crackers	70
Low Salt (Premium), 2	45
Graham, 2 regular	50
Croissant, average, 2 oz	280
Rice Cakes, average	25
RyKrisp Crispbread, Sesame, 2	100

Cookies, Cakes, Desserts
Cookies, average, 2-3 cookies, 1 oz	100
Mrs Fields', average, 2 1/2 oz	180
Baked Custard, 1/2 cup	100
Brownie, 1/4 oz piece	75
Cake, average, 3 oz piece	250
Cinnamon Sweet Roll, 2 oz	250
Danish, Apple	250
Donut, average	150
Muffins, 1 medium, 2 oz	150
Sara Lee, average, 2 1/2 oz	300
Pancakes, 3 x 4"	360
Pie, average 1/6 of 9" pie	300
Pudding, 1/2 cup	160
Jell-O (Mix), Instant, 1/2 cup	400
Waffles:	
Home-made, 7", 2 1/2 oz	350
Frozen, average, 1 1/4 oz	260
Aunt Jemima, aver., 2 1/2 oz	630

Fruit & Juices

	Sod
Fresh Fruit, average all types, 1 serving	1
Dried/Canned Fruit, 1/2 cup	1
Fruit Juice: Fresh, sqz'd, 6 fl.oz	1
Commercial, aver., 6 fl.oz	20
Carrot Juice (*Ferraro's*), 8 fl.oz	230
Tomato Juice (*Campbell's*), 6 fl.oz	570
Low Sodium (No Salt Added)	20
V8 Vegetable (*Campbell's*), 6 fl.oz	600
(No Salt Added), 6 fl.oz	45

Vegetables

Fresh/Frozen (No Salt Added), 1/2 cup

Asparagus, Bean Sprouts, Corn	3
Beets, Carrots, Celery, 1/2 cup	40
Broccoli, Cabbage, Cauliflower	10
Cucumber, Green Beans, Mushroom, Okra	3
Onions, Peas, Potato, Pumpkin, Squash	3
Peppers, Hot Chili, raw, each	3
Spinach, Turnips, 1/2 cup, ckd	40
Tomato, 1 medium, 5 oz	10
Canned: Asparagus, 4 spears	300
Beans, baked in tomato sauce	450
Beets, 1/2 cup, 3 oz	240
Corn Kernels, 1/2 cup, 3 oz	190
Creamed, 1/2 cup, 4 1/2 oz	330
Mushrooms w. butter sce, 2oz	550
Peas, 1/2 cup, 3 oz	250
Sauerkraut, 1/2 cup, 4 oz	750

Pickles, Olives

Olives, pickled: Green, 1 large	90
Ripe/black, 1 large	40
Pickles: Bread & Butter, 4 sl., 1 oz	200
Dill, 1 pickle, 2 1/2 oz	900
Sweet, 1 gherkin, 1/2 oz	130

Soybean Products

Miso (Soy Paste), 1/4 c., 2 1/2 oz	2500
Soybean Protein Isolate, 1 oz	280
Tempeh, 1/2 cup, 3 oz	5
Tofu, average, 1/2 cup, 4 oz	5

Jam, Honey, Syrups

Jam/Jelly, 1 Tbsp	2
Honey/Maple Syrup, 1 Tbsp	1
Log Cabin Syrup, 1 fl.oz	35
Lite, 1 fl.oz	90

Peanut Butter

Peanut Butter, regular, 1 Tbsp	70
Unsalted, 1 Tbsp	1

Snacks, Nuts

	Sod
Cheese Balls/Curls, 1 oz	280
Corn/Tortilla Chips, aver., 1 oz	220
Granola bars, aver., 1 bar	80
Nuts: Plain, unsalted, 1 oz	1
Lightly salted, 1 oz	80
Salted or Honey Roasted, 1 oz	160
Popcorn: Plain (unsalted), 1 cup	1
Flavored, average, 1 cup	60
Salt added, 1 cup	180
Potato Chips, plain, 1 oz	160
Flavored, average, 1 oz	250
Pretzels, regular, 3, 1 oz	450

Candy, Chocolate

Chocolate, milk, 1 oz	30
Carob Milk Bar, 1 oz	55
Fudge, chocolate, 1 oz	55
Candy Bars, average, 1 1/2 oz	60
Hard Candy, Jelly Beans, 1 oz	10
Licorice, 1 oz	30

Beverages, Alcohol

Coffee (& Substitutes), Tea, 1 cup	1
Cocoa, dry, plain, 1 Tbsp	0
Mix, average, 1 envelope	120
Quik (*Nestle*), 2 tsp	35
Soft Drinks, average, 8 fl.oz	20
Mineral Water, Perrier, 8 fl.oz	5
Gatorade Thirst Quencher, 8 fl.oz	110
Water, average, 1 cup, 8 fl.oz	5
Drier regions, 1 cup	20+
Alcohol: Beer, average, 12 fl.oz	15
Wines, average, 4 fl.oz	10
Spirits (distilled), 1 1/2 fl.oz	1

Antacids – Alka-Seltzer

	Sod
Alka-Seltzer (Per Tablet):	
Alka-Seltzer P.M., 1 tablet	500
Original (Light Blue Box)	570
Extra Strength (Dark Blue Box)	590
Flavored Lemon/Lime & Cherry	500
Antacid (yellow Box)	310
Gelatine Capsule, 1	0
Alka-Mints, chewable	0
Bromo Seltzer, 3/4 capful	760
Rolaids: All types	0
Tums: Regular/Extra Strength	0
Sodium Bicarbonate (27% sodium), 1g	270

FAST-FOODS INDEX ~ PAGE 161

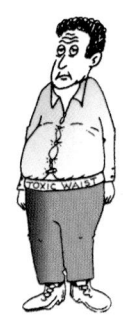

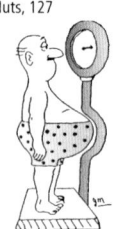

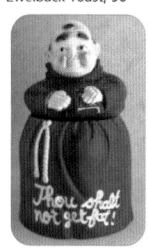

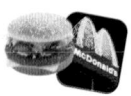

FAST-FOOD RESTAURANTS INDEX
~ SEE PAGE 161 ~

~ SEE PAGE 161 ~

Mail Order Service

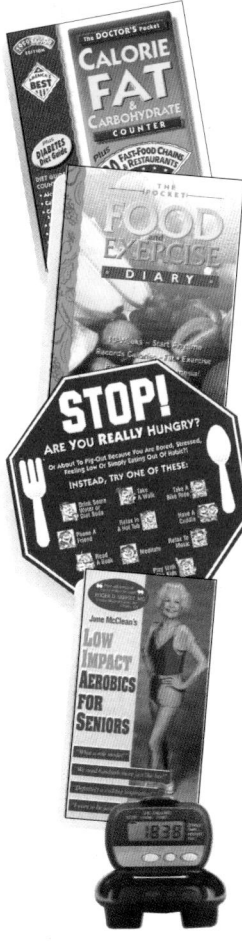

► **The Doctor's Pocket CALORIE FAT & CARBOHYDRATE COUNTER** $7.00

► **The Pocket FOOD & EXERCISE DIARY** $4.00

► **STOP! Fridge Poster**
(8"x 8" size, with magnet)
Extra Info ~ See Page 49
$3.00

► **GROOVY GRANNY VIDEO**
June McClean's Low Impact
AEROBICS FOR SENIORS
(Lively fun exercises to music)
$15.00

► **PEDOMETER**
(Measures steps, miles, calories
Includes 10,000 Step Program)
$25.00

► **TANITA BODYFAT SCALES**
Model TBF 611 - Single Users
(Other models: Phone or see Website)
$70.00

► **PERSONAL TRAINER WATCH**
Ultrak Brand - Most Sophisticated
$65.00

Shipping & Handling:
Add $3.00 for first item.
and $1.00 for each extra item.
(In California, add 7.75% Sales Tax)

Phone (949) 642-8500

www.calorieking.com

OR Mail your order with payment to:

Family Health Publications
PO Box 1616
Costa Mesa, CA 92628

Special Quantity Discounts Available

Health Professionals, Companies, Clubs,
Schools, Organizations, Fund-Raisers

NO MORE EXCUSES!!

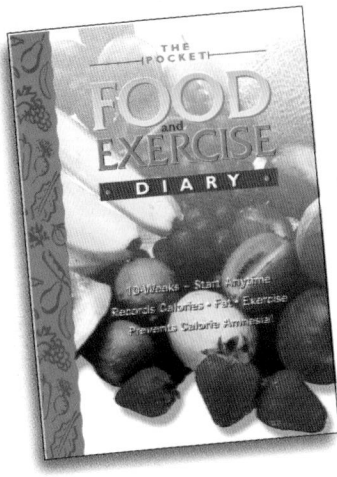

▶ Use this diary to record
your food and exercise.

▶ You'll lose more weight
and keep it off too!

▶ Records Calories, Fat &
Exercise Calories.

▶ Helps prevent
'Calorie Amnesia'!

10 Weeks (One Day Per Page)
Weekly Summary Pages
Non-Dated ~ Start Anytime
SAMPLE PAGE ~ SEE PAGE 15

**ORDER DETAILS
~ PAGE 287 ~**

University studies show that persons who use a food diary
not only lose more weight - they also keep it off!

The Pocket Food & Exercise Diary records both food
and exercise. At day's end, you simply deduct exercise
calories from food calories. Record fat grams too!

It's easy to use and most effective!

So get serious and start your diary today.
No more excuses!

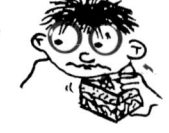

A MUST!
For Serious Weight Control

FREE SAMPLE BOOK FOR DOCTORS, CLINICS & HEALTH PROFESSIONALS
**FAMILY HEALTH PUBLICATIONS ▪ PO BOX 1616 COSTA MESA, CA 92628
PHONE (949) 642 8500 ▪ FAX (949) 642 8900**